Change One

The diet & fitness plan

Lose Weight
Simply, Safely, and
Forever

Introduction by John Foreyt, Ph.D.

Reader's Digest

The Reader's Digest Association
Pleasantville, New York | Montreal

ChangeOne Success Stories Speak!

"I started the *ChangeOne* program in March, trying to lose weight for a very special event I had in April. Little did I know that it would become a new way of life for me. I lost 25 pounds and recovered all the self-esteem that I had lost. I've made an impact in my family and friends and now give advice to others in need of a change. Your program is the best out there because it teaches you how to take control of your life. I thank you for giving back to me the beautiful and healthy woman that I had forgotten I could be and for getting me 'hooked' on exercising and enjoying every minute of it."

—Mili Henriquez

"*ChangeOne* has taught me how to eat nutritiously and still have my snacks, too. I have learned to control snacks and often don't even crave them like I used to. I tried the 'low carb' diet for three weeks before *ChangeOne* and was completely depleted of energy. I have not once been irritable, tired, or hungry on *ChangeOne*. I hope more people can enjoy the benefits of *ChangeOne* and that it will be a life-long lifestyle change! I know it will be for me."

—Teresa J. Cash

"I have lost 55 pounds on the *ChangeOne* plan since the diet appeared in *Reader's Digest*. I just entered the 'normal' BMI range a couple months ago, and I wanted to tell you that I don't recognize myself. Thank whoever came up with this plan and put together the 'latest' information. Whenever I had a rough week or felt myself slipping, I just grabbed the *ChangeOne* book and read until I got new inspiration and determination. I never gained more than five pounds before I was back on track and losing again. I seriously do not recognize myself. The sheer joy of feeling young is an everyday emotion. I began to date through an Internet dating service. I found that my photo had my future dates suspicious that I was posting my high school graduation picture. I could only laugh, because I look better now than when in high school. I have my life. I have a great man I'm seeing. The real person who was imprisoned inside me is out and very, very happy."

—Rose Lobdell

"I needed to change how I ate, and I really liked the concept of changing only one thing at a time. As a busy mother of four kids under age 11, I love that I could be on *ChangeOne* without preparing special foods or reforming my entire diet overnight. I was able to do it at my own pace, and be successful in baby steps. I've seen women from all walks of life be successful at this—if we can, you can, too!"

—Susan Miller, lost 43 pounds and 28 inches overall

"The portion control tricks are great. The easiest one for me was cutting my meal in half when I went out to dinner (except I ate all the veggies). Because it was so easy, it just became a new way of life for me. It is a real ego boost to have family and friends, even my aerobics instructor, exclaim about how thin I look."

—Kathy Bennett, lost 30 pounds and 3 dress sizes

"*ChangeOne* is a healthy lifestyle change, not a fad diet. I feel good about myself again. I have more energy and can be more active. I don't get short of breath and my heart doesn't race. I enjoy shopping and I still get a kick out of catching a glimpse of myself in a mirror. I have my life back and I love it!"

—Gail Davis, lost 50 pounds

"After considering many programs, I finally chose *ChangeOne*. I am so grateful I did. I have been on *ChangeOne* for eight weeks and have lost 16 pounds. I have dropped from a size 16-18 to a 12-14. It is the easiest weight loss I have ever had. I have changed so many habits and learned to incorporate exercise into everyday life that I already feel like a success. I also feel I am being a better example to my children. I love the recipes and ideas for food. My family loves almost everything I have prepared and they keep asking, 'Are you sure this is diet food?' "

—Lesa Crisp

"Since joining *ChangeOne* seven weeks ago, I have lost 17 pounds! I have learned to eat breakfast, which I never did before, and I have learned that it wasn't necessarily *how much* I was eating that was making me gain weight, it was *what* I was eating. I ate anything that was fast, whether it was fast food from a restaurant or microwavable foods bought from a store. They were loaded with calories. I never had the willpower to stay on an eating plan as long as I have since joining *ChangeOne*. I'm on the road to a new healthy, happy life!"

—Lori Ruiz

First printing in paperback 2007
© 2006 by The Reader's Digest Association
© 2006 by The Reader's Digest Association (Canada) Ltd.
© 2006 by Reader's Digest Association Far East Ltd.
Philippine © 2006 by Reader's Digest Association Far East Ltd.

Food photography by Elizabeth Watt
Exercise photography by Cara Howe/StudioW26
Portion guide photos by Christine Bronico
Cover photograph by Gavin Kingcome
Success Story photo portraits provided and reproduced by permission of the participants.

Address any comments about *ChangeOne, The Diet & Fitness Plan* to:
The Reader's Digest Association, Inc.
Editor in Chief, Books and Music
Reader's Digest Road
Pleasantville, NY 10570-7000

To order copies of *ChangeOne, The Diet & Fitness Plan,* call
1-800-846-2100.

Visit our website at rd.com

Printed in China
1 3 5 7 9 10 8 6 4 2 hardcover
1 3 5 7 9 10 8 6 4 2 paperback

Library of Congress Cataloging-in-Publication Data

ChangeOne : the diet & fitness plan, lose weight simply, safely and forever / Reader's Digest.--
1st ed.
     p. cm.
 Includes index.
 ISBN: 0-7621-0697-2 (hardcover)
 ISBN-10: 0-7621-0833-9 (paperback)
 ISBN-13: 978-0-7621-0833-6 (paperback)
1. Reducing diets. 2. Food habits. 3. Weight loss. 4. Physical fitness. 5. Exercise. I. Title:
Diet & fitness plan, lose weight simply, safely and forever. II. Title: Change one. III. Reader's
digest.

RM222.2.C439 2006
613.2'5--dc22

                                    2005029246

Note to our readers:

This publication is designed to provide useful information to the reader on the subjects of weight loss, healthy eating, and exercise. It should not be substituted for the advice of a physician or used to alter any medical therapy or programs prescribed to you by your doctor. Be sure to consult your doctor before proceeding with any weight-loss or exercise regimen. The use of specific products in this book does not constitute an endorsement by the author or the publisher. The author and the publisher disclaim any liability or loss, personal, financial, or otherwise, which may be claimed or incurred, directly or indirectly, resulting from the use and/or application of the content of this publication.

Acknowledgments

Most health books are conceived and written by a single person. The *ChangeOne* diet and fitness plan has taken a much different path in its three years of life. As it has expanded and grown, *ChangeOne* has drawn upon an ever-larger team of doctors, writers, food experts, fitness experts, and editors. As we go to press, *ChangeOne* has been published in 15 countries, is a major weight-loss website, and has been read about by roughly 60 million people via *Reader's Digest* magazine articles worldwide. In each case, the best experts have been brought in to adapt the *ChangeOne* approach to weight loss to particular cultures and usages.

For this major new edition, we'd like to thank the following:

John Hastings, Peter Jaret, and **Mindy Hermann** for penning the original edition of *ChangeOne*. While their names are no longer on the cover of this book, they were the founding voices of the program and shaped its fundamental message of one easy change at a time.

Christine Luff has served as Editor in Chief of the *ChangeOne* website since its inception in 2002. By interacting daily with the tens of thousands of *ChangeOne* dieters, she knows perhaps better than anyone the strengths and benefits of the *ChangeOne* approach. Christine was invaluable in this revised edition, and was the liaison for the many testimonials and success stories found in these pages.

Sari Harrar, one of the country's most gifted health writers, had the tough task of improving what was already a terrific and proven approach to weight loss. She added key sections to the book and helped make this new edition so fresh and up to date.

Selene Yeager crafted the 10-minutes-a-day exercise routines you'll find inside. Selene is not only an accomplished health book author, but she is a certified trainer, triathlete, and health-and-fitness entrepreneur.

Finally, thank you to **John Foreyt,** director of the Behavioral Medicine Research Center at the Baylor College of Medicine, who for decades has been among the most respected voices calling for sensible, incremental approaches to weight loss. Dr. Foreyt was one of the experts who originally shaped the *ChangeOne* approach and graciously contributed many summertime hours to advise us on this revised edition.

To each of you, and everyone else who has made *ChangeOne* such a successful way to lose weight, our deepest and most heartfelt thanks.

—Neil Wertheimer
Editor in Chief, Reader's Digest Books

contents

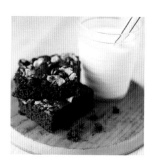

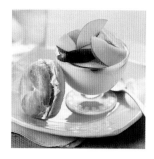

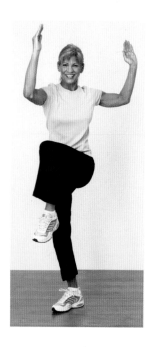

Part 3
ChangeOne Resources

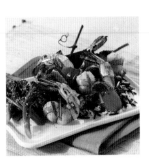

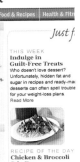

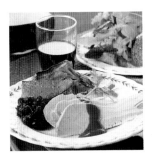

Introduction
A Program That Works

For those of us in the scientific community who spend our time in the fight against obesity, the never-ending flow of new weight-loss books is a bittersweet thing. We are certainly grateful that the people buying these books want to lose weight, since acknowledging a problem is half the battle. And many weight-loss guides do a good job of motivating and instructing people in responsible ways.

The truth is, though, that many popular weight-loss books concern us researchers. For example, it breaks our hearts to see renegade doctors hawking weight-loss programs that not only are based on weak or faulty science but also could ulti-mately hurt dieters' health. Likewise, what are we to think of weight-loss books written by celebrities, businesspeople, chefs, and athletes—books that, despite the authors' good intentions, have minimal basis in fact or research? Somehow, a fad mentality has come to dominate weight-loss advice. This week, it's the cookie diet; next week, the fried food diet; next month, a Hollywood star's weight-loss program. The public deserves better.

In 2002, I was invited to a small, private summit of weight-loss experts hosted by *Reader's Digest* magazine to discuss how to fix America's obesity epidemic. At this meeting, we spoke with complete honesty about what it takes to lose weight safely and permanently. Then we talked about how to take those truths and turn them into a weight-loss plan that was as easy and sensible as possible.

This was how *ChangeOne* was born. Based on that session, several impressive writers and nutritional experts put together the first edition of the book, and I must say, I was—and still am—most impressed. If ever there was an "anti-fad" diet, it is *ChangeOne*. Here's why I'm so supportive of it.

- It puts the focus back on how much you eat, rather than on what you eat. For all the hubbub about carbs, protein, and fat, the thing that matters most is balancing how many calories you eat in a day with how many calories you burn in a day.

- It focuses entirely on making permanent changes in how you eat and live. This is a program meant for life, not just 12 weeks.
- It is based on thoroughly sound scientific research.
- It is among the easiest, most commonsense weight-loss programs I've ever seen.

Best of all, it works. When discussing this revised edition with the editors of the book, I was given some pretty impressive statistics about how well *ChangeOne* has achieved its goals of helping people transform their lives through healthier eating and movement. Since its launch in 2003, an estimated 60 million people in 15 countries have learned the *ChangeOne* approach to weight loss through books, magazine articles, or the Internet. Read the success stories in this book, and you'll see that the response has been a resounding, "Yes! It works!"

Yet another plus: *ChangeOne* is one of the only weight-loss programs around that carefully meshes an eating program with exercise and lifestyle advice. You know it, and we researchers have confirmed it: Diet alone isn't enough to keep weight off. To make lasting changes, you need a well-rounded approach, one that bolsters your self-confidence and gets you a whole lot more active and happy.

While the first edition of *ChangeOne* featured loads of exercise advice and programs, it was based on conventional wisdom about fitness and movement. In this new edition, we've exploded much of the popular thinking about fitness and come up with an approach that's a whole lot easier, more sensible, and more intuitively appealing. You'll love our 10-minute-a-day strength and stretching plan, and you'll nod your head in agreement when we explain why how much time you spend outdoors is a top indicator of how healthy your lifestyle is.

Put it all together, and in only 12 weeks, you will get the training and practice you need to help win the weight-loss battle *permanently*. *ChangeOne* is easy. It's different. And it works. Using the ideas in this book, you can take charge of your life today, and you can succeed!

—John Foreyt, Ph.D.
Professor, Department of Medicine,
Behavioral Medicine Research Center,
Baylor College of Medicine, Houston

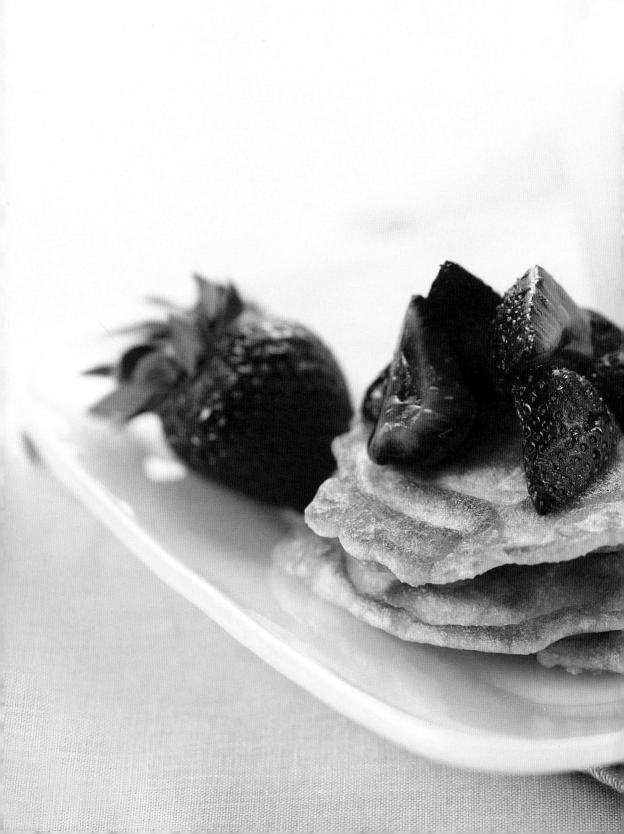

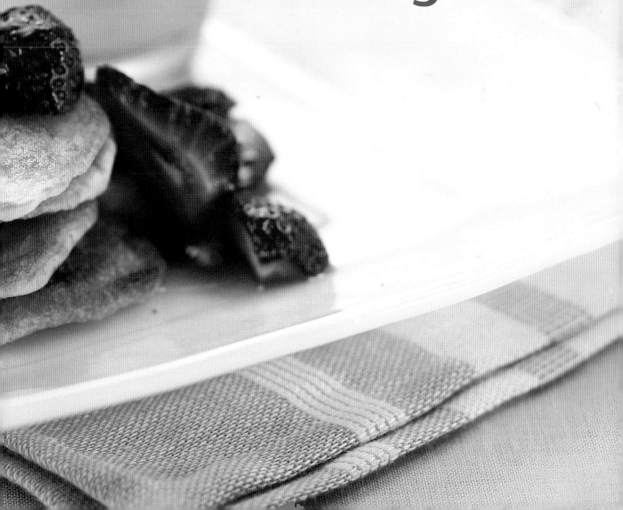

Part 1

Change One

The Eating Plan

Quick-Start GUIDE

The *ChangeOne* Eating Plan

The heart of *ChangeOne* is a 12-week program to transform how you eat. Each week introduces one new healthy diet habit to learn and practice. All foods are allowed, but in the appropriate amounts. Most people will eat about 1,300 calories a day on this plan. Larger or more active people can add roughly 300 calories through extra servings of grain or protein each day. Here's an overview of the first four weeks:

Week 1: Breakfast

Roughly 300 calories

The first task: Learn to eat a healthy break-fast every day, even if you don't normally eat anything.

The Basic Menu

- **One grain or starch**—roughly a cup (base-ball) of ready-to-eat cereal, a slice of toast, or a roll (tennis ball).
- **One dairy or high-calcium food**—a cup of milk or a cup of yogurt.
- **Fruit**—one piece, or an equivalent amount of melon or berries.

Variations: Pancakes, champagne brunches, lox and bagels, even a parfait are fine if done the *ChangeOne* way.

Week 2: Lunch

Roughly 350 calories

You'll learn to recognize a sensible lunch that fits your lifestyle and tastes.

The Basic Menu

- **One grain or starch**—two slices of sandwich bread; a tennis-ball-sized potato or roll, or serving of pasta or rice.
- **One protein**—thin palm-sized slice of cheese, a small burger patty, or three CD-sized pieces of lunch meat.
- **Fruit**—one piece, or an equivalent amount, of melon or berries.
- **Vegetables**—as much as you want.

Variations: Soups, salads, wraps, even chili, done in sensible portion sizes.

Week 3: Snacks

Up to 200 calories

Yes, you can have cake and eat it, too. In fact, you get two snacks a day.

- **Salty**—a handful of chips, microwave pop-corn, crackers, or nuts in the shell.
- **Sweet**—a palmful of M&Ms, jelly beans, malted-milk balls, raisins, or hard candy, or a mini candy bar.
- **Baked**—two small cookies, one mini cup-cake, or a 2-inch-square brownie.
- **Frozen**—2 golf balls worth of frozen yogurt, sorbet, or Italian ices; half a tennis ball worth of regular ice cream; or a Fudgsicle or juice bar.

Week 4: Dinner

Roughly 450 calories

A full day's worth of dieting begins this week, and you'll never look back.

The Basic Menu

- **One protein**—a tennis ball worth of shrimp, scallops, or crab; a deck of cards portion of chicken breast filet, beef, salmon, or tofu; a serving of light-flesh fish the size of a checkbook; 2 golf balls of beans.
- **One grain or starch**—a tennis-ball serving of rice, pasta, noodles, or bread.
- **Vegetables**—as much as you want.

Variations: Pot roasts, Chinese buffets, shish kebabs, barbecue.

ChangeOne Living

While the first four weeks cover meals, each of the next eight weeks takes on an aspect of daily life that influences how you eat:

Week 5: Dining Out

We'll ask you to go out for meals at least twice this week to practice ordering—and eating—only what you want.

Week 6: Weekends and Holidays

Plan meals or parties with family and friends. You'll not only enjoy yourself; you'll be able to resist temptation.

Week 7: Fixing Your Kitchen

Take a hard look at what's in your refrigerator and on your shelves. Is the food you see going to help you lose weight or undermine your best intentions?

Week 8: How am I Doing?

You're two months into the program, so it's time to assess your progress and clear any roadblocks.

Week 9: Stress Relief

Eating often serves as a coping mechanism for stress. We'll help you identify and relieve those hidden pressures.

Week 10: Superfoods

Yes, eat the foods you love on *ChangeOne*. But you might wish to incorporate these foods that provide particularly good weight-loss benefits.

Week 11: Keeping on Track

Pounds don't return all at once. Your goal is to devise your own "First Alert" plan to help contain the gain.

Week 12: *ChangeOne*...for Life!

You made it! So don't let boredom ruin the new you. Here's how to maintain your loss.

ChangeOne Fitness

While the heart of *ChangeOne* is the 12–week eating transformation plan, also crucial to weight-loss success is active living. In the *ChangeOne* Fitness Plan, we show you how to go from sedentary to active as easily as possible. You can do it simultaneously with the eating plan or wait until you've mastered the 12-week program to get started.

The Key Principles

1. Make one change at a time. You can't become a new person overnight—lasting change requires a measured approach.
2. The secret to weight loss is understanding portion sizes, not math. If you don't want to count calories for the rest of your life, don't diet that way.
3. All foods are allowed. Let your meals be a source of healthy pleasure and never skimp on flavor or delight.
4. Eating for a healthy weight is the same as eating for health. Think of *ChangeOne* as a way of life, and this will be the last time you have to lose weight.

Welcome to
ChangeOne

You've opened this book for one simple reason: You want to lose weight. Maybe a little, maybe a lot. Maybe you'd like to improve the reflection looking back at you from the mirror. Maybe you're hoping to fit more easily into an old pair of slacks or jeans. Or perhaps you simply want to be healthier and feel better.

Whatever your goal, *ChangeOne* will help you lose weight—and keep it off.

That may sound like a big promise. But there's really no mystery to dieting, despite the bewildering number of plans out there. Want to know a little secret? They all can work. Only one thing matters in the weight-loss game: Eat fewer calories than you burn. All diets, even the seemingly crazy ones, restrict your calories, and that's why you lose weight. Eat reasonable amounts of food, add in some calorie-burning exercise, and the pounds will melt away.

Honest, Sensible Weight Loss

You won't find any silly gimmicks in *ChangeOne*. We're not going to make you become a vegetarian, a strict carnivore, a caveman, or a goddess. But we're radically different in one crucial way: *ChangeOne* asks you to approach dieting one meal at a time, one week at a time. (*ChangeOne* means just that—one change at a time.) We won't overwhelm you on the first day. Most diets ask you to throw out the way you eat overnight and adopt a new plan. You might be Mary today, but tomorrow you're supposed to become Elle. The biggest problem with that kind of approach is people will eventually go back to their old ways—after all, you are Mary—and gain back the weight they lost.

Imagine a psychologist who expects depressed patients to be happy after one visit. Or a language teacher who announces on the first day of class that students will be able to speak French the next day. It sounds laughable because making a significant change takes time; new skills require practice. Yet instant change is what most diets ask for, and that may be why so many people end up regaining the weight they've lost.

ChangeOne slows dieting down so you can experiment and learn. (Don't worry, the pounds will start coming off right away.)

In the first week, you'll make just one change to your diet: overhaul your breakfast. To make it as easy as possible, we've provided lots of breakfast menus, several of them that can be thrown together in a matter of seconds. For the cooks among us, we've also provided some terrific recipes. In each case, we've counted the calories, so all you have to do is learn to recognize and eat reasonable portion sizes.

In the second week, while you stick with your new habit of eating a healthy, low-calorie breakfast, you'll move on to

You're Not Alone

When starting a weight-loss program, it is reassuring to know that others have found success using the same approach. So let us assure you that a *lot* of people have been down the *ChangeOne* path. In this book you'll hear the uplifting stories of a few dozen of them. But that's just the start. Some 30 million people learned the *ChangeOne* weight-loss method in a four-article series in *Reader's Digest* magazine; hundreds of thousands of people have bought this book since it was first published in 2003; untold more have visited and then subscribed to the *ChangeOne* website; and several major corporations have made *ChangeOne* their official weight-loss program. Then there's overseas. *ChangeOne* has been detailed in *Reader's Digest* editions around the world, and the book is a strong seller in 15 countries. We estimate more than 60 million people have read the *ChangeOne* diet so far, contributing to untold millions of pounds lost!

lunch. Again, we offer a variety of simple menu choices. All you do is choose one each day during the week.

In the third week, you'll focus on snacks. What do snacks have to do with dieting? Plenty. Snacks will keep you from getting too hungry, thereby strengthening your willpower. We'll offer you a variety of satisfying choices that will help your diet, not derail it.

In the fourth week, with breakfast, lunch, and snacks up and running, you'll move on to what's typically the biggest meal of the day: dinner. You'll find a tantalizing variety of great-tasting dinner menus and tried-and-true strategies for keeping portion sizes under control.

Voilà. By the end of the fourth week, you will have retooled your diet, reduced calories and fat, and discovered new ways to enjoy good nutrition and great-tasting food. And you'll be watching the pounds melt away.

This measured approach makes it easy to experiment with each meal, allowing you to incorporate the foods that you enjoy. By focusing on one meal at a time, you'll discover more about the way you eat. You may find that eating a reasonable

Making Sense of Low-Carb Mania

First, it was the Atkins Diet. Then the South Beach Diet. For several years, low-carb diets were everywhere, touting the seemingly revolutionary message that drastically cutting carbohydrates from your diet and replacing them with protein was the best way to lose weight. The message conflicted with the opinions of the medical mainstream, making for a high-profile war of words among doctors and diet proponents on television and in newspapers and magazines.

It took a few years to catch up, but the research establishment has finally put low-carb diets through rigorous analysis. The emerging message? Low-carb diets do lead to fast weight loss, especially for men. But in the long run, they are no better—and often worse—than other diets. Ultimately, cutting calories, not

changing your nutrient mix, is what counts most.

More important, recent studies comparing popular diet plans reveal that the biggest variable in weight loss isn't the diet type, but the dedication of the dieter. Those people who found a program they liked and stuck with not only lost the most weight but kept it off—no matter what program they were on! And of course, people who did a fad program for three months and then reverted back to their old habits regained the weight.

The moral of our story: Better to do a program like *ChangeOne*, which slowly, patiently teaches you lifelong healthy eating habits, than to jump on the next fad diet. Because in the end, eating fewer calories, each and every day, is the only way to lose weight for good.

breakfast and lunch is easy, but at dinner you break the bank; or maybe snacks are your biggest stumbling block. You'll also gain confidence as you succeed in getting each meal under control. And then in the following eight weeks, you'll tackle tasks that get at the deeper food issues we face—oversized restaurant portions, stress-related eating, weekend indulgences, and more.

Once you've mastered healthy eating and the pounds start falling, you'll likely be motivated and ready to exercise a little more. The *ChangeOne* approach to fitness is unique, fun, easy, and based on the same one-small-change-at-a-time method as the eating plan. You'll be amazed at how easy it is to get your body moving each day when you do it the *ChangeOne* way.

Most important, with *ChangeOne*, you'll be learning eating, exercise, and lifestyle skills that are valid for your entire lifetime. After all, losing weight is something you want to do only once. With *ChangeOne* you'll take the time to get it right.

The Numbers Behind *ChangeOne*

The meals and menus you'll find in the following pages are more than just delicious. They've been designed to offer maximum nutrition with a sensible number of calories. That's important. When you're cutting back on calories, you certainly don't want to cut back on vitamins, minerals, fiber, and the other health benefits of good food. The beauty of *ChangeOne* is that you don't have to weigh every gram or calculate every calorie. We've done that for you. The *ChangeOne* meal plans are designed to meet the following daily guidelines:

- Calories: from 1,300 to 1,600.
- Calories from fat: 30 to 35 percent.
- Saturated fats: no more than 10 percent of calories.
- Fiber: at least 25 grams.
- Calcium: about 1,000 milligrams.
- Fruits and vegetables: at least five servings a day.

The calorie target of 1,300 to 1,600 a day is the one used in most diet programs run by experts in the field of weight loss. Not everyone needs precisely the same number of calories, of

On the following pages, you'll find regular features packed with helpful tips and advice based on the latest weight-loss research, including:

Food Choices

Menus, recipes, and snacks that will help you cut calories without losing the pleasure of eating. And our photos are accurate—the portion sizes you see pictured reflect what you'll be eating.

Help!

Troubleshooting tips to help you overcome many of the most common obstacles on the path to successful weight loss.

First Person

Insights from people who have used the *ChangeOne* approach to shed pounds and keep them off.

Fast Track

Optional strategies to help you speed up your weight loss.

course. A large person uses up more calories than a small one. A very active person uses more than someone who doesn't get around much. As you'll discover, *ChangeOne* is designed to let you set your own calorie target and readjust it along the way to suit your needs.

You'll also notice that *ChangeOne* meals don't slash fat to unrealistically low levels. In fact, you may be surprised to find that some of our meal plans come in slightly higher than the American Heart Association's recommendation to get 30 percent of your daily calories from fat. The latest scientific studies show that diets with a decent amount of fat—the healthy kinds, of course—are actually more successful than diets that restrict fat to an absurd minimum.

ChangeOne is designed to help you slim down gradually, from one to three pounds a week. People who lose weight at a steady, moderate pace like this are the most likely to keep it off. But many dieters are impatient to slim down. If you are one of them, *ChangeOne* offers "Fast Track" features with suggestions to help you drop pounds faster.

Sound simple? We hope so. That's the *ChangeOne* goal—to take the mystery and frustration out of weight loss.

Getting Started

The basic *ChangeOne* meal plans you'll find in this book contain about 1,300 calories a day.

That's a reasonable goal for many people who want to lose weight. But if you're very active or heavy, you may want to set your calorie target higher. People who are physically active burn more calories minute by minute than people who are not as active. And people who are heavy burn more calories than lighter people because they use more energy carrying around the extra weight.

What's the ideal target for you? Here's what we recommend:

Aim for 1,300 calories if:

- You weigh less than 190 pounds and get less than half an hour's worth of physical activity (including walking and other everyday activities) most days.

Aim for 1,600 calories if:

- You get at least half an hour's worth of vigorous exercise most days of the week.
- You weigh more than 190 pounds.

Keep in mind that you can always adjust your calorie target up or down during the program. If you aren't losing weight as quickly as you'd like, you can decrease your calorie level. (We don't recommend going below 1,300 calories a day, however, because a diet that skimpy is likely to fall short on vitamins, minerals, and other nutrients you need.) If you feel too hungry on most days, you can increase it. What's key is that you do not feel hungry. Researchers have found that dieters quickly adjust to a lower calorie level, so if after a few weeks you're still starving, eat a little more. Once you reach your weight goal, we'll help you find a calorie target that balances the energy you take in with the energy you burn. (For more help on this, check out www.changeone.com.)

ChangeOne Fitness

The *ChangeOne* approach to eating is based on sensible, proven principles that transcend fads and trends. The *ChangeOne* approach to exercise is equally sensible and equally honest. And in the spirit of honesty, it needs to be acknowledged: While it is possible to lose weight through dietary changes alone, for long-lasting health and weight loss, exercise is essential. Research proves it, and common sense acknowledges it.

Water, Water...

What can you quench your thirst with? Here's the *ChangeOne* approach to drink:

- Coffee or tea is fine. If you take either with milk or sugar, choose skim or a non-dairy (low-calorie) creamer, and use an artificial sweetener.
- Drink water, and lots of it. Seltzer, mineral water, and diet sodas are also acceptable. All quench your thirst—and reduce appetite—at no additional calories.
- Avoid regular soda, with all its sugar and empty calories.
- Fruit juice is healthy, but adds calories without fiber, so you're better off with the whole fruit and a glass of water.
- One glass of wine or beer per day is acceptable. They add more than 100 calories to your day, but there's debate whether those calories will slow your weight loss.

Look at it this way: How many hours of your day are spent sitting or lying down? For many adults today, it is as high as 23 out of 24 hours! Often, our daily routine moves us from one resting spot to the next—bed to TV to kitchen table to car to work desk, and then nine hours later, through the same routine in reverse. But we weren't built for such sedentary living. From prehistoric times to just a few decades ago, the typical person spent much of his day on his feet, doing calorie-burning, heart-enhancing labor. It is no coincidence that the beginning of the obesity epidemic in America coincides almost perfectly with the emergence of modern conveniences that have removed most any need to exert ourselves.

The 1,600 Club

If you opt for 1,600 calories a day instead of the *ChangeOne* basic plan of 1,300, don't worry about counting every extra calorie. Here's all you have to do:

■ At breakfast, double your starch or grain serving.

■ At lunch or dinner, double your portion of protein (that is, your meat, chicken, fish, or tofu serving); or at dinner, double your portion of starch or grain again.

Society's answer to the sedentary lifestyle has been the billion-dollar fitness industry. But it hasn't helped us much. For one thing, the exercise establishment makes things too complicated, with all its jargon and measurements and quotas and programs and costly gear. Put simply, it is guilty of imposing a fitness approach meant for athletes on everyday folks like us.

The *ChangeOne* approach to exercise is a whole lot simpler. It is based on the premise that healthy movement should happen all the time, not in 30-minute workouts a few times a week. Specifically, we define healthy exercise as:

■ Walking for relaxation and energy, each and every day;
■ Stretching and strengthening a few muscles, each and every day;
■ Getting outdoors as often as you can;
■ Living with a high-energy, upbeat attitude, and letting it influence your daily choices.

Notice that there are no wardrobe changes, no gyms, no big-time commitments, no special gear involved with any of that. Rather, the *ChangeOne* approach to fitness says exercise can and should be embedded in all that you do. Live the high-energy way, and you'll burn more calories, strengthen your heart, and help keep the weight off—for good.

You'll find great advice and directions in Part II to help you shift from sedentary to active living, one small step at a time.

Real Rewards

Most people on a diet want to see changes on the scale. That's natural. We recommend that you weigh yourself once a week, preferably every Monday (it will help you stay honest over the weekend). Use the same scale and choose the same time of day. Keep a log of your weight.

But remember, logging pounds on the scale is only one way to measure your progress, and not necessarily the best way. If you're losing fat and adding muscle, for instance, your weight may remain the same, but you'll look and feel a lot better (and your waistline is likely to slim down). One *ChangeOne* participant actually stopped lifting weights when the numbers on the scale weren't dropping as fast as he would have liked. But he looked great, and the strength training had a lot to do with that. We convinced him to start exercising again and to pay less attention to the scale.

That's good advice for anyone beginning a diet. Keep an eye on your image in the mirror, your clothing size, your energy, and the notches on your belt, and you'll enjoy all the rewards of slimming down.

Week **1**

Breakfast

How does this sound? This week you'll start _ChangeOne_ by eating breakfast every morning.

Maybe you don't eat breakfast. Plenty of hopeful dieters forgo the first meal of the day. What better way to make my diet work, the thinking goes, than not eating? People figure they'll end up taking in fewer calories that way.

In fact, it works the other way around. People who skip breakfast often end up consuming more calories during the day. Those who start the day with a healthy meal, meanwhile, are more likely to stick to healthy eating throughout the day.

In this chapter, you'll find the secret to eating healthy, pleasurable breakfasts. We provide several, and then tell you simple ways to adapt them to your own tastes. Every day this week, help yourself to whichever _ChangeOne_ breakfast strikes your fancy. Experiment— and don't worry if you try something that doesn't fill you up. The rest of the day you can eat the way you normally do. That's all there is to taking your first step toward losing weight—and keeping it off.

Why Breakfast Is Key

If you usually skip the morning meal, you may need a little convincing to get you to eat it. Many successful followers of *ChangeOne* didn't start out as breakfast eaters, either. What they discovered was that beginning the day with a healthy meal was the single most important change they made. "I was amazed, really amazed," one *ChangeOne* adherent told us. "Starting to eat breakfast changed the way I ate all day long. It really made the difference."

Don't just take our word for it. Scientific evidence comes from experiments like one conducted at Vanderbilt University in Nashville, Tennessee. Researchers recruited overweight women who typically missed breakfast. All the women were put on a 1,200-calorie-a-day diet. One group divided calories between just two meals, lunch and dinner. The second group ate those meals plus breakfast. Twelve weeks later the breakfast eaters had lost 17 pounds; the women who didn't eat breakfast had shed 13.

Wait a minute, you might say: Weren't both groups consuming the same number of calories? No, the researchers concluded. The women who ate breakfast were better able to stick to the 1,200-calorie diet. Those who went hungry until lunch were more tempted to cheat a little.

Breakfast Portions

To help you assess portion sizes, we use both standard measurements and the *ChangeOne* portion-size guide. Make it a point to get the items we use as guides and hold them in your hands to get a clear sense of correct portion sizes. In the breakfast portions below, members of the 1,600 Club can double the starch or grain serving.

Type of food	Example	Amount	*ChangeOne* guide
One starch or grain	Ready-to-eat cereal	1 cup	Baseball
	Hot cereal	½ cup	2 golf balls
	Toast	1 slice	
	Roll	Small	Tennis ball
One dairy or high-calcium food	Milk	1 cup	Diner coffee cup
	Yogurt	1 cup	
One piece of fruit	Orange, apple	1	
	Berries, cut fruit	½ cup	
Optional	Butter, jam	1 teaspoon	Thumb tip
	Nuts	1 tablespoon	Thumb

If you pass up breakfast, this study showed, you're likely to eat more, not less, than if you start the day with a meal.

The role of a healthy breakfast isn't limited to people seeking to lose weight. Skipping breakfast puts even *thin* women at risk for gaining weight. A new study finds women who didn't have breakfast ate more during the day.

The reason for these results is pretty obvious when you think about it. The longer you go without eating, the hungrier you get. And the hungrier you get, the more likely you are to gobble down anything you can get your hands on. When you open the day with breakfast, you begin by taming the hungry beast inside and make it easier to keep cravings in check.

This is such an important point that it deserves elaboration. Hunger is in good part related to blood sugar, which is to the human body what gasoline is to a car—its primary fuel source. Eating a good breakfast makes sure there is plenty of blood sugar in your bloodstream available for your body to convert into energy. When blood sugar dips, your body responds with food cravings—and for many people, the cravings are for sugary foods, since sugary foods convert so quickly to blood sugar. But this wreaks havoc on your body's chemistry, particularly your insulin levels, and leads to unhealthy eating patterns.

The short of it: You want generally stable blood sugar and insulin levels for both healthy weight and overall health. And the way to achieve that is to eat small amounts frequently. A healthy breakfast not only sets you up for good eating patterns for the rest of the day, but immediately takes care of the lower blood sugar level that is natural after a night's sleep.

One other good reason why the *ChangeOne* program kicks off with breakfast: It's an easy success. Of the three meals, a healthy, sensible breakfast is the simplest to pull off. That will help you stay on track for the day. Psychologists say that levels of two brain chemicals that give us a sense of control—cortisol and adrenaline—peak right after we get up. The confidence they provide may make it easier to stick to our good intentions, such as a healthier diet. These chemicals ebb later in the morning, so it can be tougher to say no to the doughnuts

Help!

"I'm just not hungry in the morning. Do I really have to force myself to eat if I'm not hungry?"

Give it a try. One reason you're not hungry may be that you're unaccustomed to eating so early. So try this: Start off with a few bites of something that sounds appealing—toast, say, or a cereal bar—for five mornings in a row. After two or three mornings, you might start to notice your early morning appetite increasing. Also, schedule dinner a little earlier than usual if you can, and eat only enough to feel satisfied without being stuffed. This will increase the chances of your appetite waking up when you do. If you're still struggling, eat just one item from a *ChangeOne* break-fast—a piece of fruit, for instance—and save the rest for a midmorning mini-meal.

The Perfect
ChangeOne Breakfast

Need some guidance on what a healthy breakfast looks like? If cereal isn't your thing, here's an egg-based breakfast that works perfectly. New studies show that eggs make you feel full longer than many other foods, lowering calories eaten the rest of the day. For that reason, eggs are one of the superfoods prescribed in Week 10.

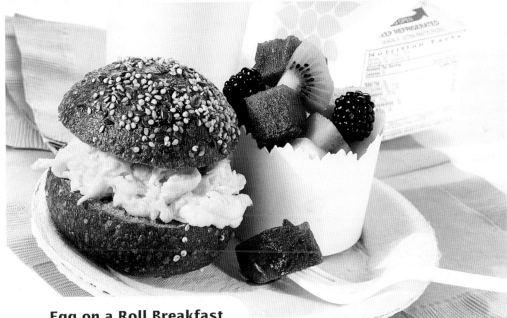

Egg on a Roll Breakfast

1   egg, scrambled, poached, or hard cooked

1   small whole wheat roll (size of a tennis ball)

½   cup fresh fruit salad (2 golf balls)

1   half-pint (8 ounces) skim or low-fat (1 percent) milk

Calories 300, fat 8 g, saturated fat 2.5 g, cholesterol 215 mg, sodium 340 mg, carbohydrate 41 g, fiber 4 g, protein 19 g, calcium 400 mg.

■ SUBSTITUTIONS

Instead of	Try
1 egg	½ cup scrambled egg substitute, or ½ cup low-fat cottage cheese
1 small roll	1 English muffin 1 small pita 1 slice wheat toast
½ cup fruit salad	6 ounces orange juice 1 orange 1 banana 1 apple

Time-Saver

This is a breakfast you can buy on the road as easily as make at home. If you have a favorite diner or coffee shop, let them know this is "the usual" and that you'll be by often to order it. Or ask a fast-food outlet such as McDonald's or Dunkin' Donuts to make it for you on an English muffin.

someone brings into the office—especially if you're starving because you skipped breakfast.

Here's a compelling argument: Most successful dieters eat breakfast. Since 1993 researchers at the University of Colorado and the University of Pittsburgh have been gathering data on people who lost 30 pounds or more and then kept the weight off. The project, called the National Weight Control Registry, is designed to learn what it takes to shed pounds permanently. Four out of five say they eat breakfast every day.

Making the Change

Choose a *ChangeOne* breakfast each day this week. Mix and match the meals any way you like. The important thing is to start your day with a good breakfast and then go on with life—and the rest of your day's regular meals. Don't worry that you'll end up consuming more calories than usual. Like a lot of breakfast converts, you're likely to feel less hungry in mid-morning and at lunchtime.

Don't let the morning rush get in the way. Putting breakfast together doesn't have to require more time than it takes to put cereal in a bowl, scatter a little fruit over it, and pour the milk. If you're really in a hurry:

- Set the table for breakfast before going to bed. You'll save time, and the table will be a reminder when you get up.
- Take care of one or two morning chores the night before. Instead of deciding what to wear after you get up, for example, select the next day's outfit before bed.
- Prepare a fruit salad on Sunday so that you can quickly spoon up some every morning of the week.
- Set the alarm clock 10 minutes early.

If all else fails, keep a box of breakfast bars and plenty of fresh fruit around for a handy, easy-to-pack breakfast.

Behind the *ChangeOne* Breakfast Menu

Each *ChangeOne* breakfast is designed to contain 300 calories or less. That's enough energy to power your morning and still get you started on losing weight.

(Continued on page 30)

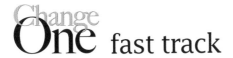

ChangeOne fast track

Hoping to drop a size before your upcoming class reunion? Determined to cut a slimmer figure when you hit the beach come summer? To speed your progress, choose one or more of these Fast Track changes this week:

Eat breakfast twice

Instead of having your usual lunch, make your midday meal another ChangeOne breakfast. Eating breakfast twice during the day isn't our idea. Lately several big cereal manufacturers have been touting it as a novel weight-loss method.

Help yourself to a bowl of their flakes for breakfast and lunch, they promise, and you can have a full dinner and still shed pounds. It works, especially if high-calorie lunches are your downfall.

Get walking

A core component of the *ChangeOne* approach to weight loss is walking. If you've mastered breakfast and are willing to take on a small change in your life not related to food, then make it to get outside and walking at least 20 minutes everyday. Take a brisk stroll in the neighborhood, a quick circuit of the office complex, or up and down a few flights of stairs if they're handy.

The scientific support is clear: If you weigh 180 pounds, you burn about 2.2 calories a minute sitting in a meeting or in front of the TV. Get up and walk, and you more than double that number, to 4.7 calories. Quicken your pace to a brisk walk and your metabolism knocks off 7.2 calories a minute. The benefits can add up fast.

Keep a food diary

People who are asked to keep close track of what they eat during the day, researchers have found, almost always begin to lose weight—even if they don't consciously go on a diet. There are several reasons for this.

When you're keeping a food diary, you become more aware of what you actually eat. And when you know you have to write down every nibble, you think twice before you grab that extra treat.

Keeping a food diary also reveals eating patterns you may not have been aware of—the fact that you snack more than you imagined, for instance, or that most of your eating occurs late in the day. Those insights can help you shape the best strategy for losing weight. You'll find a handy Daily Food Diary form and instructions on page 341. Track your eating every day this week.

Speed up the program

Though participants generally like the week-by-week pace of *ChangeOne*, you could do the first four weeks' assignments in less time to speed your weight loss. For example, give yourself three days for breakfast, four days for lunch, three days for snacks, and four days for dinner.

That would get you through the first four weeks and have you dieting from breakfast to bedtime in two weeks, instead of the four we recommend. The tradeoff is that you won't have as much time to experiment with meals to find the foods that satisfy you, and you could miss out on the opportunity to discover—and solve—problems in your eating patterns. But your goal is to look stunning for your beach vacation, and you don't have a lot of time.

The Story of Cereal

A good bowl of cereal, cold or hot, is one of the smartest breakfast choices you can make, as long as you choose wisely. Try to find cereals with lots of dietary fiber—at least 3 grams per serving. And check the ingredients for whole grains like oats or wheat. Pictured at right are the most familiar breakfast cereals in portions that contain 100 calories. Add milk and fruit, and you'll have a complete meal.

ABOUT MILK

Still drinking whole milk? Now's the time to lighten up. Take it one change at a time: Step down from whole milk to 2 percent, then from 2 percent to 1 percent. It won't take long before lower-fat milk tastes as good as what you were drinking before. Here's what you'll save in artery-clogging saturated fat and calories:

Type of milk	Saturated fat per cup	Calories
Whole (3.5% fat)	5.0 grams	149
Reduced fat (2%)	2.9 grams	122
Low fat (1%)	1.6 grams	102
Skim (nonfat)	0.3 grams	86

TIPS FOR TOPPINGS

Staring down the same old bowl of flakes can be daunting. Here are five toppings that can liven up your breakfast flakes for an additional 30 to 50 calories:

- 1 tablespoon shredded coconut
- 2 teaspoons chopped peanuts
- 1 teaspoon cinnamon-sugar
- ½ teaspoon cocoa powder
- 2 teaspoons mini-chocolate chips

A Perfect Bowl of Cereal

- ⅔ cup bran flakes
- 2 tablespoons raisins
- 2 teaspoons chopped nuts or sunflower seeds (optional, but adds 30 additional calories)
- 1 half-pint (8 ounces) skim or low-fat (1 percent) milk

Calories 260, fat 3 g, saturated fat 1.5 g, cholesterol 15 mg, sodium 360 mg, carbohydrate 51 g, fiber 5 g, protein 13 g, calcium 300 mg.

HOT CEREALS

When it's cold outside, there's nothing like a steaming bowl of hot cereal. Oatmeal and farina are classics, but there are many others to choose from:

- Cracked wheat*
- Cream of rice
- Grits
- Malt
- Maple wheat*
- Oat bran*

*Extra high in fiber

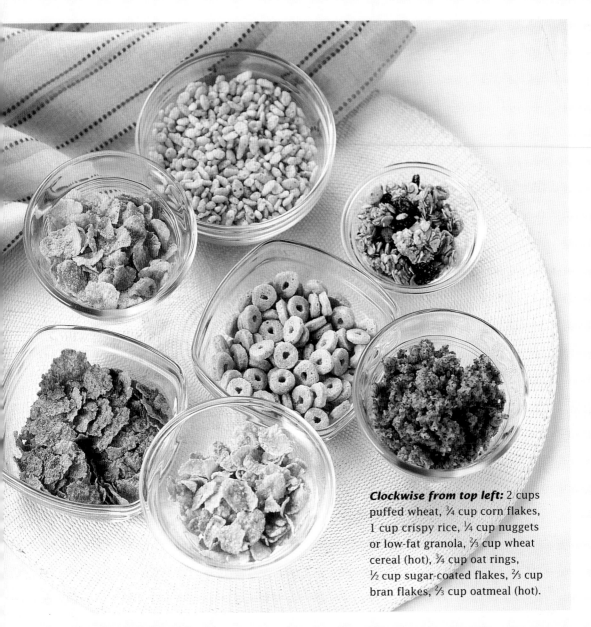

Clockwise from top left: 2 cups puffed wheat, ¾ cup corn flakes, 1 cup crispy rice, ¼ cup nuggets or low-fat granola, ⅔ cup wheat cereal (hot), ¾ cup oat rings, ½ cup sugar-coated flakes, ⅔ cup bran flakes, ⅔ cup oatmeal (hot).

MAKE YOUR OWN

You can create your own signature breakfast cereal by mixing two or more different types. Here's a combination that will last for days:

- 4 cups puffed wheat cereal
- 1½ cups oat rings
- ½ cup low-fat granola
- 1½ cups bran flakes
- ½ cup sliced almonds

Mix and store in an air-tight container. One serving equals ¾ cup. You'll have a little left over after 10 servings.

Calories 130, fat 4 g, saturated fat 0 g, cholesterol 0 mg, sodium 115 mg, carbohydrate 21 g, fiber 3 g, protein 4 g, calcium 40 mg.

What's more, each *ChangeOne* breakfast includes at least one food that's high in fiber. There are several good reasons for this. The biggest shortfall in most people's diets is fiber, experts say. We should get about 25 to 30 grams a day to be our healthiest; we average a mere 15.

Fiber's an important defense against several common health problems. It's also a key player in a healthy weight-loss diet. Because it's filling, fiber makes a meal feel more satisfying on fewer calories. One form, called soluble fiber, absorbs water to form gels that slow digestion, so high-fiber foods stay with you longer than other kinds of food, keeping you from getting hungry.

And by slowing down digestion, fiber also helps keep blood sugar steady, which cuts cravings and evens out insulin levels. This has several benefits, including signaling to your body to cut down on the amount of fat it is storing.

All this fiber talk sounds scientific, but you've probably experienced the difference between a low- and high-fiber breakfast many times. Just think about how you feel a few hours after having a doughnut and coffee for breakfast (virtually no fiber and lots of insulin-spiking refined sugar) versus having whole grain cereal and milk (loads of fiber and low refined-sugar levels).

In fact, to test the hunger-taming effects of high-fiber foods, scientists at Australia's University of Sydney compared two seemingly similar breakfasts: a bowl of bran flakes, which are high in fiber, and a bowl of cornflakes, which are not. Volunteers in the bran group reported feeling less hungry later in the morning than those who ate cornflakes. In a similar experiment, researchers at the New York Obesity Research Center at St. Luke's-Roosevelt Hospital recently pitted a sugary, low-fiber breakfast cereal against oatmeal, among the highest-fiber cereals. When volunteers ate the sweetened flakes, they tended to eat as much at lunch as if they'd had nothing but a glass of water at breakfast. When they sat down to a bowl of oatmeal, they felt fuller longer and ate as much as 40 percent less for lunch.

(For more on why high-fiber foods are so terrific, see "More Good Reasons to Fill Up on Fiber" on page 33.)

Help!

"What if I can't find a cup of yogurt with only 80 calories? Or a granola bar that has 120 calories? How exact do I have to be?"

Don't get too hung up on exact calorie counts. If you can come within 10 to 20 calories of the recommended amount in the target food, you'll be fine. Remember, the *ChangeOne* program is more about recognizing healthy foods and eating reasonable servings than it is about counting calories.

Change One success stories

Winning the Battle Against Temptation

When Debra Outlaw first started *ChangeOne*, she knew immediately that it was different from other diets.

"I never had to go through the awful 'consuming hungries' that I had experienced on other plans. When you phase in major changes over four weeks, it gives your system plenty of time to adjust to the new calorie levels for each meal."

Now 116 pounds lighter, she is much healthier and more in control of her eating than ever before. "Staying with the plan consistently is key," she says. "With dedication and perseverance, every temptation does not become a war."

Debra found that one of the most helpful changes she made was to eat breakfast. "I had always skipped breakfast unless we were going out to eat," she says. "I didn't realize how it affected my energy level. One Sunday morning I was late for church and had to go without breakfast. By the time I finished my duties, I was so weak! I now have a full appreciation for breakfast and enjoy it so much."

Debra also tried not to look for excuses to eat. "If the plan was a good plan, and I knew that it was, then it would serve me well for every meal, every day," she says. "I could not see special events as a time for indulging. I had to focus on the joy and celebration and not the food. I could no longer use stress as an excuse to eat, either."

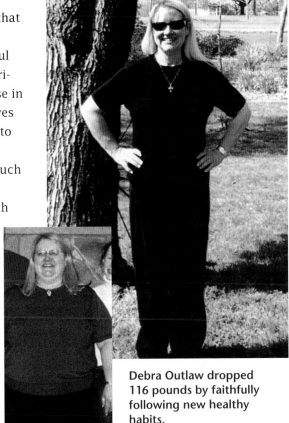

Debra Outlaw dropped 116 pounds by faithfully following new healthy habits.

For Debra, the trick is faithfully following her new healthy habits. "If you truly want to develop new habits, you need to be consistent," she says. "People tell me they could never stick to the plan every day, as though that would be such a burden. I think it's just the opposite. When you go on and off the plan, losing weight seems much harder. Temptations really do lose their power with consistency."

For more ChangeOne *success stories, go to www.changeone.com/successstories*

A Fruitful Choice

ChangeOne breakfasts also include at least one serving of fruit. Fruit, like whole grains, is a terrific source of fiber. One apple has almost six grams of fiber, which is 20 percent of the recommended daily amount. Also, the lion's share of people who hit the recommended goal of five servings of fruits and vegetables every day got at least one of those at breakfast.

When we say fruit, we mean fruit you can chew. Fruit juice is fine now and then, but many are surprisingly high in calories, especially if they've been sweetened. A cup of cranberry juice cocktail contains a hefty 140 calories. Even a cup of apple juice weighs in at 116 calories. Ounce for ounce, that's more than cola. What's more, most fruit juices don't have nearly as much fiber as the fruit from which they're made. Compare three of the most popular:

Orange juice (1 cup)	An orange
Calories: 100	**Calories:** 64
Vitamin C: 80 mg	**Vitamin C:** 80 mg
Fiber: 0.4 g	**Fiber:** 3.3 g

Apple juice (1 cup)	An apple
Calories: 116	**Calories:** 81
Vitamin C: 2.2 mg	**Vitamin C:** 7 mg
Fiber: 0.2 g	**Fiber:** 4 g

Grapefruit juice (1 cup)	Half a grapefruit
Calories: 115	**Calories:** 60
Vitamin C: 67 mg	**Vitamin C:** 62 mg
Fiber: 0.2 g	**Fiber:** 1.3 g

ChangeOne encourages you to help yourself to fruit not only at breakfast but for snacking, too. We stop short of saying you can eat as much fruit as you want because most fruit contains a fair amount of sugar, which means it adds calories to your diet. But we've never met anyone who got fat eating too many mangoes. Certainly, if the choice is between a candy bar and a piece of fruit, reach for the fruit.

Pop a Pill

For years researchers were divided on the value of taking a multivitamin. Now there's a growing consensus that popping a one-a-day-type pill is a smart move.

In 2002, in fact, the *Journal of the American Medical Association* published a landmark article that recommended taking a multivitamin daily. We think that's especially smart advice when you're trying to cut back on calories. Even the best-planned diet, after all, can fall short on essential vitamins and minerals. A multivitamin will fill in any gaps.

Weight Loss Potential from the Dairy Case

Something else you'll notice about *ChangeOne* breakfasts: Most of our meal plans include milk or yogurt. Nonfat or low-fat dairy products are a terrific low-calorie source of calcium, which you need for a key trio of health reasons: It helps keep bones strong, it reins in blood pressure, and recent studies suggest it may lower the risk of colon cancer.

Calcium may also turn out to have a weight-loss benefit, although this has not been fully substantiated. The evidence first showed up in a study designed to test whether men who added two cups of yogurt to their diet every day would lower their blood pressure; their readings did drop. They also lost weight—11 pounds in a year, on average. Another study showed that dieters who ate three to four ser-vings of dairy products daily lost 70 percent more weight in six months than people on the same diet who were not eating dairy. And better still, those in the dairy group also lost more fat from around their middles.

More Good Reasons to Fill Up on Fiber

With all the attention being given to carbo-hydrates, protein, and fat, it's easy to forget fiber. But when you're dieting, fiber could well be the part of food most worthy of focus.

Fiber, which is the indigestible part of plant-based food, gives whole grains, fruits, and vegetables their snap, crunch, and crispiness. And since your body can't digest fiber, it passes through without adding calories.

Here are a few more reasons why fiber is great for you:

Long-term weight loss: In a 1999 study published in the *Journal of the American Medical Association,* scientists tracked the diets of 2,909 men and women over the course of 10 years. Those who chose high-fiber foods ended up weighing almost 10 pounds less, on average, than those who got very little fiber.

Better cholesterol levels: High-fiber foods have been shown to lower LDL cho-lesterol, the bad stuff. A study by University of Toronto researchers recently showed that a diet that gets more than one-third of its calories from high-fiber foods like fruit, vegetables, and nuts can lower LDL cholesterol by 33 percent. Volunteers on a high-fiber diet saw their LDL numbers drop within the first week.

Diabetes prevention: In two major studies conducted by researchers at the Harvard School of Public Health, people who ate the most fiber from whole grains had the lowest risk for type 2 diabetes: High-fiber grains cut their risk for the disease by 30 percent.

Reduced cancer risk: Many studies show a lower risk of several kinds of cancer among people who include lots of fiber in their diets. By eating a healthier diet based on plant foods, most of us could cut our cancer risk by at least one-third, experts say.

The magic ingredient in dairy products seems to be calcium. One two-year study found that college-age women who ate a low-calcium diet gained weight; women who got plenty of calcium in their diets maintained a steady weight or even lost a few pounds.

Why? Experts have found that getting too little calcium triggers the release of a hormone called calcitriol, which tells the body to store fat rather than burn it. When calcium levels are high, calcitriol levels remain low and the body burns fat instead of storing it. Calcium's not quite the whole story, since subjects who took a calcium supplement pill in the diet studies didn't lose quite as much weight as people who got the mineral in their meals. That finding suggests that something else in dairy products may help spur weight loss.

Okay, what if you're allergic to dairy? You're not alone. As many as 30 percent of people are lactose intolerant, which means they do not have enough of the lactase enzyme, crucial for the digestion of milk sugars. But even with low lactase, experts say, you may be able to digest milk with no stomach discomfort thanks to sugar-processing microbes we all carry in our intestines. If you're lactose intolerant and want to find out if these microbes will help your body tolerate dairy on a small level, try adding milk gradually to your diet, rather than all at once. Start with a half cup a day.

Of course, you don't have to drink milk or eat other dairy products to be healthy or lose weight. You can substitute low-fat soy milk or rice milk and get calcium other ways—from a supplement, for example, or in calcium-fortified foods. The *ChangeOne* menu includes several foods with added calcium to help you hit the target level. Other nondairy sources rich in calcium include tofu, oatmeal, beans, and dark leafy green vegetables like collards, spinach, and mustard greens.

ChangeOne Breakfast Recipes

Of all the meals of the day, breakfast is the one in which we use the most ready-to-eat foods. But a delicious home-cooked breakfast is such a nice way to launch a day! So on your next calm morning, consider making one of our *ChangeOne* breakfast recipes: They're quick, easy, and oh-so-delicious.

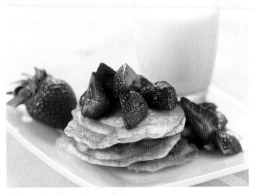

Silver Dollar Pancakes
page 277

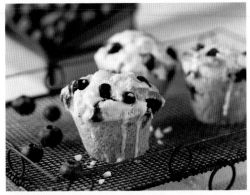

Blueberry Muffins with Lemon Glaze
page 279

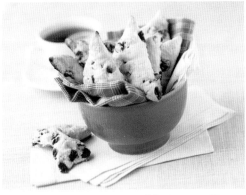

Dried Cranberry Scones with Orange Glaze
page 278

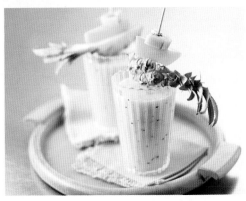

Tropical Smoothie
page 284

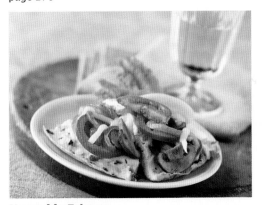

Vegetable Frittata
page 282

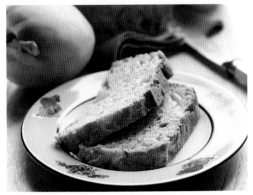

Peach Quick Bread
page 280

Lunch

Contrary to what you've heard, the single biggest problem Americans face in the battle of the bulge isn't what they eat, it's how much. We now annually gobble up 140 pounds more food per person, on average, than we did in 1990. How is that possible? Take a look at lunch.

Giant cheeseburgers with strips of bacon, 64-ounce jumbo drinks, super-size fries: Runaway inflation has hit the luncheon counter.

This week sanity prevails. You'll eat delicious lunches that satisfy without crazy excess.

For many people, lunch presents the biggest challenge of the day. We grab our midday meals in the middle of crowded schedules, work, errands, and distractions. And because lunch is the meal we're least likely to eat at home, we typically have less control over what's on the menu.

But that's all the more reason for you to learn ways to make lunch a great-tasting, sensible meal. With some advance planning, and using the lunches in this chapter and on pages 286-291, you'll be able to keep your calories in line and still keep the midday meal an event to enjoy.

Change One quiz

Ready for Lunch?

Thinking over the food choices you made last week will help you find the best ways to master the midday meal this week. Complete these nine questions by circling the number to the right of the appropriate answer.

1. Last week how often did you know in the morning what you'd have for lunch?

Never	1
A few days	2
Most days	(3)
Every day	4

2. How often did you know at least where you would have lunch?

Never	1
A few days	2
Most days	(3)
Every day	(4)

3. How often did you grab whatever happened to be handy?

Most days	1
Several days	(2)
Rarely or never	3

4. Which phrase best describes the choices available to you at lunch?

Very little choice	1
Some choice—same three or four things	(2)
Ample choice—varied and interesting	3

5. How would you rate your typical lunch?

Not very healthy	1
Healthy enough	2
Very healthy	(3)

6. How many servings of vegetables did you typically eat at lunch? (French fries don't count.)

None	1
1	(2)
2 or more	3

7. What was your usual choice for a sandwich bread?

White or French roll	1
Whole wheat, rye, or other dark brown bread	2
Seven-grain or other whole grain bread	(3)

8. How often did you eat lunch at home this past week or bring lunch to work?

Never	1
1-2 times	2
3-4 times	3
5-7 times	(4)

9. What was your usual beverage at lunch?

Regular soft drink	1
Sweetened fruit drink	2
Milk, sugar-free soft drink, or water	(3)

Turn to next page to tally your score.

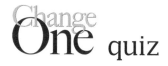 quiz

Score

Add up the numbers you've circled in the right-hand column.

A score of 24-30: You're already well on your way to eating a good lunch.

A score of 19-23: A few simple strategy changes could help make the switch to a *ChangeOne* lunch easier.

A score of 9-18: Okay, you've got serious work to do. By improving your lunches, you can take a giant step toward trimming calories and slimming your waistline. Put checks beside questions that scored a 1 or 2. Then look for the corresponding answers in the key below for tips that will help you this coming week.

1, 2, 3. If you have no idea where you'll have lunch—or what you'll choose—you're at risk of grabbing whatever's handy when lunchtime rolls around. That could spell trouble for your diet. Study the tips on pages 290 and 291 to master lunch by planning ahead.

Of course, not all of us always know ahead of time where we'll eat lunch. If that sounds like you, then it's time to keep a very close watch on portion sizes, wherever lunch hour finds you.

4. When your choices are limited, your best option may be to bag it—lunch, that is. You'll find several tasty packable lunches in the *ChangeOne* menus. If you're pressed for time in the morning, put your lunch together the night before.

5. Is your lunch falling short on good nutrition? Most of what's available at fast-food restaurants and other lunch spots is high in saturated fat and sugar and low in fiber and nutrients. If your typical lunch rarely sees a green vegetable, it needs work. If there's a huge cheeseburger on your lunch tray—well, you already know there's work to do. If the lunch spots available don't offer much choice, your best bet is to bring your own meal.

6. What, no vegetables? You're missing out on one of the best health and diet foods around. Follow the *ChangeOne* menu this week, and you'll get at least one serving at lunch, usually two.

7. Breaking the white bread habit can be tough, but you'll get more nutrients—and feel fuller longer—when you eat breads that are made from whole wheat or rye flour. You'll get even more fiber, plus healthful vitamins and minerals, from breads that contain whole grains like oats.

8. Don't dismiss the idea of brown-bagging your lunch. This week give it a try for a day or two. There's no better way to control exactly what and how much you eat. Many people find that packing a lunch relieves them of the pressure of having to choose the food they'll have when they're hungry. Not to mention the fact that it will save you a lot of money.

9. Sugary soft drinks and fruit-based beverages pack a load of calories. Some experts place much of the blame for the country's growing weight problems on the popularity of colas. No wonder: The sugar and corn syrup in soft drinks, added to juices and laced in sports drinks, now supply more than 10 percent of our total calories.

That's an awful lot of calories from foods that don't supply much else in the way of nutrition. Switch to a sugar-free beverage or help yourself to a glass of plain or sparkling water, and you'll shave 150 calories from your diet just like that.

Low-fat milk is another smart choice. Sure, milk contains calories, but it's also loaded with protein and calcium. Calcium is essential for healthy bones. And as you discovered last week, there's evidence that it also helps speed weight loss.

Don't Let Lunch Blindside You

Let's face it: Food corporations have our number. Super-size it! Two sweet rolls for the price of one! A free bucket-size soda when you order the giant fries!

We're conditioned to look for a good deal, and more food for less money sounds about as good as it gets.

But consider the numbers. A double cheeseburger with bacon weighs in at a massive 600 calories. Add on the large fries, and you get another 500 calories. With a small drink— or what passes for small these days—you're up to about 1,300 calories.

That's the basic *ChangeOne* calorie target for a whole day, all in one meal!

Of course, most dieters know better than to order a huge, fatty meal. But even healthy-sounding lunch selections can hide a surprising number of calories. Crispy chicken?

"I always thought chicken was the healthiest choice," one *ChangeOne* adherent told us. Then she learned that at one leading restaurant chain, a single such serving packs 550 calories. An individual-size pizza? Throw on the toppings and the calories can exceed 800. Taco salad? Order one at another well-known lunch spot, and you'll help yourself to more than 900 calories. Even with an increase in the number of healthy choices, fast-food restaurants are dangerous to

Lunch Portions

These meal plans use both standard measurements and the *ChangeOne* portion-size guide. Here's what a standard serving looks like (members of the 1,600 Club can double your protein portion at lunch or dinner; or double your starch or grain at dinner):

Type of food	Example	Amount	*ChangeOne* guide
One starch or grain	Potato	Medium	Tennis ball
	Roll	2 ounces	Tennis ball
	Pasta, rice	⅔ cup	Tennis ball
One protein	Cheese	¼ cup grated	Palmful
	Lunch meat	2–3 ounces	2–3 CDs
One fruit	Orange, apple	1	
	Berries, cut fruit	½ cup	Cupped handful
Vegetables		Unlimited	

your weight. People eat 200 more calories on days they eat fast food, according to a new study from the U.S. Department of Agriculture.

Unless you have a clear idea of what to choose—and make sure that you can get it—you could find yourself having to pick between going hungry during the day or going overboard on calories.

Making the Change

This week, while you keep up the good work at breakfast, help yourself to a healthy, delicious lunch, *ChangeOne* style. *ChangeOne* lunches contain about 350 calories. That includes everything—eats and drinks. Compare that to the calories in most fast-food and deli meals, and you'll see why sticking to the *ChangeOne* menu will speed your weight loss.

Eat a typical fast-food lunch, and you've exceeded your nutritional needs by hundreds of calories.

The meal plans you'll find here include lunches you can make at home, lunches you can pack, lunches you can order at a good deli or sandwich shop that's willing to do it your way, and even a fast-food meal that will work for you. Mix and match them any way you like. If you prefer to have pretty much the same lunch every day, go for it. If variety is the spice of your life, there are plenty of options here. What matters is sticking as closely as you can to the *ChangeOne* lunch plan every day this coming week.

As much as possible, decide in advance what and where you're going to eat. Right off the bat, you're in control. No more putting yourself at the mercy of the burger hut because it's the only thing you can find. No more searching the vending machine for something, anything, that looks halfway healthy. No more raiding that bag of tortilla chips because you're famished and it's the only edible item in the drawer.

Instead, consider some other options.

If you eat most of your lunches out: Make a list of the *ChangeOne* lunches that you'll be able to order at your favorite lunch spot or company cafeteria. Try to choose a place that really will do it your way, including keeping portion sizes under control. When in doubt, eyeball the serving sizes in this chapter for a rough idea of what a *ChangeOne* lunch should look like. Keep the handy visual equivalents in mind. Before you dig into lunch, make sure that what's on your plate matches up. At some lunch places, you may end up eating just

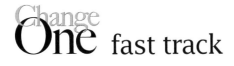

Change One fast track

If you're anxious to speed your progress, choose one or two of the following Fast Track changes and you're likely to see pounds melt away faster:

Turn off the TV

At least three times this week, turn off the television and walk for half an hour when you would otherwise have sat in front of the tube. It doesn't take a genius to figure out that sitting around watching television is bad for anyone's waistline. Yet even researchers have been surprised by the link between TV viewing and tubbiness.

Women who watch three hours of television a day have an average body mass index (BMI) that is 1.8 points higher than those who watch just one hour a day, according to a recent study by University of Utah researchers. For a 5-foot-7-inch woman, that's an extra 12 pounds. (To calculate your BMI, check out page 344.)

Hate to miss your favorite shows? Tape the ones you really want to see. By fast-forwarding through the commercials, you'll save at least eight minutes per half-hour show—extra minutes you can grab to do something active and keep off the couch.

Put down your fork

When you eat too fast, you deny your body the time it needs to signal that you're full. Experts say it takes about 20 minutes from the time you start eating for your stomach and brain to coordinate on these so-called satiety signals.

This week during lunch and dinner, lay your utensils down between each bite. Take notice of what happens when you slow down. Savor what you're eating. And try another tactic: The minute you feel satisfied, get up from the table.

Pour it on

This week carry a bottle of water with you and take a swig whenever you feel thirsty. That way you'll be less tempted to grab a sugary, calorie-filled drink. And drink one 8-ounce glass of water with lunch and dinner. When you include a glass of water with your meal, you get some calorie-free help on quenching your hunger.

Use the 50 percent solution

Dinner portions, like lunch, are often bigger than most of us want or need. And since dinner's usually the biggest meal of the day, giant portions can really pile on the calories. This week downsize your dinner entrées. Serve up half of what you would normally eat. After you're done, take a few minutes to relax and savor the meal. If you're still hungry, help yourself to half of what's left over. Otherwise, get up from the table.

Create a diversion

Identify one time of the day when you're eating for no other reason than because that's when you typically eat. This wouldn't be a regular mealtime, but perhaps a mid-morning coffee break, afternoon snack, or late-evening splurge.

Now instead of eating at that time, do something else—something that really appeals to you. Read the paper, take a brief stroll, pursue a hobby, call a friend—anything that gets you through that period. You may find that the reason you ate at that time was habit, not hunger.

half of what you're served and taking the rest home. Ask for a to-go container when you place your order, and enjoy what's left over tomorrow. Think of it as two meals for the price of one. Now, that's a bargain.

If you usually eat at home: Choose the meals you think you'll like the best from the *ChangeOne* lunch suggestions. You may find that something you wouldn't normally eat tastes great and really fills you up. Remember, there's little risk. If you feel ravenous by midafternoon, you can have a snack and your usual dinner later. Eventually you may want to stick to one or two particular meals (see "Keep It Simple," below). If you end up going for a wide variety, consider writing each day's lunch menu on your calendar the way fine restaurants post their menu du jour. When you begin to feel hungry as the noon hour approaches, you'll know exactly what's coming.

If you plan to pack a sack: Make up your shopping list and buy what you'll need at the beginning of the week. Don't forget lunch bags and storage containers. If your early mornings are crazy, do as much preparation as you can the night before; until you get in the swing of packing your lunch, it's easy to rush out the door empty-handed. Write "Got Lunch?" on a note and stick it on the refrigerator or front door to make sure you won't forget.

Help!

"I don't have a refrigerator at work to store my bag lunch. Should I worry about food going bad?"

No. The packable lunches on the *ChangeOne* menu will keep just fine for five hours in a coolish spot on a shelf or in a desk drawer. To be on the safe side, try a few simple preparation tips:

- Freeze a small plastic bottle of water to use as a sandwich chiller and then as a drink.

- Use a refreezable ice pack.

- Buy an insulated lunch box.

- Peel eggs only when you're ready to eat them.

Keep It Simple

Many people prefer not having to decide every day what they're going to eat. They find it comforting to open up the lunch sack to the same peanut butter and jelly sandwich with an apple and an oatmeal raisin cookie. And talk about being in control: If you eat the same lunch every day, you never have to wonder about how many calories you're getting. Some diet experts even recommend monotonous meals. In one study, volunteers who were offered a four-course meal consumed 44 percent more calories than those offered just one course.

Still, not everyone wants to sit down to the same thing every day. And variety will give you this: By trying out several *ChangeOne* lunch options, you'll find the ones that work best for you. All that really matters is arriving at a plan for lunch that you can stick with.

Behind the
ChangeOne Lunch Menu

You may be surprised by some of the choices you find on the *ChangeOne* lunch menu. Like avocado slices. Peanut butter. Cheese. Nuts. None of these would make its way into a low-fat diet. Yet we've included them in *ChangeOne* for a very good reason. The latest evidence demonstrates that you don't have to cut way back on fat to lose weight. New data even show that most people shed pounds more successfully on diets containing moderate amounts of fat than they do on very low-fat regimens.

Surprised? For years nutritionists have told us to cut back on fat—all fat. Too much fat on the menu makes people fat, they said. Gram for gram, fat contains twice as many calories as protein or carbohydrates. Just as bad, it puts our hearts and arteries at risk by increasing cholesterol. Or so the experts said.

And we listened. Over the past three decades, the total percentage of calories from fat in the American diet has fallen by a remarkable 6 percent.

But now, in a stunning reversal, the experts are offering very different advice. Some fats are actually good for our hearts, they say. What's more, slashing fat from your diet, rather than helping you lose weight, may actually make it harder to maintain a healthy weight. Very low-fat diets could even be unhealthy.

Good Fat, Bad Fat

Truth is, experts have long known that there are various kinds of fat. The two main categories are saturated fat and unsaturated fat. Saturated fat comes mainly from animals, either in the form of meat or the fat in cheese, milk, and other dairy. Unsaturated fat comes mainly from plants and fish. One of the biggest sources in our diets is vegetable oils such as corn, safflower, olive, peanut, and canola.

When it comes to heart disease, the culprit is saturated fat. Because of its chemical makeup, saturated fat causes the body to churn out extra LDL cholesterol, the harmful, artery-clogging kind.

Unsaturated fat, in contrast, has been shown to lower LDL. Further, it can also raise HDL cholesterol, the friendly form

(Continued on page 46)

d a Better Sandwich

dieter's best friend, believe
options are endless, and if
you can craft a satisfying
ndwich.
you're ordering over the
ng your own, keep an eye
n the supposed lightweight
, tuna, even meatless
n easily overstuff a sandwich
ces of meat (twice as much
swallow in a meal) or drown
aise (as much as 700 calories
worth in a tuna salad sandwich).

What you get, the experts point out, can
be a day's worth of calories between two
slices of bread. Not only will that blow
your diet, it will also put you to sleep by
midafternoon.

What you want is what you see here.
Check out these *ChangeOne* tips for
building a better sandwich.

BREAD

- Whole grain roll (tennis ball)
- Rye bread, 2 slices
- Pumpernickel bread, 2 slices
- Italian, French, or sourdough
  bread, 2 slices
- Tortilla, medium
- Sub roll, 3 inches

MEATS

- Turkey, 2 ounces (2 CDs)
- Deli ham, 2 ounces
- Lean roast beef, 2 ounces
- Corned beef, 1½ ounces
- Tuna salad (with low-fat mayo),
  ½ cup (2 golf balls)

MEAT ALTERNATIVES

- 2 tablespoons peanut butter
  (2 thumbs)
- 2 tablespoons soy nut butter
- 2 tablespoons tofu cream cheese
- 3 tablespoons hummus (3 thumbs)
- ¼ avocado, sliced

DRESSINGS

- Yellow mustard, unlimited
- Dijon mustard, unlimited
- Honey mustard, 2 teaspoons
  (2 thumb tips)
- Low-fat mayonnaise, 1 tablespoon
  (thumb)
- Apple butter, 2 teaspoons
  (2 thumb tips)
- Fat-free salad dressing, 2 tablespoons (2 salad-dressing caps),
  or reduced-fat dressing (adds
  about 30 calories)

COMPLEMENTS

- Reduced-fat cheddar or jack cheese,
  ⅔ ounce (palmful)
- Pickles, unlimited
- Lettuce, tomato, grilled vegetables,
  unlimited
- Spinach, arugula, watercress leaves,
  unlimited
- Thinly sliced apple, 3 slices
- Jam for peanut butter, 2 teaspoons
  (2 thumb tips)
- Hummus, 1 tablespoon (thumb)

SANDWICH SIDES

Stumped by side salads? Choose one of
these—and keep in mind that pickles are
freebies:

- Green salad topped with chopped
  veggies (tomato, cucumber, peppers,
  broccoli, etc.), two tablespoons
  sliced olives, a couple shakes of
  olive oil, and vinegar
- Three-bean salad, ½ cup

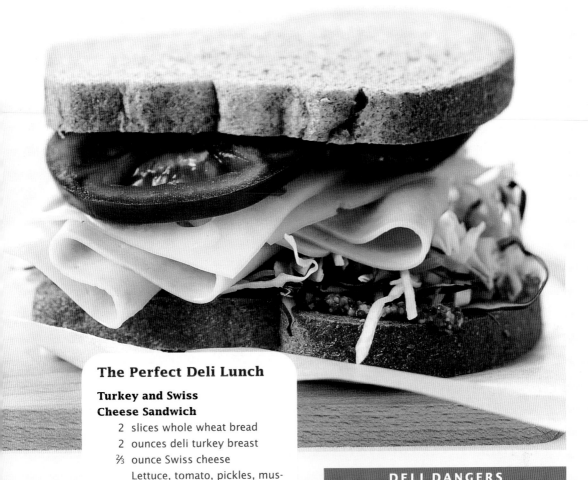

The Perfect Deli Lunch

**Turkey and Swiss
Cheese Sandwich**

    2 slices whole wheat bread
    2 ounces deli turkey breast
   ⅔ ounce Swiss cheese
       Lettuce, tomato, pickles, mus-
       tard, onion, peppers, unlimited

and ...

   ½ cup Italian pickled vegetable
       salad (cupped handful)
   ½ cup melon

Calories 330, fat 10 g, saturated fat 4 g,
cholesterol 40 mg, sodium 1,750 mg,
carbohydrate 43 g, fiber 7 g, protein 23 g,
calcium 250 mg.

■ "Clear" coleslaw, made with vinegar
  and a touch of sugar rather than
  mayo, ½ cup
■ Italian-style pickled vegetables,
  unlimited
■ Grilled vegetables, unlimited
  (but not too oily)
■ Sliced or diced tomato, unlimited

DELI DANGERS

Okay, you can enjoy your deli favorites
if you keep to a modest 2 ounces of
filling (2 CDs). That said, here are
popular lunch meats ranked from
best to "wurst" based on calories and
artery-clogging fat. There's no harm
in enjoying them once in a while, but
keep in mind that they're all higher
in calories than leaner fillings like
turkey breast.

■ Prosciutto   ■ Cotto salami
  di Parma   ■ Beef bologna
■ Turkey salami   ■ Liverwurst
■ Beer salami   ■ Beef pastrami
■ Corned beef   ■ Genoa salami
■ Beef salami   ■ Dry salami

that removes dangerous cholesterol from the body. Remarkably, getting plenty of unsaturated fat actually protects your arteries from hardening. Studies around the world bear it out: The less saturated fat and the more unsaturated fat people eat, the lower their risk of heart disease.

In particular, an unsaturated fat found in deep-water fish and some plants is proving to have amazing health benefits. Called omega-3 fatty acids, these compounds are not only great for your heart and arteries, but they battle inflammation through your body and help prevent several major diseases. They can even help lift mild depression, contributing to feeling more energized. Omega-3 fatty acids are abundant in salmon, mackerel, tuna, and flaxseed oil. Because these are not frequently eaten foods, more and more people are taking them in supplement form. What a change—doctors recommending a type of fat pill!

So why did so many nutritionists recommend cutting back on all fat? Because some of them thought the good fat/bad fat message was too complicated for people to understand. By telling people to cut back on all fat, the thinking went, saturated fat levels would fall. And with the nation's waistline expanding, cutting back on total fat didn't seem like such a bad idea.

Carbohydrates Aren't So Simple

When we dutifully cut back on fat, we replaced it largely with carbohydrates, mostly the simple kind found in French fries, white bread, crackers, and sugar. That's bad news for two reasons. First, it turns out that a high-carbohydrate, low-fat diet of this kind increases levels of triglycerides, a form of fat in the blood. Higher triglyceride levels are strongly linked to a greater danger of heart disease.

Second, a diet low in fat and high in simple carbohydrates may actually make it harder, rather than easier, to lose weight. Simple carbohydrates, because they are so easy for the body to digest, send blood sugar levels spiking up. The surge in blood sugar triggers a surge in insulin from the pancreas. That's normal. As mentioned back in the breakfast chapter, one of insulin's jobs is to move blood sugar into muscles, where it provides fuel for movement. But another of its roles is to prompt the body to store excess energy as fat. That's normal, too. But if blood sugar and insulin levels continually

Friendly Fast Food

Can't avoid a trip through the drive-thru at the local burger joint? Here's what to order. Notice: No soda! If you don't have a drink available, get a cup or bottle of water.

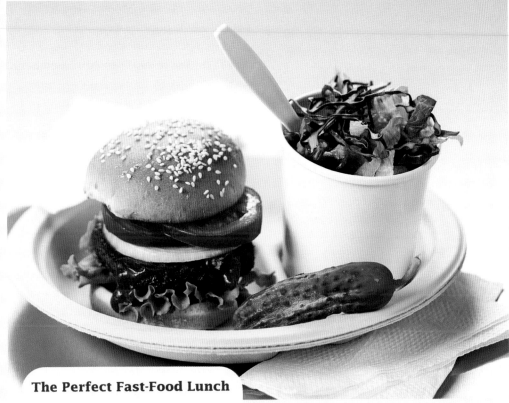

The Perfect Fast-Food Lunch

- 1 regular hamburger, with desired condiments (but no mayo!)
- 1 green salad, unlimited, topped with chopped vegetables (tomato, red cabbage, green pepper)
- 2 tablespoons fat-free dressing (2 salad-dressing caps), or reduced-fat Italian dressing (adds about 30 calories)

Calories 310, fat 14 g, saturated fat 4 g, cholesterol 30 mg, sodium 660 mg, carbohydrate 36 g, fiber 3 g, protein 14 g, calcium 150 mg.

TIPS FOR ORDERING

The nation's favorite fast-food chains offer some lower-calorie picks. Ask the restaurant where they've posted their nutrition information. Be sure to choose entrées that fall between 260 and 310 calories. Here are some safe choices:

Taco Bell: Tostada, Gordita Supreme, Soft Taco Supreme
Burger King: Hamburger, Whopper Jr. (no mayo)
McDonald's: Hamburger, Chicken McGrill (no mayo), any salad (fat-free dressing)
Wendy's: Jr. hamburger, grilled chicken sandwich, small chili with cheese
Subway: Any "7 Under 6" sandwich

Help!

"Last week I was so hungry by the middle of the morning that I felt almost light-headed. Is that normal?"

Well, the light-headed part is. Hunger can make you feel woozy. It can also make you feel distracted or grumpy. If you get that hungry, however—at any time of the day—it's time to eat something. If you're especially heavy or active, you may simply need more calories. Your body is burning more to keep you moving.

We're not talking about scarfing down doughnut holes. In a reduced-calorie diet like *ChangeOne*, it's important to make every calorie count for nourishment. Choose snacks that do what they're supposed to do: take the edge off hunger. Next week we'll take a closer look at snacks. For now, consider helping yourself to one of the following if hunger threatens:

- A piece of fruit
- A handful of nuts (about one ounce)
- All the celery or carrot sticks you like
- As big a glass of tomato or vegetable juice as you want
- Popcorn (skip the butter and you can help yourself to 2 cups worth)
- A cup of chicken or miso soup
- A cup of nonfat or low-fat milk, or a cup of nonfat or low-fat yogurt

Don't be afraid to reach for a snack. One recent survey found that snacking wasn't the downfall of most failed dieters; what got most of them into trouble was losing control at one of the three big meals of the day. Tame your hunger, and you'll stay in control.

spike and then drop, it can spell trouble. And that's what seems to happen when you eat a lot of simple, easy-to-digest carbohydrates. When blood sugar slumps, we feel hungry. Naturally, we reach for something to eat. And if that something is another simple carbohydrate, up go the blood sugar levels. The resulting roller coaster, researchers are beginning to think, makes people hungry more often during the day, and the surges of insulin prime the body to store fat.

There's still much unresolved about the roles of carbohydrates, insulin, and blood sugar levels. But one thing is certain: Cutting back on total fat and filling up on simple carbohydrates like low-fat crackers and cakes hasn't made us thinner. We're fatter than ever. And evidence is accumulating that a diet with moderate amounts of fat in it may make it easier to shed pounds.

Eat Fat, Get Slim

Consider the surprising results of an experiment conducted at Brigham and Women's Hospital in Boston. Thirty overweight people followed a low-fat diet. Another group of 31 people followed a diet with a moderate amount of fat—very much like the *ChangeOne* diet. The total calorie target was the same for both groups. Six months later, volunteers in the two groups had lost the same amount of weight. But after 18 months, a telltale difference surfaced: Only 20 percent of the people in the low-fat group were still following the diet, compared to 54 percent of those in the moderate-fat group. What's more, the moderate-fat dieters, as a group, had lost more body fat and slimmed their waistlines more than the low-fat dieters.

A Sample *ChangeOne* Lunch

Sandwiches are the great American lunch, and on page 44 we show you exactly how to build them, *ChangeOne* style. But for variation, here's a soup-and-salad lunch that perfectly meets the criteria of a healthy lunch: lots of vegetables and modest portions of healthy grains, proteins, and fruit that add up to about 350 calories.

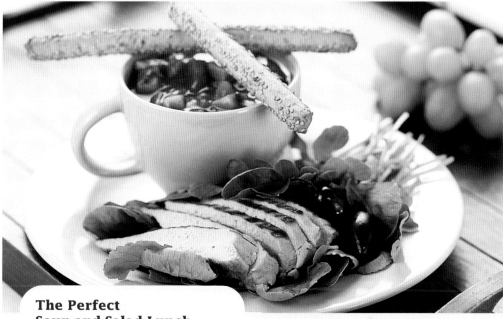

The Perfect Soup-and-Salad Lunch

1   cup vegetable soup (diner coffee cup)

2   breadsticks, medium

1   green salad, unlimited, topped with:

2   ounces grilled chicken

2   tablespoons olives, or 1 tablespoon chopped nuts, or 1 tablespoon grated cheese

2   tablespoons fat-free dressing (2 salad-dressing caps), or reduced-fat Italian dressing (adds about 30 calories)

½   cup grapes (cupped handful)

Calories 350, fat 10 g, saturated fat 2.5 g, cholesterol 60 mg, sodium 1,680 mg, carbohydrate 39 g, fiber 5 g, protein 26 g, calcium 100 mg.

■ SUBSTITUTIONS

Instead of vegetable soup (1 cup, 72 calories), consider:

- Gazpacho (1 cup, 46 calories)
- Beef barley (1 cup, 67 calories)
- Chicken noodle (1 cup, 75 calories)
- Manhattan clam chowder (1 cup, 78 calories)
- Minestrone (1 cup, 82 calories)
- Tomato (1 cup, 85 calories)

POWER SOUP

Soup is great for staving off hunger. Researchers at Penn State University discovered that chicken rice soup was more filling than the same amount of chicken and rice with a glass of water. Why? Soup is satisfying because it brings out all the flavors of its ingredients. Also, it may linger longer in your stomach, which will keep you feeling full.

Why? One reason, researchers say, is that a diet with moderate amounts of fat is simply more satisfying than a harsh low-fat regimen. It's a healthy diet people can live with. And that's the only kind of diet that really works over the long term. Another reason may be that people consuming moderate amounts of fat are less likely to overdo simple carbohydrates and will find it easier to keep hunger in check.

The new advice is the same whether you hope to protect your heart or shed excess weight. Replace saturated fat with unsaturated fat wherever you can. Switch from butter to olive or canola oil, for instance, and eat less meat and more fish. (Fish is abundant in polyunsaturated fats, particularly a form that contains omega-3 fatty acids, which have been shown to protect the heart.) Keep portion sizes under control so you don't overdo calories. And steer your diet away from simple carbohydrates like sugar and white bread and toward more complex carbohydrates like those in whole grain breads and cereals. These recommendations are the basis of the *ChangeOne* menu because they are the surest strategy for slimming down and keeping pounds off—not just for a few weeks, but for good.

The Perfect Diet Food

Something else you'll notice about the *ChangeOne* lunch menu: It features plenty of vegetables. Every meal includes at least one serving, often two. No other food fills you up on fewer calories while delivering more nutrients. Vegetables are rich not only in fiber but also in disease-fighting antioxidants. They're mostly complex carbohydrates, the kind that keep blood sugar levels off the roller coaster. Vegetables are so good in so many ways that they're free on *ChangeOne*—with the exception of potatoes, which are high in simple carbohydrates.

And as any chef will tell you, nothing brightens up a plate like dark leafy greens, red or yellow peppers, a luscious ripe tomato, or rich orange carrot slices. On the *ChangeOne* lunch menu, you'll find plenty of clever ways to add a serving or two of vegetables to your favorite sandwiches and soups to make them not only more filling but more flavorful...without piling on calories.

ChangeOne Lunch Recipes

Few of us cook in the middle of the day. Yet eating lunch at fast-food restaurants and company cafeterias spells nothing but trouble. Many of our *ChangeOne* lunch recipes can be made in advance, and the rest are super easy and fast. Time to upgrade your midday meal!

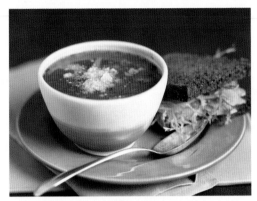

Hearty Split-Pea Soup
page 286

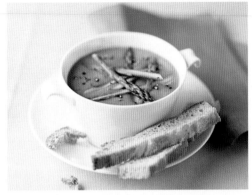

Cream of Asparagus Soup
page 287

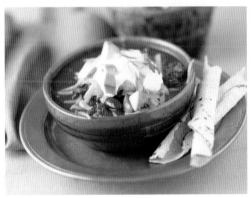

Meatless Chili Pots con Queso
page 288

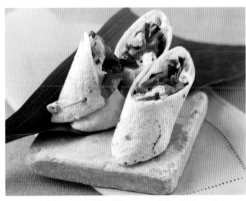

Roasted Vegetable Wraps with Chive Sauce
page 289

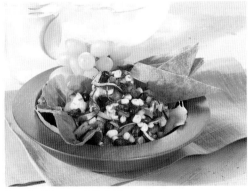

Pete's Chopped Salad
page 287

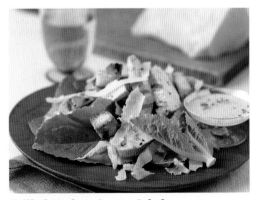

Grilled Turkey Caesar Salad
page 289

Snacks

An entire chapter on snacks? In a book about losing weight? Are we serious? You bet we are.

Over the next several days, you'll learn how to use two snacks a day to take the edge off hunger and make losing weight easier.

We think you'll be surprised at what you'll learn. In fact, one *ChangeOne* follower told us he chose to repeat the snacks week. "It wasn't until I filled in a food diary that I realized how often I snacked during the day," he explained. "And it wasn't until we tackled snacks that I saw how often I grabbed something when I wasn't even all that hungry." After two weeks of focusing on munchies, he really began to drop the pounds.

The same may be true for you. For years, nutritionists wagged their fingers and told us not to eat between meals. But now a new way of thinking about snacks has emerged. The two snacks a day you get on *ChangeOne* will help you stay on track. Eating something between meals can be one of a dieter's smartest strategies.

Savory Surprises

In the pages ahead, we'll explain the best approaches to healthy, fun snacking. But to get you started, here are a dozen fresh and delicious alternatives to the usual chips and candy bars. Each is just 100 calories—the perfect amount for a snack. Remember: with *ChangeOne*, we want you to enjoy food!

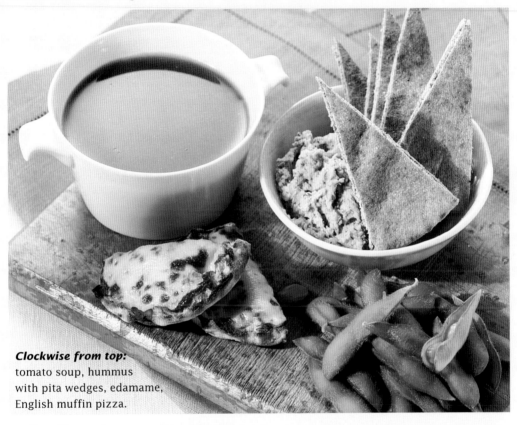

Clockwise from top:
tomato soup, hummus
with pita wedges, edamame,
English muffin pizza.

- Soup (minestrone, vegetable, tomato, chicken noodle), 1 cup (diner coffee cup)
- Edamame (soybeans ready to eat from the shell), 4 ounces (deck of cards)
- V-8 juice, up to 2 cups
- Three-bean salad, ½ cup (2 golf balls)
- Hard-cooked egg, 1
- Beef jerky, 1 ounce (a 1- by 6-inch piece)
- String cheese, low fat, 1 piece
- Hard cheese, ⅔ ounce (thumb)

- Peanut butter, 1 tablespoon (thumb), on a regular-size rice cake
- Corn tortilla topped with grated, reduced-fat cheese, 2 tablespoons (2 thumbs)
- Hummus, 2 tablespoons (2 thumbs), and ½ pita, cut into wedges
- English muffin pizza: half muffin spread with 1 tablespoon pasta sauce and 2 tablespoons grated cheese, baked at 350°F until cheese bubbles.

Make Snacks Work for You

When we ask people new to *ChangeOne* to describe the single biggest fear they face in dieting, many of them declare "hunger." That's not surprising. Dieters often think they have to resist hunger in order to lose weight. This week we want you to pay close attention to hunger cues. And instead of resisting them, we want you to feed them...with a healthy snack. Here's why.

Hunger is an extremely powerful force. Getting enough fuel for our bodies is essential to survival. It is a matter of life and death, literally, so the body has a variety of internal signals that alert it when its energy stores are dipping low. Some come from the belly. Some originate in the brain.

The longer we go without eating, the more powerful those signals become. It doesn't take long before they're so urgent that almost all we can think about is food. As hunger intensifies, willpower weakens. If you get hungry enough, you'll reach for anything.

That's where smart snacking comes in. Help yourself to something sensible when you feel hungry, and in doing so, you'll help ensure that hunger doesn't rise up and devour your determination to lose weight.

Worried that snacking will make it harder to lose weight? Worry not. Surprisingly, several large studies have found no link at all between how many snacks people eat and how much they weigh. Even people who snack before bedtime—once considered a big diet taboo—don't seem to be any more likely to be overweight than people who skip late snacks.

Eating more often than just three times a day might actually have advantages over the three-meals-a-day pattern when it comes to health. In a study at St. Michael's Hospital at the University of Toronto, researchers tested two nutritionally identical diets. One group of volunteers ate their allotted food

Check-In

Last week you added lunch to your *ChangeOne* menu. If you went off the plan for a day or two, don't worry. Change takes time. People sometimes take two steps forward and one step back. That's no cause to get discouraged. Take a deep breath, remind yourself of what matters most to you, then resolve to take two more steps forward starting tomorrow. This is an approach to eating that will last your entire life, so messing up a day or two is no big deal over the long run. If you feel frustrated because you don't quite have breakfast and lunch under control, consider taking another week with them before moving on.

Change One success stories

Benefits Far Beyond Just Weight Loss

Last year Lyndel Walker was feeling pretty overwhelmed by the amount of weight she needed to lose.

"My husband's doctor had told him to try the Atkins Diet, and I just couldn't be convinced that the high-protein, high-cholesterol approach could be healthy in the long term," she says. Once she found out about *ChangeOne*, she "knew that it could really help me do what I already knew I needed to do."

Lyndel has already lost 105 pounds and plans to lose another 30.

Besides her weight loss, Lyndel lists other benefits from *ChangeOne*. "I can now fit into airline seats, bend over to tie my shoes or paint my toenails, climb up into the kids' wooden fort without worrying that I will crash it, and shop in the 'regular' clothes sections. I have truly enjoyed being more physically active and just having a sharper mind and much more energy. Two of my grandchildren were visiting this summer from France, and I could go to the zoo, bike, swim, and just play so much better than in the past."

Lyndel is thrilled about her family and friends' reactions to her weight loss. "My husband never made me feel bad about my weight, but he has enjoyed being able to get his arms around me again," she says. "My children know that it means I will have more years to be a grandmother to their children and are happy about that."

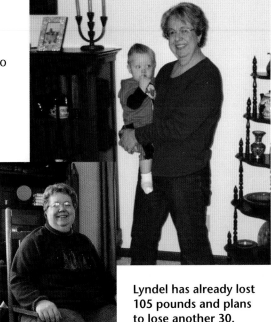

Lyndel has already lost 105 pounds and plans to lose another 30.

She also hears many comments about the amazing changes in her appearance. "When I see casual acquaintances that I haven't seen for quite a while, they seem to respond strangely to me, and then I realize they do not even recognize me."

Lyndel advises anyone trying to lose a significant amount of weight to be patient. "When I started, I knew that it would take at least a year to really get anywhere with my weight, but I also knew that it would take the rest of my life to stay at a reasonable weight," she says. "*ChangeOne* has helped me make changes that can last a lifetime."

For more ChangeOne *success stories, go to www.changeone.com/successstories*

How We Snack

Almost everyone grabs at least one snack a day. Half of the people in a survey conducted by Columbia University researcher Audrey Cross snacked two to four times a day. Afternoons were their favorite snack time, when they were most likely to reach for something salty. The next favorite was before bedtime, when many people's taste buds yearn for something sweet, like chocolate or ice cream.

in three square meals. The others ate the same food in the same amounts but divided it among 17 snacks. Compared to the three-meals-a-day group, the snackers actually saw their cholesterol levels drop. Eating smaller meals more frequently, the experts concluded, kept blood sugar and insulin levels down, which in turn reduced the body's output of cholesterol. That's good, of course, and for anyone who wants to lose weight, those results hint at even more good news: Holding blood sugar and insulin levels steady can also keep hunger in check.

While eating 17 snacks might be going a bit overboard, one or two during the day is vital to weight loss. Just ask the successful dieters in the National Weight Control Registry. A majority of them report they eat five times a day: three small main meals and two snacks.

This week help yourself to a snack when you feel hungry. But before you reach for it, we're going to ask you to do one simple thing: Make sure you're really hungry.

Learn to Spot Hunger Cues

In this chapter, we've grouped snacks and desserts together. One of our reasons is that the same foods often serve both purposes—frozen yogurt, fruit, a piece of chocolate, an oatmeal cookie—depending on when we eat them. Another reason is that most of us think of snacks and desserts as optional foods, a treat that's not part of our basic diet. On *ChangeOne*, we welcome you to help yourself to sensible portions of snacks and desserts. All we ask is that you reach for them to satisfy genuine hunger.

Isn't that the reason most of us eat in the first place? Surprisingly, no. Weight-loss experts say we typically eat for reasons that have nothing to do with genuine physical hunger. We take a tub of buttered popcorn or a box of chocolate-covered raisins to our seat at the movies simply because that's what we've always done. We eat because someone just brought a coffee cake into the office, and who can resist? Often we take up our forks simply because it's mealtime, or because everyone else is eating.

(Continued on page 60)

ChangeOne fast track

To speed your progress, choose one or two of the following optional Fast Track changes this week.

Downsize your dishes

Portion sizes aren't the only things that have grown bigger in recent years. So have the sizes of the plates and bowls on which those portions are being served. If you have a tendency to pile your plate high and finish it all, try switching to smaller dinnerware.

Use a bread plate instead of a dinner plate for your entrée. Ditch the giant pasta bowls and use a smaller cereal bowl to serve spaghetti. If the plates you already have won't do, buy an inexpensive set of downsized plates and bowls for everyday use. Another clever way to make a little less food seem like more: Try using a salad fork instead of a regular fork at your next meal and a teaspoon instead of a tablespoon for your soup and cereal.

Slim your sips

Plenty of people look to a cola for a pick-me-up in the midafternoon. If you're still reaching for soft drinks or other beverages sweetened with sugar, you're drinking a lot of calories that aren't doing much to satisfy hunger.

Studies show that beverages slip right down without triggering fullness signals. If you drink a 16-ounce cola, you'll consume 160 calories or more before you know it. This week, switch to sugar-free versions of your favorite beverages. Or try sparkling water flavored with a squeeze of lemon or lime.

Get stronger

Part of the *ChangeOne* approach to fitness is to spend 10 minutes a day strengthening and stretching your muscles. The weight-loss benefits are huge, and when broken down to just 10-minute routines, strengthening is easy, fun, and habit-forming. So if you are willing to step up your fitness levels at the same time you are making changes to your eating, turn to page 240 for our 10-minute routines.

Not ready for strength training just yet, but still want to get more active? Then pick up the pace of your regular walks!

The quicker your pace, the more calories you burn each minute. A 180-pound person burns 4.7 calories per minute walking at a leisurely 20-minute-mile pace (three miles per hour). Speeding up to a 15-minute mile (four miles per hour, about as fast as most people can walk comfortably) increases the calories burned to 7.2 per minute.

And disregard the fitness advice about slowing down to burn more fat. Research has proven that's a myth.

Hold the butter

Accustomed to slathering butter on bread or dinner rolls? One pat of butter contains a whopping 36 calories and four grams of fat, most of it saturated. If you smear a bunch on bread, you can easily tally up 120 or more calories on butter alone.

This week enjoy the unadulterated flavor of bread without all those extra calories. Choose whole grain varieties. The extra fiber these contain will slow digestion and make you feel fuller, and you'll get so much extra flavor that you may not miss that butter—at least not terribly.

Salty Snacks

Lusting for potato chips? Then have some—just not too many. The following lists show you 100-calorie portions for some favorite snacks:

CHIPS
- Potato chips, 12
- Tortilla chips, 8
- Baked tortilla chips, 10
- Corn chips, 15 (If you can't bear counting, serving size for all is roughly a handful.)

PRETZELS
- Pretzels, 20 thin sticks
- Soft pretzel, about ⅓ of a pretzel
- Peanut butter-filled pretzel nuggets, 6

CRACKERS
- Ak-Mak, 4
- Rye wafers (such as Ryvita), 4
- Wheat Thins (reduced fat), 15
- Ritz Bits, 25
- Triscuits, 4
- Peanut butter-filled crackers, 2 sandwiches
- Rice cakes, 2 regular size

Tips for Choosing Crackers
Looking for great taste and the benefits of fiber and low fat? Try Ak-Mak, lavosh, or rye wafers. Generally of Scandinavian or Middle Eastern origin, these are made with whole wheat or rye, meaning there's more fiber to fill you up and very little fat. Enjoy them plain or topped with hummus, roasted pepper dip, peanut butter, or reduced-fat cheese.

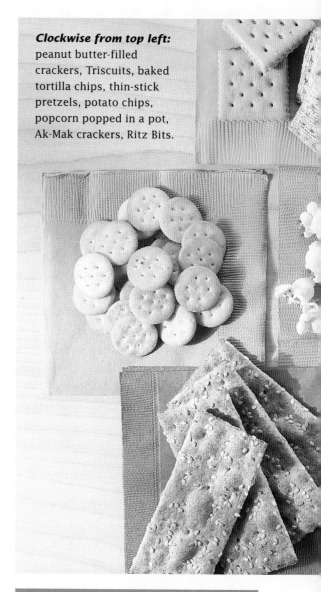

Clockwise from top left: peanut butter-filled crackers, Triscuits, baked tortilla chips, thin-stick pretzels, potato chips, popcorn popped in a pot, Ak-Mak crackers, Ritz Bits.

BAKED VS. FRIED
Many brands of crackers and potato chips boast that they're "baked, not fried." The implication, of course, is fewer calories. But the calorie difference isn't always that great. The baked brands still use some fat, and their calorie count is often close to the fried products. So don't simply buy because the label says "baked." Look for brands that supply at least 1 gram of fiber and less than 3 grams of fat per serving.

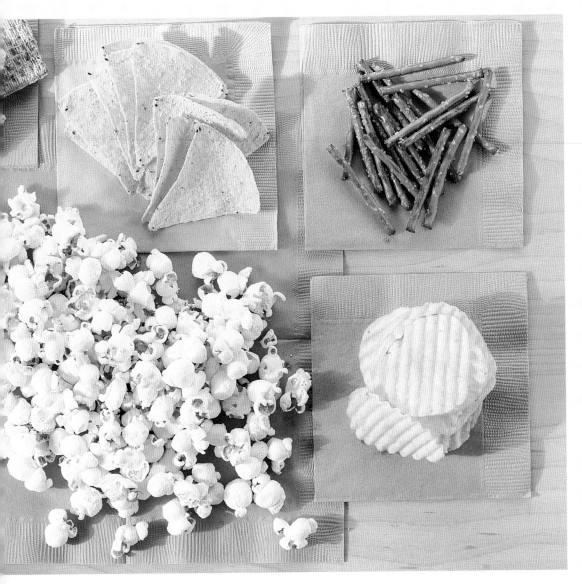

POPCORN

- Air-popped popcorn or popcorn popped in a pot, 3 cups (three handfuls)
- Microwave popcorn (butter flavor), 1 cup (handful)
- Cheddar cheese popcorn, 1 cup
- Popcorn cakes, 2

Spicing Up Popcorn

First, pop it on the stove or in a regular corn popper, adding a couple of tablespoons of vegetable oil to help heat up the kernels and prevent them from burning. Most of the oil stays behind in the pot, but enough gets onto the kernels to help salt and other seasonings stick. Next, sprinkle lightly with salt (if desired) and your choice of seasonings. Try chili powder, Italian seasoning, or a sprinkle of Parmesan cheese, or create your own flavor combos.

The experts call these reasons for eating environmental cues. Something in our surroundings gives us the urge to eat. You may not be hungry in the sense that your body is running short of fuel. In fact, you may have just finished a big, filling meal. But the sight, smell, or memory of past occasions prompts the urge to eat, and you help yourself, often without thinking.

Emotional Eating

Environmental cues are just some of the reasons we eat when we're not really hungry. Many of us eat for emotional reasons, too. After all, food can be comforting. It's an integral part of being sociable. Getting together over a meal with friends or family can be a pleasant way to relax after a long day. And there's no need to get too fancy about it: Food simply tastes good.

Pleasure we get from food has a biochemical basis, researchers say. When we eat something delicious, the experience triggers the release of endorphins in the brain, the same feel-good chemicals once associated with "runner's high." Certain foods may have their own mood-enhancing effects. Carbohydrates are thought to increase the absorption of an amino acid called tryptophan, which in turn boosts levels of serotonin, another brain chemical associated with mental well-being.

There are other reasons why eating is linked to emotions. If your parents comforted you or rewarded you with food, for instance, you may tend to reach for something to eat when you're feeling low or want to give yourself something for a job well done. If you get into the habit of eating something when you're feeling bored, you'll find yourself feeling hungry every time boredom strikes.

The same can be true for those feeling lonely. "I'd get home from work at the end of a long day, which was a hard time for me anyway after being divorced," a *ChangeOne* participant told us. "I'd have dinner. And then, maybe because I was feeling lonely, I'd just go on eating and eating. Dessert. Cookies. I wasn't hungry. Somehow it just seemed to make me feel better. Recognizing that pattern made a big difference for me."

Unlimited Snacks

Some foods are so low in calories that you can help yourself to as much as you want. Here are a few:

- Jicama slices
- Raw bell pepper slices
- Cherry tomatoes
- Carrot and celery sticks
- Sugar-free Jell-O

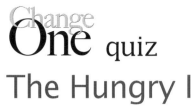 quiz

The Hungry I

What drives your snacking—emotions, environment, or just plain old hunger? Check only the shapes with the statements that apply to you.

○ When I go to the movies or a concert, I almost always get popcorn, candy, or some other treat.

☐ When I'm very busy, I sometimes don't even notice that I'm hungry.

◇ On stressful days, I often find it relaxing to eat something.

◇ If I'm bored and there's food around, I'll eat it.

☐ It's no big deal for me to say no to treats if I'm not really hungry.

◇ There are certain foods I really crave, like chocolate or salty snacks.

☐ I like the feeling of being really hungry when I sit down to a meal.

○ I have a tendency to clean my plate even if I'm not really that hungry.

◇ If I'm feeling a little down or blue, eating something can really help.

○ If there's a plate full of cookies or chips in front of me, I won't be able to resist taking some.

○ I have to be careful about having junk food around the house. If it's there, I'll eat it.

☐ My way of dealing with stress is to get up and do something.

☐ As long as I know I'll be sitting down to a meal soon, I can deal with feeling hungry.

○ Dinner just doesn't seem to be dinner without dessert.

◇ I definitely don't like the feeling of being hungry.

Score

Tally up the number of colored shapes you checked according to color.

☐ green _____
○ red _____
◇ yellow _____

What your score means:

☐ If you checked mostly green boxes, at least you're not snacking because you're bored or stressed. This week choose from among the recommended *ChangeOne* snacks, and you'll keep calories under control.

○ If you checked mostly red circles, you tend to be an "on cue" snacker. You reach for a snack not necessarily because you're hungry but because of cues in the environment around you. Recognizing those

cues—and asking yourself if you're really hungry—could help you avoid gobbling up calories you don't really want.

◇ If you checked mostly yellow diamonds, you tend to be an "emotional" snacker. You have the urge to eat something when you're feeling anxious, sad, lonely, or under stress. Many people do. Recognizing what real hunger feels like—and finding ways other than eating to deal with your emotions—will help you control calories and eat more healthfully.

If your score was divided evenly among greens, reds, and yellows, you're halfway to becoming a smart snacker. The tips in this chapter will guide you the rest of the way.

Help!

"My husband lost five pounds in two weeks. I've barely lost one. And we seem to be eating the same amount of food. What gives?"

You're different people. Some people can eliminate one thing from their diet—sugary colas, for instance—and begin dropping pounds immediately. Others have to watch everything they eat, and still the progress seems slow. There are many reasons. Some people's metabolic rates are higher than average, so they burn more calories even when they're just sitting around. Some people do a lot of fidgeting during the day, which also burns calories. One study found that fidgeters can burn more than 500 calories a day jiggling their legs or pacing around.

If you're feeling frustrated by the pace of your weight loss, consider making an additional Fast Track change. (You'll find Fast Track suggestions on page 57.) And hang in there. Remember the tortoise and the hare. Even with weight loss, slow starters can be the first ones across the finish line.

The problem with environmental and emotional eating is obvious. If you eat when you're not genuinely hungry, you'll almost certainly consume more calories than your body needs. There are healthier ways than overeating to deal with stress, boredom, or loneliness. Simply distracting yourself by doing something else you enjoy—listening to music, calling a friend, reading a book, watching a movie, going for a walk, or doing a crossword puzzle—often works. So how do you know if environmental or emotional cues are controlling when and how much you eat? The first step is paying attention to what genuine hunger feels like.

Last week you began to be more aware of times during the day when you felt hungry between meals—and what you did about it. Using what you learned, take the "Hungry I" quiz to learn more about your own hunger profile.

Knowing When You're Genuinely Hungry

One day early this week, try a simple experiment. If you typically have either a midmorning or midafternoon snack, skip it. Push the next meal about an hour later than usual. Then pay attention to how you feel. After you've gone four or five hours without eating anything, your body will begin to send out physical hunger cues. Some of these come from a part of the brain called the hypothalamus. When blood sugar levels fall, the hypothalamus senses an impending energy crisis and begins to issue "feed me" orders by way of the central nervous system. Your stomach growls. Your thoughts zero in on food. You may find yourself getting cranky.

This physical hunger is different from the emotional or environmental kind, and it is not the same as a food craving. Food cravings target specific foods. You may crave chocolate when you're feeling lonely. You may find yourself craving a fast-food hamburger when you're on a car trip. Cravings are almost always responses to emotional or environmental cues.

(Continued on page 66)

ChangeOne success stories
Feeling Better About Herself

When Teresa Williamson first read about *ChangeOne*, she was intrigued by its simple and sensible approach. She gave the diet a try and has lost 75 pounds and 38 inches.

"I feel so much better about myself and more self-confident because of the weight loss itself and the fact that I have done it on my own," she says.

Teresa's weight loss is not the only benefit she's gotten from *ChangeOne*. "I feel good physically. I'm not out of breath all the time anymore from physical exertion," she says. "I have also had a noticeable improvement in my asthma. I used to use an inhaler regularly, but now I use it seldom, because my body is not having to work as hard." She adds, "I can shop in the regular-size clothing section, something that I haven't done in many years. That is very exciting!"

Teresa loves the commonsense approach of *ChangeOne*. "I know that I'm not doing any harm to my body by doing this diet. Diet pills can cause harm, as can fad diets. There are no special meals that must be bought—just good food from the store. That means for me that if I continue throughout my life to follow *ChangeOne* principles, I should easily be able to maintain weight loss once I achieve my goal weight."

The *ChangeOne* portion-size guides have helped Teresa keep her servings in check. "Also, knowing that I should

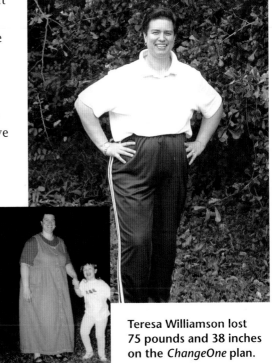

Teresa Williamson lost 75 pounds and 38 inches on the *ChangeOne* plan.

eat breakfast, a snack, lunch, a snack, and dinner helps me tremendously. Now I eat because I'm hungry, whereas before, I ate whenever and whatever I wanted to."

Teresa's friends and family are amazed by her progress. "My sister-in-law told me that I am just melting away!" she says. "At church, people are always commenting on how good I look now and how much slimmer I look! My husband is proud of me and is constantly telling me that I am doing great and look good."

For more ChangeOne *success stories, go to www.changeone.com/successstories*

Sweet Snacks

Love sugary sweetness? As long as you trust your willpower enough to stick to our portion sizes, then *ChangeOne* has some sweets for you. Here are 100-calorie helpings of some favorites:

FRUIT

Fruit would be a perfect food except for one problem—it has lots of natural sugars, making it much higher in calories than vegetables. An example: A cup of raw orange sections has 14 grams of sugar, compared to 1 gram of sugar in a cup of raw broccoli. We recommend getting small or medium fruit when possible, but having a portion that's a bit larger won't undo your *ChangeOne* plan.

- Dried apricots, about 6 to 8 (palmful)
- Raisins, 3 tablespoons (3 thumbs)
- Grapes, ¾ cup (tennis ball)
- Apple, 1
- Orange, 1
- Fruit cocktail in juice, ½ cup
- Banana, 1
- Melon balls, 1 cup (baseball)
- Pineapple chunks, ½ cup (2 golf balls)

Our Daily Recommendation

ChangeOne suggests two mealtime servings of fruit a day—one at breakfast and one at lunch—with the option of a third fruit portion for a snack. Eating more than three servings a day is good for general nutrition, but keep in mind that the extra calories could slow down your weight-loss efforts.

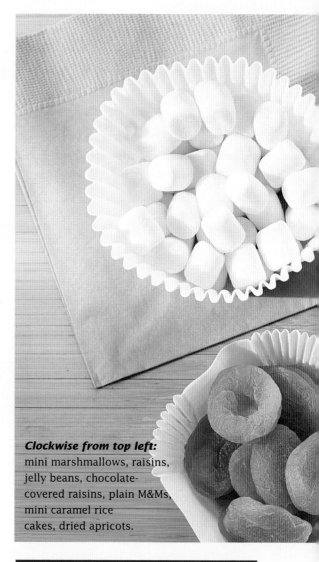

Clockwise from top left: mini marshmallows, raisins, jelly beans, chocolate-covered raisins, plain M&Ms, mini caramel rice cakes, dried apricots.

SWEETS

- Hard candy, 4 pieces
- Cracker Jack, ⅓ cup (palmful)
- M&M's, plain, 30 (palmful)
- M&M's, with peanuts, 10 (palmful)
- Caramel-peanut chocolate bar, trick-or-treat size, 1
- Chocolate and wafer bar, trick-or-treat size, 2
- Flaky peanut butter chocolate bar, trick-or-treat size, 2
- Mini rice cakes, caramel-corn flavor, 10

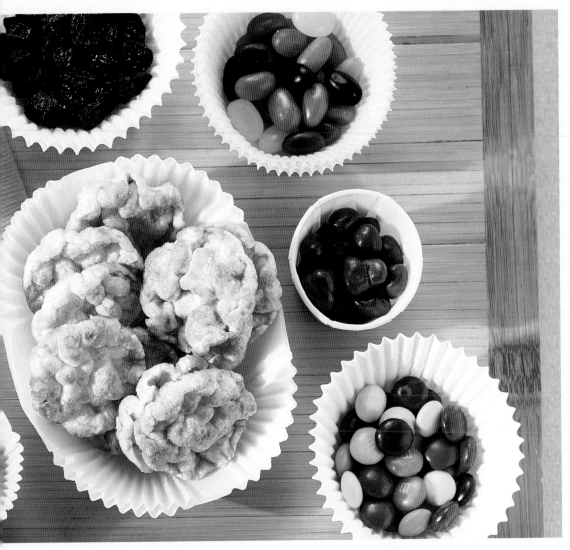

- Raisins, 3 tablespoons (palmful)
- Jelly beans, 25 (palmful)
- Licorice, 3 twists
- Marshmallows, large, 5
- Marshmallows, mini, 40 (palmful)
- Chocolate-covered raisins, 20 (palmful)
- Malted-milk balls, 7 (palmful)
- Yogurt-covered raisins, 2 tablespoons (2 thumbs)

Tips for Candy

When nothing but candy will do:

Buy high-quality treats or candy that you really like. When the flavor is intense or when you're eating a favorite, you'll be satisfied with less.

Minis are in. Buy the smallest pieces you can find. From the label figure out how many pieces equal 80 to 100 calories (or about ⅔ ounce). Eat them one by one, taking time between bites to enjoy each one.

Trick or treat year-round. Bags of fun- and bite-size candies are easy to find any month of the year. A portion is one or two pieces. Put them in an awkward, out-of-the-way spot—say, high in a cupboard behind the wineglasses—and then go there only to take out what you'll eat for the day.

Calcium Choices

Not only does calcium build strong bones, now there's research that shows it also helps the body burn fat. Some favorite calcium-rich snacks, in 100-calorie portions, include:

- Low-fat or nonfat yogurt, plain or artificially sweetened (one cup)
- Yogurt smoothie: In a blender, mix ½ cup yogurt, ½ cup skim or low-fat milk, and one cup frozen unsweetened strawberries until mixture is smooth
- Low-fat or skim milk (one cup)
- Skim or low-fat milk flavored with sugar-free syrup (one cup)
- Reduced-fat cheese
- Skim or low-fat latte (medium size)
- Hot cocoa made with skim or low-fat milk (one cup)
- Calcium-fortified orange juice (one cup)
- Juice pop made with calcium-fortified juice
- Sugar-free pudding made with skim or low-fat milk (one cup)

Physical hunger isn't so specific. When your body needs more energy in the form of food, you don't focus on the taste of a particular food. What you want is food to fill you up. Any food at all.

Two Essential Questions

As part of your hunger test this week, try another experiment. When you finally sit down to eat, make a point of slowing down and paying close attention to how you feel as you eat. Notice what it feels like as your hunger sensation gives way to a feeling of satisfaction.

During the rest of this week, each time you feel the urge to grab a snack between meals, pause for as long as it takes to ask yourself these two simple questions: Am I really hungry? Can I wait until my next meal to eat?

If the answers are a resounding "Yes!" and "No!" help yourself to a snack. But if your answer is a lukewarm "Well, maybe," take five—get up and change what you're doing. Some options:

- Take a quick stroll.
- Drink a tall glass of water.
- Make a phone call.
- Complete a chore that needs doing—dusting, tidying up, pushing papers.
- Wash your face or hands.
- Brush your teeth.
- Practice a relaxation technique like deep breathing.
- Work on a crossword puzzle.
- Page through a magazine.

With any luck, you'll be distracted enough that if you weren't hungry, you'll forget about snacking. Food cravings typically disappear as quickly as they come, and hunger from environmental or emotional cues lasts only as long as the cues are right in front of you.

(Continued on page 70)

Baked Desserts

A baked dessert is a time-honored tradition. Here are 100-calorie portions for several popular choices, plus three make-your-own ideas:

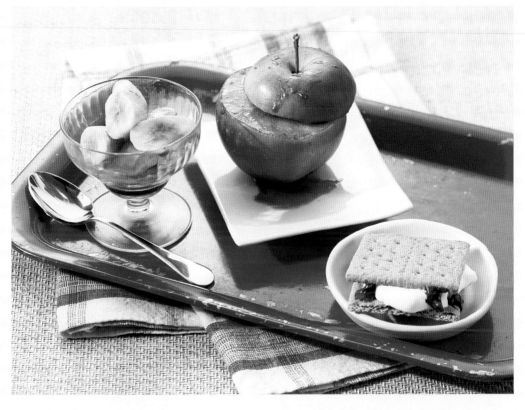

- Angel food cake, 1 slice, or about ¹⁄₁₂ of the cake
- Fruit pie (apple, berry, strawberry, etc.), as thin as you can slice it and still see it, about 4 forkfuls
- Brownie, 2-inch square
- Chocolate cake with frosting, 1 slice about ½-inch thick
- Cupcake with frosting, 1 mini, half-dollar size across
- Pumpkin pie filling, without crust, ⅓ cup, about 5 forkfuls

BANANAS FOSTER

Slice a small banana into 1-inch pieces. Sprinkle with ½ teaspoon brown sugar and add ½ teaspoon butter. Microwave until bubbly, about 1 minute.

BAKED APPLE

Core a medium apple (not a Red Delicious—it gets too watery). Sprinkle inside with cinnamon and sugar. Cover and microwave for 3 minutes, or until soft.

MICROWAVE S'MORES

On each of two graham cracker squares, place 5 chocolate chips and 1 large marshmallow. Microwave for 10-15 seconds, until marshmallow gets puffy.

Frozen Desserts

In summertime or anytime, everyone loves a frozen treat. Here are lots of 100-calorie choices. The trick is to indulge and enjoy, without going overboard. Remember, it's a treat.

COLD AND CREAMY TREATS

- Nonfat frozen yogurt, ½ cup (2 golf balls)
- Light or fat-free ice cream, ½ cup
- No-sugar-added ice cream, ½ cup
- Italian ice, ½ cup
- Chocolate ice cream, ⅓ cup (½ tennis ball)
- Super premium chocolate ice cream, 4 tablespoons (golf ball)
- Sorbet, ½ cup
- Fudgsicle

Tips on Toppings

If you could have a tablespoon of topping on your ice cream, what would you choose? Here are tasty picks rated from lowest to highest in calories per tablespoon. Those over 50 calories are pushing out your second snack of the day.

Whipped cream	10
Raisins	27
Granola	28
Chocolate syrup	41
Chopped almonds	47
Butterscotch topping	52
Chocolate chips	52
Strawberry topping	53
Hot fudge topping	70
M&M's	71
Chocolate sprinkles	72
Peanut butter candies	75

Choosing Flavors

Ice-cream fruit flavors—strawberry and peach, for example—are lowest in calories because the fruit takes the place of higher-calorie, higher-fat ingredients such as whole milk and cream. Highest-calorie ice creams are vanilla, French vanilla, and varieties with mix-ins such as cookie pieces or nuts.

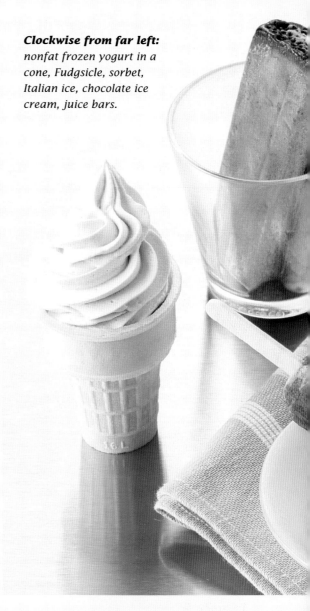

Clockwise from far left: nonfat frozen yogurt in a cone, Fudgsicle, sorbet, Italian ice, chocolate ice cream, juice bars.

FROZEN FRUITS

- Frozen grapes, ¾ cup (tennis ball)
- Frozen banana
- Frozen strawberries, 1 cup (baseball)
- Fruit/juice pop, 1
- Homemade sorbet, 1 cup

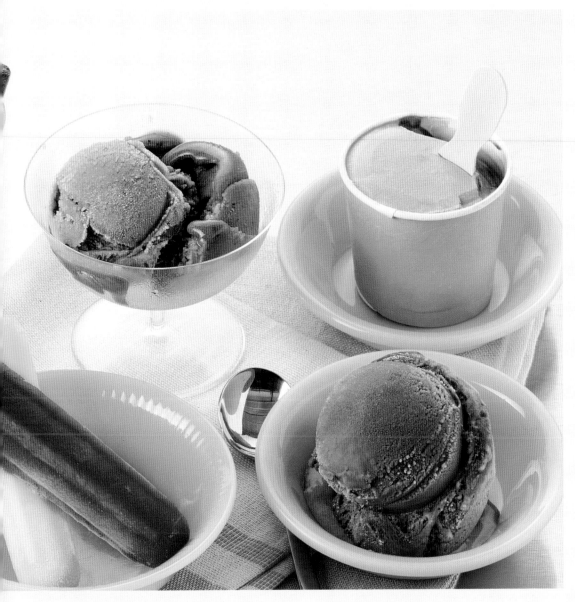

To make sorbet:

1. Freeze an entire can of fruit packed in heavy syrup.

2. Take out of the freezer 30 minutes ahead of time and place on the counter. After 30 minutes open the can on both ends and push out contents into a food processor. Add ½ cup apple juice and process until smooth.

3. Serve soft, or refreeze. One portion is ½ cup.

About Freezing Fruit

Fruit is easy to freeze and refreshing to eat. Start with your choice of ripe fruit—grapes, bananas, berries, melon, pineapple, peaches, mangoes, nectarines, plums— whatever you like. Cut whole fruit into bite-size pieces. Place on a baking sheet and freeze until firm. Remove from sheet and place in a resealable plastic bag or container. Store in freezer until needed.

But if after five minutes or so you're still hungry, then by all means, it's time for a snack.

Reach for a Snack That Satisfies

Snacks seem to be everywhere these days. Vending machines are crammed with them. Grocery stores have entire aisles devoted to them. There are snacks at the checkout counter, at the movie theater, where you pump gas—snacks almost wherever you turn.

And like so much else on the food landscape, many of these so-called snacks are oversized, fat-laden, calorie extravaganzas. The cookies on sale at delis these days are the size of saucers. Family-size bags of potato or tortilla chips could feed a village. And as the Tufts University Health & Fitness Letter discovered, even the venerable *Joy of Cooking* has felt the pressure. In the 1960s and 1970s, the book's recipe for brownies suggested 30 servings; in the latest edition the exact same recipe now suggests 16 servings. The fact is, even what passes for an individual-size portion these days can spell big

8 Tips to Control Hunger Cues

1. Instead of buying snacks at a movie, a ball game, or other event, chew a stick of sugar-free gum. Pretty soon you'll associate the taste of gum, rather than high-calorie food, with that setting.

2. At parties, stand as far away as you can from the bowls of chips, dips, and other munchies.

3. On car trips, plan ahead by bringing a few *ChangeOne* snacks. If you have a tendency to munch in the car, bring just a single serving, not the whole box. Put the rest in the trunk.

4. Buy snacks in small packs. If you buy the giant size to economize, divide it into single-serving bags or containers as soon as you get home.

5. Put the healthiest snacks where you'll see them when you first open a kitchen cabinet or the refrigerator. Hide the others behind them.

6. Don't snack in your office. (And definitely don't keep bags of chips or pretzels in your desk drawer.) Go somewhere else— kitchen, cafeteria, lounge, or outside. That way you won't associate your office with food.

7. At home, enjoy your snacks in the kitchen—and nowhere else.

8. Don't eat to relax. Relax, then eat. Stress is such a big factor in diet that we've devoted a whole chapter to it. Look ahead to Week 9, which begins on page 148, for stress-busting tips.

Nuts and Seeds

Nuts and seeds are filled with proteins and good fats, making them healthy but dense in calories. They are also filling, so it doesn't take too many to quell hunger.

All of the snacks in this chapter equal about 100 calories (the size that *ChangeOne* recommends), starting with this selection:

- Pistachios, in shells, 30 (handful)
- Pumpkin seeds (handful)
- Peanuts, in shells, 10 (handful)
- Almonds, 16 to 20 (palmful)
- Sunflower seeds, in shells (palmful)
- Peanut butter, 1 tablespoon (thumb)

SNACKING TIP

Buy your nuts with their shells still on. Opening them takes time and effort, so you're less likely to eat too many. And for many people, the mindless play of cracking, splitting, picking, and sorting is as satisfying as eating the nuts themselves.

ABOUT PEANUTS

Peanuts—actually a legume rather than a true nut—and peanut butter have become a trendy diet food. A Harvard University study showed that dieters eating peanuts and peanut butter found it easier to stick to their diets. More good news—peanuts may also be good for your heart.

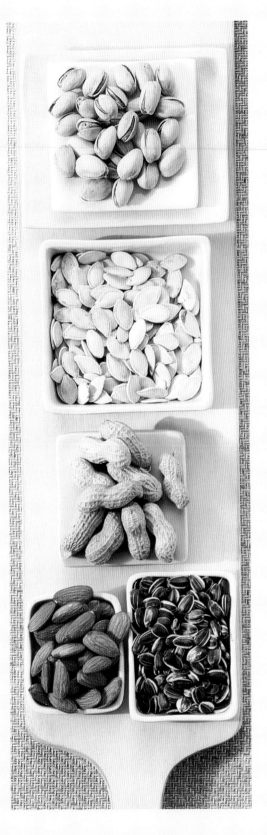

From top: *pistachios, pumpkin seeds, peanuts, almonds (left), and sunflower seeds.*

trouble when you're trying to lose weight. A seven-ounce package of tortilla chips can easily contain more than 1,000 calories. And sure, you could stop eating when you start feeling satisfied. But who among us can do that with these nutritional booby traps?

Nibblers, take heart. We've put together a menu of good-tasting, low-calorie snacks that will tame your hunger without scuttling your diet. Of course you'll find carrot and celery sticks on the list, simply because they make terrific munchies. But you'll also find some surprises, like wheat crackers with hummus, Fudgsicles, a melted-cheese tortilla, pistachios, and even s'mores.

Behind *ChangeOne* Snacks

Nutritious snacks tend to be more satisfying and filling than junk food– and often contain fewer calories.

Every *ChangeOne* snack contains about 100 calories— enough to ease hunger pangs and still keep you within your calorie guidelines. We've chosen snacks that offer plenty of flavor. It may be a no-brainer, but it's worth repeating: If something doesn't taste good, don't eat it. Why waste calories on a fat-free cracker that tastes like sawdust when you can help yourself to a handful of rich-tasting nuts or a piece of pita with sizzling salsa?

Beyond good taste, a snack worth its calories should also be satisfying in other ways. If it's 95°F in the shade, you want something cool and refreshing, like a real fruit sorbet. If you're just in from shoveling snow, hot chocolate might be the pick. Naturally, a snack should also satisfy your hunger long enough to tide you over until the next meal. Research shows that snacks that take up a lot of volume per calorie—popcorn or fruit-and-yogurt smoothies, for instance— tend to make people feel fuller on fewer calories.

Snacks that pack a lot of nutrition also turn out to be more satisfying and filling than those with a lot of empty calories. Remember the nuts we mentioned earlier? One recent study found that snacking on nuts might actually help people keep their weight down. The reason: Nuts are loaded with protein, vitamins, and, yes, fat. With all of that content, it doesn't take very many of them to satisfy your appetite.

Munch on low-fat crackers, which are made up mostly of simple carbohydrates, and you can go on eating and eating,

Cookies

Cookies are a special treat, whether homemade or store-bought. Here are 100-calorie portions that work for snacks or desserts:

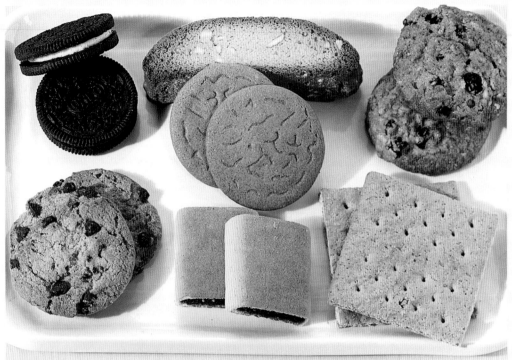

Clockwise from top left: *cream-filled sandwich cookies, biscotti, oatmeal raisin cookies, graham crackers, fig bars, chocolate chip cookies, ginger snaps (center).*

- Chocolate chip, two 2-inch cookies
- Oatmeal raisin, two 2-inch cookies
- Cream-filled sandwich cookie, two 2-inch cookies
- Fig bars (like Fig Newtons), two
- Graham crackers, two squares
- Ginger snaps, two 2-inch cookies
- Biscotti, one

For more about cookies—and some tasty recipes—see pages 318-328.

TIPS FOR BUYING COOKIES

Don't rush to buy fat-free versions of regular cookies: They just don't taste as good, they tend to cost more, and most shave off few if any calories. And be careful of portion sizes when it comes to cookies bought at bakeries—not only are they huge in circumference, but they are often thicker than a normal cookie. One-third of a large cookie is all you need; save the rest or share.

Health Tip

You can trim calories off your favorite cookie recipes—just take out a third of the sugar and butter or margarine; if the recipe calls for 1 cup, use ⅔ cup instead. Or look for recipes that call for light margarine, applesauce, and other calorie-lowering ingredients.

hoping you'll find some flavor in the next bite, piling on calories before you begin to feel satisfied. A few nuts, on the other hand, can give you that satisfaction.

Choosing a nutritious snack is important for another reason: When you're on a low-calorie diet, it's just good sense to make those calories count. As we've said, a lot of us tend to think of snacks as a little something extra—a treat we allow ourselves that isn't really part of our diet. We're kidding ourselves. In fact, treats are a surprisingly big part of what we eat during the day. According to one survey, about 20 percent of our total calories on average comes from snacks—all the more reason to make sure those calories deliver essential nutrients as well as good taste.

On *ChangeOne,* snacks will make up about 15 percent of your total calorie intake. Naturally, since no one expects a snack to be a balanced meal, we're including some less-nutritious favorites just because they taste good. After all, it's not about avoiding candy, cookies, and other treats for good. It's more about eating them less often and in reasonable portions—and learning to enjoy them more.

Fitting Snacks into Your *ChangeOne* Program

You can choose two snacks, a snack and a dessert, or two desserts during the day. You can also serve up slightly larger portions of food at your meals, especially if you find yourself getting too hungry. As often as possible, try to make sure that one selection comes from the "Calcium Choices" on page 66. You already know the evidence linking calcium to weight loss. And getting enough calcium is important for strong bones.

Use snacks this week to help manage your hunger. If you get ravenous in the morning, it's okay to munch on something. If your appetite roars to life in the midafternoon, then grab a snack. But before you do, remember to take the hunger test. Ask yourself: Am I really hungry? Can I wait until my next meal?

ChangeOne Snack Recipes

Bad weather was made for good cooking! So the next time you are house-bound by rain or snow, whip up a batch of *ChangeOne* cookies or other snacking treats. They're yummy, filling, sweet, yet completely within your *ChangeOne* eating guidelines.

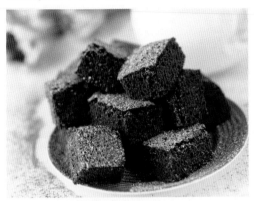

Chocolate Snacking Cake
page 318

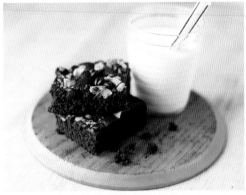

Brownie Bites
page 319

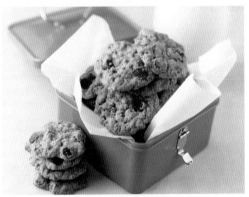

Chocolate Chip Oatmeal Cookies
page 321

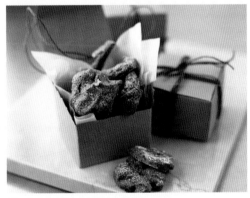

Meringue Nut Cookies
page 323

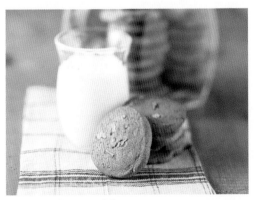

Pecan Icebox Cookies
page 322

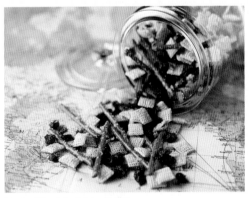

Ruby-Studded Trail Mix
page 324

Dinner

Pull a chair up to the table. It's dinnertime.

For most of us dinner comes at the end of a long day of work or errands. It's the time we relax and reward ourselves. If you've been following *ChangeOne* week by week, this chapter will complete a month of determination and healthy changes. Good going! You've taken control of breakfast, lunch, and snacks.

This week we'll show you how to make dinner a daily celebration. You'll slow down, savor the flavors, and enjoy the company. And by doing so, you'll actually eat less.

Dinners are typically the biggest meal of the day and the source of the most calories. That's why taking charge of dinner can have the biggest weight-loss payoff. Many of our *ChangeOne* volunteers saw their weight loss accelerate when they got dinner in shape. By being sensible about portions and using the meals and tips in this chapter and on pages 292-317 as a guide, you'll discover that you, too, can enjoy delicious dinners while melting the pounds away.

Slow Down. Relax. Enjoy.

In this book, and at www.changeone.com, you'll find a tantalizing selection of *ChangeOne* dinner suggestions, with plenty of ways to tailor them to your own tastes. We've made the menus as varied as possible to take advantage of the extraordinary culinary diversity available to us—from Chinese stir-fries to Italian pasta dishes to good old American beef on a bun. Of all the meals of the day, dinner is the one that most reflects our family history, culture, and special tastes.

(If you eat a lot of dinners out, you may want to glance ahead to Week 5, in which we take a look at strategies you can use to eat smart at restaurants. But first take a few minutes to look over the dinner meal plans on these pages. They'll give you a good idea of what a *ChangeOne* dinner contains and what sensible portion sizes look like.)

When you sit down to dinner this week, there's one simple change you'll want to make no matter what's on the table: Slow down and savor the meal. Too often these days we're doing a mad dash from here to there, gobbling down meals without really taking the time to taste what's in front of us. And eating too quickly is one reason so many of us find ourselves struggling with weight.

So this week give dinner your attention. Set aside enough time that you don't feel rushed. You may not be able to treat yourself to a leisurely dinner every night, but if you can make

Dinner Portions

These meal plans use both standard measurements and those from the *ChangeOne* portion-size guide; members of the 1,600 Club can add an extra serving of starch or grain here or double your protein portion at lunch or dinner:

Type of food	Example	Amount	*ChangeOne* portion
One starch or one grain	Rice, pasta, noodles	⅔-1 cup	Tennis ball—baseball
	Roll	Medium	Tennis ball
One protein	Chicken, beef	3-4 ounces	Deck of cards
	Tofu	3-4 ounces	Deck of cards
	Light-flesh fish	6 ounces	Checkbook
	Salmon, shellfish	3-4 ounces	Deck of cards
	Beans	½ cup	2 golf balls
Vegetables		Unlimited	

sure you enjoy an unhurried dinner at least three times during the coming week, you'll begin to see why savoring a meal is one of the simplest and smartest dieting strategies around.

Here's why: Just as a body sends signals for hunger, research shows, it also signals when it's had enough food. Those cues, called satiety signals, are the body's way of balancing calories we consume with calories we burn. They work effectively as long as we take the time to notice them.

If you've ever stood up from a holiday feast feeling as if you're as stuffed as the dinner bird, though, you know that it's easy to eat more than you really need—sometimes a lot more. Studies show that it takes up to 20 minutes after food reaches your stomach for satiety signals to kick in.

Hence the problem with fast food, and fast eating in general, regardless of what's on the menu. Scarf down food in a big hurry, and you don't give your body time to tell you, "Hey, all right already, I've had enough!" You can end up consuming way more calories than you need or even want.

"I realize now I was like a feeding machine," one *ChangeOne* participant told us. "Hand to mouth, hand to mouth—I never paused. I just plowed through whatever was in front of me. I never stopped to think about what it tasted like. Or how I felt. The change that made the biggest difference for me was learning to put my fork down every few bites and just stop for a minute." As she learned, a leisurely meal gives your body and brain time to catch up with your fork. Slow down and you will end up feeling satisfied on far fewer calories than if you rushed through dinner.

One of the best ways to eat less is to eat slower.

Making the Change

We know, we know: Given how crowded life is for many of us, taking time for dinner isn't always easy. You may have to rearrange your schedule a bit. You may need to let that rerun of *Frasier* or *Friends* wait for later. You may have to reschedule an appointment or two.

Even so, give it a try. Make it a goal that everyone in your house who plans to eat dinner sits down together. You'll find it's worth the effort, not only for the opportunity to relax and savor the meal but also for the new chance to spend time with your friends and family. If you're used to an eat-and-run approach to dinner, you can rediscover its pleasures—and make yourself a smarter eater—with these seven simple changes:

1. Arrange your schedule so you have at least 30 quiet minutes for dinner.

2. When you have dinner at home, always have it in your dining area. That way you won't associate food with other parts of the house—the couch in front of the television, for instance.

3. If the menu allows, divide your meal into courses—for instance, main course and vegetables, salad, and dessert. Choose the order that works best for you.

4. Make the meal the focus of dinnertime. Turn off the television. Put away the newspaper. Let the answering machine take your calls. A little dinner music is fine, as long as it doesn't distract you from the meal.

5. Serve an eight-ounce glass of water with dinner. Between each bite, put down your fork and take a small sip of water. Sipping water forces you to slow down. Water with dinner also makes a meal more filling without adding any calories. Many people find that it helps them clear their palate and more fully experience the flavors in a meal.

6. Pay attention to how the food tastes. Notice how the flavors complement or contrast with one another. Take small bites and let them linger in your mouth long enough so that the full flavor is released.

7. Between courses take a minute or two to relax, chat, and savor what you've just eaten. It may sound paradoxical, but lingering over dinner could help you drop pounds and maintain a healthy weight.

Check-In

Last week you added snacks to your *ChangeOne* menu. You'll find that low-cal snacks help you manage hunger and stay in control of what you eat. Still mastering the art of snacking? Struggling with breakfast or lunch? Then by all means, take another week. If you find yourself too rushed in the morning to put together a *ChangeOne* breakfast, look back to Week 1 for some time-saving tips. If you're having trouble controlling portion sizes when you go out to lunch, try packing it a few times this week. Still grabbing a candy bar from the vending machine when you suffer a midafternoon snack attack? Select a smarter snack from the *ChangeOne* suggestions in Week 3 or from the additional ideas on pages 318-328. And plan ahead to make sure the snack is handy when hunger strikes.

Knowing When Enough Is Enough

Paying attention to satiety signals is just one more way to make sure that you keep portion sizes under control. And in the end, portion size is really the key to the success of any diet. Consider, for example, a study from researchers at the National Cancer Institute in Bethesda, Maryland. Their investigation showed that people underestimate portions all the time. In the study, men underreported daily calorie intake by 12 to 14 percent; women by an even worse 16 to 20 percent! These weren't white-lie errors, but honest misjudgments of how much they were eating. The implication: Merely getting better at knowing proper portion size could cut daily calorie intake substantially.

Some dieters discover that once they learn to stop eating when they're no longer hungry—before they're too full—they automatically eat reasonable portions. Learning the art of knowing when you're satisfied takes time, though. And it doesn't work for everyone. So practice memorizing those portion sizes. We've suggested everyday objects for comparison, but another way to get a sense of how much a cup or an ounce contains is to prepare meals at home as often as you can this week.

To follow the *ChangeOne* recipes you won't need anything more exotic than a set of measuring cups and spoons. If you want to get fancy, invest in a kitchen scale that can be adjusted to zero after you place a bowl or plate on it. A scale makes it quick and easy to weigh three-ounce portions of pasta, for instance, or five ounces of fish. But it's not essential. You can also divvy up a 12-ounce package of pasta into four equal servings. A variety of individual portion-size storage containers will also come in handy.

Behind the *ChangeOne* Dinner Menu

Each of the suggested *ChangeOne* dinners contains between 400 and 460 calories. By following *ChangeOne* breakfast, lunch, snack, and dinner recommendations, you'll tally roughly 1,300—or 1,600—calories a day. As we promised before, that's a level that will guarantee you'll lose weight at a reasonable, healthy pace.

How can *ChangeOne* dinners be so thrifty with calories? A big reason is that each dinner includes at least two servings of vegetables. Vegetables are so low in calories—a half-cup of

Change One fast track

In a hurry to see more pounds come off? Choose one or two of the following Fast Track changes to speed your progress:

Turn in early

Surprisingly, insomnia, or even chronically falling short on sleep by an hour or two, may keep you from reaching your goal. Some researchers suspect that overtired people unwittingly compensate for their lack of energy by eating more.

New research suggests that staying up late also prompts your body to store more calories. Losing sleep can also make people more susceptible to stress, and thus more likely to overeat. Whatever the reason, weight-loss experts recommend trying to get seven or eight hours of sleep every night.

If you've been burning the candle at both ends lately, say good night to late nights a little early this week. If you find yourself repeatedly waking up in the night no matter when you go to bed—especially if you're a heavy snorer—talk to your doctor. You could have sleep apnea, a common problem that can be treated easily. Being overweight is a common risk factor for this condition.

Have some fun

This weekend set aside time to do something fun that also involves moving around. Hiking, badminton, touch football, gardening—anything that strikes your fancy, as long as it's active. Make it a family outing, if you'd like. Invite a friend. Or choose something you want to do just for yourself. Set aside at least an hour for activity.

Open your diary

Keep a food diary, again or for the first time. We've recommended it before, and we're recommending it again for one simple reason: It's the single best way to jump-start your diet, research shows.

Now that you're adding dinner to the other *ChangeOne* meals, keeping a log of what you eat will help you see how far you've come in changing your diet. It's also a great way to spot trouble: certain times of the day when you eat more than you'd like, or certain situations that trigger hunger cues. You'll find a sample food diary form on page 339.

Chew on this

Pick up some packs of sugarless gum and place them everywhere: your kitchen, your desk, your car, your purse. When you're tempted to reach for a snack, grab a piece of gum instead. You may find that the act of chewing relieves your snacking impulses. Also, try chewing a stick while you're cooking meals—there's no way you can sample your wares while you're blowing bubbles.

Energize yourself

Many people—including doctors—think of exercise in terms of formal periods of high exertion. We disagree. While scheduled, high-intensity workouts are great for those who can take the time and have the interest; the rest of us have lives to lead. So stop thinking of exercise as a task, and instead, think of it as a lifestyle. That means bounding up steps, sitting less, walking more, being more playful. We offer loads of ways to sneak activities in your life in the Get Active chapter. Give it a read and get started!

spinach contains only 27, for instance, and the same amount of sliced carrots just 30—that you can think of them as "free" foods and help yourself to as much as you want.

One exception is vegetables that are creamed or sautéed in butter or oil. Another is fried vegetables. In these cases, you do need to pay attention to serving sizes. Ounce for ounce, the fat in butter, cream, or cooking oil has more than twice as many calories as either protein or carbohydrates. So even small amounts can drive up the calorie total fast. A teaspoon of butter packs 34 calories. A teaspoon of cooking oil contains 40.

Including fat in your diet is a good thing– particularly when you use plant-based fats, such as olive oil.

While the *ChangeOne* menus on these pages are relatively low in fat, we've been careful to include some fats, especially the unsaturated kinds that can improve cholesterol levels. Fat adds flavor and enjoyment to food. Diets with a moderate amount of fat offer much more variety and flexibility than strict low-fat diets. As long as you keep portion sizes under control, you can eat any kind of food you enjoy, even if it contains fat.

Remember, new research findings show that when you're trying to lose weight, diets with moderate amounts of fat work the best. Sure, it's wise to eliminate fatty foods that you don't really like or want. It's smart, too, to replace saturated fat with unsaturated fat. You can do this easily by using olive oil or canola oil instead of butter, for instance, and choosing a mayonnaise made with canola oil. But don't get hung up on fat. Managing portion sizes is a much smarter way to keep calories under control.

About High-Protein and "Low-GI" Diets

For over a decade, there's been nonstop buzz over high-protein diets. It's easy to see why they've proved so popular. Any diet that invites you to live on steak and eggs is going to attract attention.

But most doctors remain very skeptical of most high-protein diets. It's not that these regimens don't help people lose weight. They do. A study by Arizona State University scientists published in 2002 showed that young women who ate a meal high in protein burned more calories during the next several hours than women who ate a high-carbohydrate, low-fat meal. The reason, researchers surmise: Protein requires more energy to digest than carbohydrates do. That extra energy consumption showed up in slightly elevated body temperatures for the women consuming high-protein meals. Another study, this one from 1999, found that volunteers were more satisfied after eating a meal with 29 percent of its calories from protein than after a meal with only 9 percent of its calories from protein. They also burned more calories to digest the higher-protein meal.

Before you get too excited, though, keep this in mind: You'll burn a lot more calories by taking a 15-minute walk after dinner than you will consuming extra protein. And while it's true that high-protein foods seem to satisfy hunger well, complex carbohydrates do the same, often with fewer calories.

High-protein diets may also pose long-term risks if you don't choose the foods in them wisely. Many foods high in protein, like meat, are also high in saturated fat, which can be rough on your arteries. Probably more important when you're controlling calories is the fact that overloading your diet with protein raises the risk that you'll come up short on other nutrients, such as the essential vitamins, minerals, and fiber in vegetables. Over the long haul, a very high-protein diet could lead to nutritional deficiencies.

If you follow weight-loss trends, you also know that "low-glycemic-index" diets are hot as well. The glycemic index (GI) is a measurement of how fast foods are converted into blood sugar by your digestive system. The approach is simple: Foods that convert quickly into blood sugar (in other words, high-GI foods, primarily dietary sugars and simple carbohydrates) are bad for you; slow-to-digest, low-GI foods are good for you.

There's some validity to this premise as well, and indeed, most high-protein diets are low-GI, since protein is very low-GI food. One recent study showed that people on low-GI diets burned 80 calories more per day that dieters on a regular low-fat diet. Plus, they reported feeling more energetic and less depressed and hungry. The problem here is that it is extremely hard to monitor the glycemic index for all the foods you eat. A long-term eating program shouldn't be so mathematically complicated.

Help!

"I often don't get home from work until late—which means I eat dinner just before going to bed. I've heard eating before bedtime causes food to go right to fat. Is that true?"

Worry not. As long as you eat sensible portions at dinner, it won't magically appear on your thighs tomorrow. Despite what some fad diets tell you, the timing of meals makes almost no difference in whether the calories are burned up or stored as fat. It's the number of calories a meal contains that matters, not what time you eat.

Of course, many people don't like the feeling of going to bed on a full stomach. If you're one of them, try moving your dinner schedule up an hour. Choose meals that take a little less time to prepare. Do as much advance preparation as you can, either the day before or over the preceding weekend. After dinner take a walk. Many people find that walking helps them digest a meal and encourages sounder sleep.

Also problematic is that the glycemic index of a food can change based on what is being eaten with it.

Bottom line: There are kernels of truth in many of the popular weight-loss theories. But why put all your weight-loss hopes in one narrow scientific theory, particularly given that your goal is a *lifetime* of healthy weight—and good health as well? *ChangeOne,* by pairing plenty of protein with good fats and complex carbs, is sensible, easy to track, and provides all the protein and low-GI food you need to garner their benefits. And there's evidence that this triple combo of nutrients keeps people feeling so much better that they don't want to overeat!

The watchword is moderation. Familiar? Sure. But it's still the best advice around. Protein, carbohydrates, and fat—you need them all. Tipping your diet too far in the direction of one or another forces you to cut way back on the variety of foods you get to eat, which makes it harder to stick to a diet. And by loading up on one constituent of food, you'll inevitably fall short on another that may be just as important. We've made sure that the *ChangeOne* plan contains all the protein you need to be healthy and feel satisfied after a meal, but not so much that it bumps other essential nutrients off the menu.

Cutting back on calories is what really matters when you're trying to lose weight, after all. For most of us, that simply means eating less. That's all there is to it. No magic. Just good common sense about portions.

What If I'm Losing Weight Too Fast?

Yes, it sounds crazy—everyone on a diet wants this problem. But there's a danger to dropping pounds too fast. Experts recommend losing no more than three pounds a week.

Why? Because losing weight faster than that means you're burning off muscle as well as fat. Losing muscle tissue will leave you weaker than when you began your diet. It can also lower your basal metabolic rate—the rate at which your body burns fuel to sustain itself—because muscle tissue requires more calories for maintenance than does fat. The result: The less muscle, the fewer calories you'll burn, and the harder it will be to maintain weight loss.

If you've lost a lot more than three pounds a week on average— more than 10 pounds in your first three weeks—it's time to slow down. Add 200 to 300 calories to your diet by eating an extra snack or two, or increasing portion sizes slightly. And to make sure you don't lose muscle tissue, increase your exercise. You'll find details about an easy eight-week fitness program beginning on page 198.

Change One success stories
Living Healthy Together

Moderation is the key to a full life for Betsy and John Larimer. Since they decided to decrease serving sizes at the dinner table, they not only feel healthier, they've also dropped a few clothing sizes.

"In our house, we monitor the portions of everything we eat," Betsy says. Shortly after they were married, she gained what she liked to call "wedding weight," and John was diagnosed with rising blood pressure and increasing cholesterol levels.

"When John's cholesterol skyrocketed, I knew it was time to start eating right," Betsy says. "We needed a new way of life, not a temporary diet or a quick fix. We read *ChangeOne* and learned how to make weekly improvements in our eating habits and lifestyles. In just three months, I lost 12 pounds, and John lost 17. At first, eating healthy wasn't easy, but as our weight dropped, we were motivated to stick with it."

To reduce calories, fat, and sodium, the couple trimmed their dinner portions in half. "We found that we didn't need the large quantities of food we were accustomed to eating," says Betsy. "I began asking our butcher to cut salmon and steak into sensible sizes for us, and at the deli counter, I ordered reduced-fat cheese and lean lunch meats sliced thin.

"We learned to eat slowly, taking time to enjoy our food, and soon we recognized when we felt satisfied as opposed to feeling stuffed. Eventually, John and I could differentiate between being truly

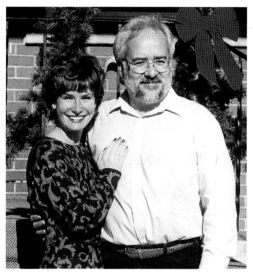

John Larimer lost 17 pounds in 3 months on *ChangeOne*. His wife, Betsy, lost 12 pounds in that time.

hungry and merely craving food as an emotional response.

"We limited our visits to restaurants, knowing that we could prepare healthy food ourselves," Betsy explains. "Salads became a regular staple. The fiber filled us up, helping to limit our portions at dinner. We also ate nutritious breakfasts, lunches, and snacks.

"My husband and I continue to eat right, motivating each other along the way," she confirms. "Checking in on one another during the day is easy, since I'm an administrative assistant at the same company where John works as an engineer. Eating healthy can be tough at times, but we know that the benefits are immeasurable."

For more ChangeOne *success stories, go to www.changeone.com/successstories*

Help!

"I've been putting in lots of time being active, and I haven't seen big results on the scale. What's wrong?"

Nothing. By being as active as you can, you're doing the right thing. The frustrating fact is that it takes a lot of exercise to lose even a small amount of weight.

So why bother? Here are three very good reasons:

1. Physical activity does burn calories—and those extra calories will help you lose weight over time.

2. You'll be much more likely to keep the weight off. Almost all the successful dieters in the National Weight Control Registry say that a big part of their success comes from exercise.

3. Being physically active has been shown to improve people's mental outlook and boost their self-confidence—two changes that can make it much easier to stick to a diet.

Don't stop exercising because you're not losing weight. Stay active and take another look at your diet. Make sure you're not consuming a lot of empty calories in the form of sweetened beverages. Recalibrate portion sizes to make sure yours are still within the *ChangeOne* guidelines.

Goal-Setting: It's Finally Time

Chances are you had in mind the number of pounds you wanted to drop back when you started *ChangeOne*. That's great. In fact, this week we want you to put your goal in writing—and sign your name to it.

Now it might seem puzzling that we have waited until the fourth week of the program to get to the topic of goals. But there are two reasons we waited.

First is that it is impossible to set a reasonable goal when you are just embarking on a new skill. If you never played golf, for example, how can you predict how good a golfer you can be in 12 weeks? You need to learn some of the skills and practice them before assessing that. Only then can you determine a reasonable path to success.

The same is true for *ChangeOne*. These first four weeks you have been learning new skills and practicing them every day. We assume you have been losing weight and also reaping other personal rewards. Now that you know your weight-loss strengths and weaknesses, isn't it a smarter time to set a realistic goal?

The second reason for the delay is that goal-setting is serious business. Rightly or wrongly, your performance against your goals defines success for you, motivates you, and, too often, lets you down. Goal-setting is so important, in fact, you'll discover that we revisit the subject a month from now. But until then it's time for some basics.

Take that initial weight-loss goal you set for yourself and think about it for a few minutes. Ask yourself three questions:

1. Is my goal a reasonable one, something I can achieve based on the progress I'm making so far?

2. How long is it likely to take to reach my goal?

3. What weight would I be satisfied with if I can't quite hit my ideal goal?

After you've given these weighty questions some thought, set out your goals for the coming months. We recommend having a goal in mind for the end of the

12-week program about two months from now. If that's not your ultimate goal, set another target on a longer time frame.

Think TRIM

As you think about workable goals for the coming two months and beyond, keep in mind the acronym TRIM. It stands for:

Time-bound: An effective goal should have a deadline—a time when you expect to reach it. Choose a date two months from now, when you will have completed the 12 weeks of the *ChangeOne* program. Select the day and mark it on the calendar.

Realistic: We've said it before, but it's worth repeating: If you set a goal you can't reach, there's no point in setting it. Choose a target that you're pretty sure you can hit. Odds are you won't go from a size 20 to a size 12 in the next few months. But you could get to a size 16, or even 14.

Inspiring: Your goal should be something that really matters to you—attainable, but ambitious enough to excite you. Maybe you don't really care all that much about pounds on the scale, for instance; what you're concerned about is getting into shape so that you can keep up with the kids on hikes and bike rides.

Measurable: A worthwhile goal has to be measurable. The first step is to make it as specific as possible. The next is to describe exactly how you plan to measure your progress. Here are a few examples.

Instead of	Make your goal to
Lose as much weight as I can before summer begins	Drop 10 pounds over the next two months
Be better about my diet	Follow *ChangeOne* at least six days out of seven each week
Get back into shape	Jog for 45 minutes at least three times a week in preparation for a 10-K charity run
Try to be more active	Walk at least 30 minutes five days a week over the next two months
Eat fewer sweets	Treat myself to just one dessert a week over the coming month
Feel less embarrassed by the way I look	Lose 10 pounds and join a water aerobics class by Memorial Day

In addition to pounds on the scale, give yourself at least two other goals. Dropping several dress sizes, for example, or fitting into a pair of jeans you wore two summers ago.

It's Not All About the Scale

Why have another goal in addition to pounds on the scale? Because while weight is the measure that most people use, it's not necessarily the best one. Who really cares what the bathroom scale says? What most people really want is to look better. And the scale can lie.

For example, let's say you're doing a great job on your diet, dropping calories and burning fat. At the same time, you've gotten so gung-ho about exercise that you've started going to the gym. You're tightening up flabby muscles and even adding some strength. You look great! You feel terrific!

But when you step up on the scale, oops: Your weight has barely budged. Why? As we've pointed out before, you're replacing fat with muscle, which actually weighs more than fat, volume for volume. You're changing your body composition for the better. The reflection in the mirror shows it. Maybe you've dropped a waist size or two as well. You feel stronger and fitter. But if you have no other gauge than pounds on the scale, you'll be disappointed.

Once you've settled on realistic and measurable goals, fill out the *ChangeOne* Contract on page 339. Why a contract? Because while it's one thing to decide on a set of goals, it's another to really commit to them. Make a deal with yourself in writing. The form even includes a place for you to sign. And while you're at it, have someone witness the contract. Telling people your goals can often serve as essential extra motivation.

If all that sounds silly, you may be surprised. There's something powerful about putting your John Hancock on any agreement, even one you make with yourself. Before you sign it, make sure the goals you've set for yourself pass the TRIM test. Check again to be sure they're goals you are willing and able to work toward over the next few months.

Your Healthy Weight?

One target worth keeping in mind is your healthy weight. Since height and weight are related, experts don't rely on pounds alone. Instead they use a formula called body mass index (BMI). On page 344 you'll find information on how to calculate your current BMI and the number of pounds you'll need to lose to reach a healthy BMI.

Because individual body types differ, the official BMI chart offers a recommended range, not a single magic number. Having your healthy weight in mind can often serve as a great motivator.

But keep your perspective. If you're overweight, losing just a few pounds will make you healthier. Studies show that people who drop 5 percent of their body weight significantly improve their blood pressure and cholesterol numbers, thereby reducing the strain on their hearts and arteries. They also lower their risk of diabetes. The closer you get to your recommended BMI, the healthier you'll be.

ChangeOne Dinner Recipes

Sure, we like to try new things for dinner. But most of us have favorites that we eat regularly—dishes like meat loaf and roasted chicken. Our *ChangeOne* recipes mix everyday classics with fresh ideas. Enjoy these great-tasting dinners, knowing each will help you lose weight.

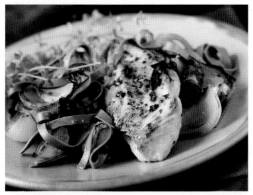

Sautéed Chicken with Caramelized Onions
page 293

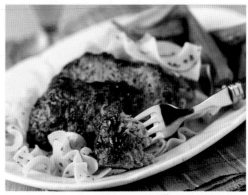

Heartland Meat Loaf
page 300

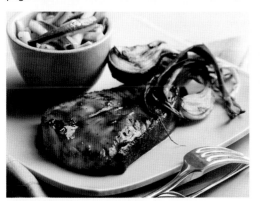

Barbecued Halibut Steaks
page 299

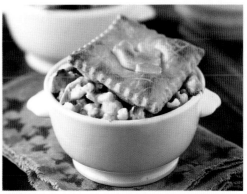

One-Crust Chicken Potpie
page 294

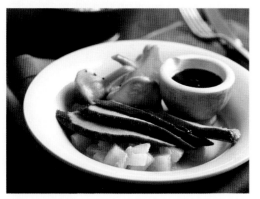

Sweet-and-Sour Glazed Pork with Pineapple
page 299

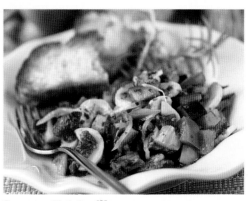

Summer Ratatouille
page 306

Dining Out

Even though you're watching what you eat, that's no reason to deny yourself the pleasure of eating out. Yes, the serving sizes surpass imagination, and in many restaurants the notion of cooking light means one stick of butter in the sauce instead of two. But if you approach dining out with common sense and a little bit of nerve, you can have a great meal while sticking with your plan.

This week dine out at least twice. Order exactly what you want, and don't take no for an answer!

Who knows? You might find it great fun getting the waiter and chef to deliver a more personalized meal to you. Remember, there's no need to fear a restaurant. You are the customer, paying to get what you want. So enjoy it, take your time, and savor the flavors—as you desire them.

A *ChangeOne* Evening Date

Dining out has become one of the great national pastimes. In 1970, the average American spent about one-quarter of the household food budget dining out. Today it's more like one-half. And why not? Never before have we had so many mouthwatering choices, from spicy Thai stir-fries and sizzling Mexican rice dishes to exotic Japanese sushi and good old American comfort food.

But there is a downside to dining out. Restaurant food typically contains 22 percent more fat than food consumed at home, experts say. And portion sizes? They've spiraled out of control at many eateries.

Portion creep happened gradually enough that most people didn't realize exactly how big those entrées had become until an organization called the Center for Science in the Public Interest (CSPI) began conducting clever sting operations a few years ago. The group rounded up meals from restaurants like the kind many of us dine in regularly. In one operation, CSPI sampled almost two dozen Chinese restaurants. In another, its investigators ordered from the menus of a variety of Italian restaurants, including several well-known nationwide chains.

What they found made headlines. Portion sizes and fat content at many of the nation's eateries have become so bloated that many meals border on health hazards. In some cases,

Dining-Out Portions

These meal plans use both standard measurements and those from the *ChangeOne* portion-size guide; members of the 1,600 Club can add an extra serving of starch or grain here, or double your protein portion at lunch or dinner:

Type of food	Example	Amount	*ChangeOne* portion
One starch or one grain	Rice, pasta, noodles	⅔-1 cup	Tennis ball—baseball
	Roll	Medium	Tennis ball
One protein	Shrimp, scallops, crab	4 ounces	Baseball
	Chicken, turkey	3-4 ounces	Deck of cards
	Beef, veal	3 ounces	
	Salmon	3 ounces	
	Light-flesh fish	6 ounces	Checkbook
Vegetables		½ cup if with oil or butter; unlimited if steamed or raw	2 golf balls

CSPI found, a single entrée exceeded what many of us should eat in a whole day. At some Chinese restaurants, for instance, an order of kung pao chicken packed 1,400 calories. Love Italian food? A spaghetti-and-meatballs meal at some restaurants measured in at almost 1,000 calories.

Fettuccine Alfredo, or pasta in a cream sauce, soared to almost 1,800 calories in a single serving. Even half of one of these entrées puts you over your *ChangeOne* dinner target. Garlic bread to go with that? Eat a couple of pieces of the butter-soaked bread in many restaurants, and you could tally up an additional 350 or more calories.

If you dine out a lot—and most of us have about four meals a week in restaurants or fast-food places—numbers like those can be discouraging. But even though the chef rules the kitchen, remember that you rule the table. You're the one footing the bill, after all. You choose what to eat and how much of it you want. You determine how quickly or slowly to enjoy a meal. You say when you've had enough. In some restaurants, you can even give the chef specific directions for how you want your meal prepared.

The chef may rule the kitchen, but you rule the table. Order *exactly* what you want.

Many of the strategies you'll use to take charge in restaurants are the same ones you've already been practicing: planning ahead, keeping an eye on portion sizes, and monitoring hunger and fullness signals. This week keep them in mind when you take yourself out to dinner. They'll help you sit down to a *ChangeOne* meal you'll enjoy without regrets.

Do Your Menu Homework

If you're considering a restaurant you've never tried before, stop by and look over the menu before you go in to make sure you'll be able to order the meal you want. Most establishments display their menus outside. Some even post them online. You won't be able to learn much about portion sizes, of course, but at least you'll know whether the menu includes some decent options. You could even pick the safest bets before you go in. That way you won't have to look at the menu and be tempted by steak smothered in hollandaise sauce or deep-fried cheese blintzes.

If you dine out frequently, keep your own personal list of diet-friendly restaurants in your area—places where you know you'll be able to get a great-tasting, low-calorie meal.

But there are some kinds of restaurants you should avoid altogether—unless you have an iron will. All-you-can-eat joints, buffet-style restaurants, even sprawling salad bars pose a hazard. Salad bars sound healthy enough, but many of them are stocked with calorie-rich dishes like creamy pasta salads. Better to order a simple garden salad with salad dressing on the side. Fried-chicken eateries and barbecue joints? Most of what's on the menu is so high in calories and fat that you'll bust your calorie budget before you satisfy your hunger.

Fast-food restaurants have made some progress in offering healthier alternatives to their usual fare, such as grilled chicken sandwiches and salads. But menus change all the time, as chains constantly seek offerings that sell better. And even as they test healthier fare, fast-food restaurants keep adding bigger, unhealthier fare as well. (Aren't triple cheeseburgers bad enough without several slices of bacon?) So while fast-food restaurants offer convenience and familiarity, you'll need to be extra careful when eating at them. And remember, you're shooting for at least two servings of vegetables. At the local burger joint, you'll be lucky to get a piece of lettuce and thin slice of tomato.

But don't worry. There are still plenty of places where you can sit down to a good meal, as you'll discover paging through the suggested menus we review this week.

On the following pages, we'll guide you through the good and not so good of some popular restaurant cuisines.

But at the restaurant, you'll need to be specific about your desires, or you'll end up with piles of high-calorie food on your plate. Take control from the start, and don't let the restaurants dictate your dining experience. Beginning on page 94 you'll find some advice for getting exactly what you want—and nothing you don't want.

(Continued on page 100)

Check-In

What meal do you typically eat out? Breakfast? Lunch? Dinner? All of the above? If you dine out a lot, take a fresh look at the portion sizes in the first four weeks of *ChangeOne* so that when that plate of pasta or a burger lands in front of you, you'll know just how much to eat and how much to take home for later.

Many dieters find that keeping a visual equivalent in mind helps prevent portion creep. If you treat yourself to a restaurant meal once or twice a month, definitely use the tips in this chapter to guide you when you open the menu. But enjoy yourself, too. Have that steak and eat it, too. If dinners out are an occasional treat, you don't have to worry. Still, pay attention to how full you feel. When you're satisfied, push your chair back and savor the feeling of being in control of what and how much you eat.

Italian Restaurants

Appetizer, pasta, main course, dessert—that's a standard meal in many Italian restaurants. Can you fit it into *ChangeOne*? Certainly, when you pay close attention to portions and include lots of vegetables. Check out our sample meals below.

MENU 1 (Photo on opposite page)
  Green salad dressed with balsamic vinegar and a drizzle of olive oil
  Spaghetti with red clam sauce (baseball)
  Sautéed broccoli
  Piece of fruit, or fruit salad (2 golf balls)

Approximate serving info (based on *ChangeOne* sizes): Calories 440, fat 11 g, saturated fat 1.5 g, cholesterol 15 mg, sodium 240 mg, carbohydrate 70 g, fiber 12 g, protein 20 g, calcium 200 mg.

MENU 2
  Cup of minestrone soup (diner coffee cup)
  Chicken breast cacciatore (deck of cards)
  Plain pasta (tennis ball)
  Spinach with garlic
  Cup of fresh berries (2 golf balls)

Approximate serving info (based on *ChangeOne* sizes): Calories 440, fat 13 g, saturated fat 3 g, cholesterol 45 mg, sodium 1,140 mg, carbohydrate 56 g, fiber 12 g, protein 29 g, calcium 250 mg.

CHOOSING YOUR MEAL

Soups

Italian soups are hearty, almost filling enough to be a meal if paired with a slice of crusty Italian bread and a green salad. Minestrone—a tomato-based soup with vegetables, beans, and pasta—is a great choice. Pasta e fagioli features a fiber-rich combination of beans (fagioli) and pasta in a savory broth. Top either with a sprinkle of Parmesan cheese for richer flavor.

BEWARE

- **Pasta primavera:** Unless it's made the *ChangeOne* way (see page 303), this may be the biggest impostor of all; many restaurants make this dish with lots of cream.
- **Eggplant parmigiana:** Breaded and fried eggplant soaks up the oil.
- **Stuffed mushrooms:** Stuffing is usually a combo of cheese, fatty sausage, and cream.
- **Antipasto salad:** Mostly cheeses and salami slices.

Appetizers

Often listed as "antipasto" on the menu, appetizers run the gamut from fresh seafood salads to fried mozzarella, eggplant, and zucchini. To get the biggest bang for your buck, stick with the nonfried seafood or a virtually calorie-free fresh vegetable salad. If you're wondering how some of your current favorites stack up, here's a list of portions around 100 calories, ranked from best to worst in terms of calories and nutrition:

Appetizer	Serving size
Minestrone soup	1 cup (diner coffee cup)
Marinated shrimp	½ cup (2 golf balls)
Pasta e fagioli	1 cup (small coffee cup)
Fried calamari	⅓ cup (½ tennis ball)
Fried eggplant	½ cup
Mozzarella sticks	1 (1 thumb)

Main meals

Portions in many Italian restaurants are big enough to feed at least two. To keep your meal size in check, limit your pasta portion to about ⅔ cup (tennis ball). Here's a sampling of Italian dishes that all deliver about 250 to 300 calories:

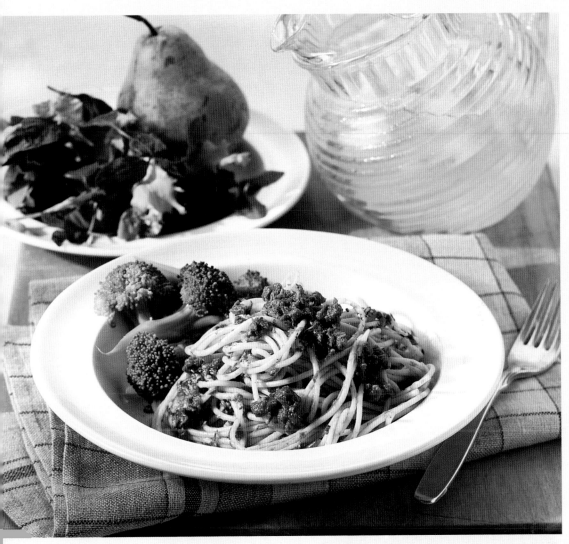

Entrée	Serving size
Chicken cacciatore*	3 ounces chicken (deck of cards)
Veal marsala*	2 ounces veal
Veal scaloppine*	2 ounces veal
Chicken or egg-plant parmigiana*	3 ounces chicken or eggplant
Cheese lasagna	About 1 cup (baseball)
Ravioli and tomato sauce	About 1 cup
Baked ziti	¾ cup (tennis ball)
Fettuccine Alfredo	¾ cup
Spaghetti and meatballs	¾ cup

*Plus ⅔ cup cooked pasta

TIPS FOR ORDERING

Out with your spouse or children? Here's how to order for four, family style:

- One large salad, dressing on the side
- One appetizer
- Two pastas
- Two nonpasta main dishes
- Two vegetable sides

Chinese Restaurants

Most of us can't go long without Chinese food. It's hard to resist dishes like crispy egg rolls, wonton soup, and tangy stir-fries. While some Chinese dishes can break your calorie bank, smart choices can be enjoyable additions to your weight-loss plan. Take the guesswork out of ordering with one of these menus.

Menu 1 (Photo on opposite page)
> Cup of wonton soup (diner coffee cup)
> 1 small egg roll (deck of cards)
> Chicken chow mein (baseball)
> Steamed mixed vegetables
> Cup of pineapple chunks (baseball)

Approximate serving info (based on *ChangeOne* sizes): Calories 470, fat 19 g, saturated fat 4.5 g, cholesterol 130 mg, sodium 1,010 g, carbohydrates 52 g, fiber 8 g, protein 25 g, calcium 200 mg.

Menu 2
> Cup of egg-drop soup (diner coffee cup)
> Moo goo gai pan (tennis ball)
> Brown rice (baseball)
> Steamed broccoli
> 1 fortune cookie
> 4 orange wedges

Approximate serving info (based on *ChangeOne* sizes): Calories 420, fat 16 g, saturated fat 4.5 g, cholesterol 95 mg, sodium 1,590 g, carbohydrates 47 g, fiber 6 g, protein 26 g, calcium 150 mg.

CHOOSING YOUR MEAL

Soups

Chinese soup is a terrific starter. Your best bets are egg-drop soup or wonton soup. Hot-and-sour soup has about twice the calories of those. Likewise, velvet corn chowder and other hearty soups are more calorie-rich.

Appetizers

You can say yes to appetizers. Look for marinated vegetables or favorites that can

BEWARE

- **Tangerine or orange beef:** The citrus is hard to find—it's just fried peel with breaded, fried beef.
- **With walnuts:** Nuts are great, but not with the extra fats and calories they pick up when they're caramelized (sugared and sometimes fried), as is done in many Chinese restaurants.
- **Spicy eggplant:** This is one vegetable that soaks up lots of oil.

be steamed rather than fried—wontons, dumplings, and spring rolls, for example. Here are some common choices in serving sizes that are around 100 calories, ranked from best to worst in terms of calories and nutrition:

Appetizer	Serving size
Marinated spinach salad	1 cup (baseball)
Dumplings, steamed	2 small or 1 medium
Spring roll, steamed	1 medium
Egg roll, all types	1 small
Spring roll, fried	1 small
Fried wonton	1 small

Main meals

Sharing entrées is half the fun at a Chinese restaurant. To avoid overdoing it, try to limit yourself to a couple of bites from each entrée and pick dishes with more veggies and fewer fried ingredients. We've ranked several favorites from lowest to highest calories, ranging from about 250 to 300 calories:

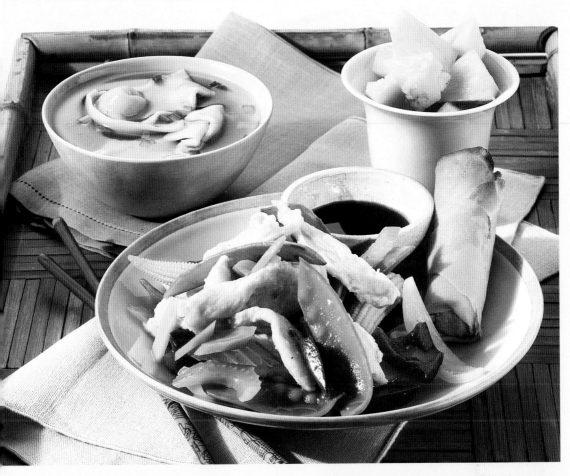

Entrée	Serving size
Moo goo gai pan	¾ cup (tennis ball)
Chicken chow mein	¾ cup
Sweet-and-sour pork	¾ cup
Chicken egg foo yung	¾ cup
Beef egg foo yung	¾ cup
Pork egg foo yung	¾ cup
General Tso's chicken	⅔ cup (tennis ball)
Shrimp egg foo yung	⅔ cup
Chicken or beef fried rice	⅔ cup
Kung pao chicken or pork	½ cup (2 golf balls)
Moo shu pork	⅓ cup (half tennis ball)
Cashew chicken	⅓ cup

TIPS FOR ORDERING

- Order a one-pot soup. The portion is generous, with lots of soup broth to fill you up.
- Order a side of steamed vegetables to mix in with a saucy main course. The extra veggies add fiber and other nutrients to your meal and make your portion look more generous.
- Ask for dumplings steamed rather than pan-fried. They taste just as good and have fewer calories.

Surf and Turf

Steak houses and fish restaurants are an excellent dining-out choice.

Many entrées are available grilled—a cooking method that lets fat drip away—and plainer side dishes help you control calories. But steaks that hang over the edge of the plate and fish fillets that make side dishes look like garnishes hardly fit the *ChangeOne* strategy. Get your doggie bags ready!

Menu 1 (Photo on opposite page)
Grilled portobello mushroom
Green salad with fat-free dressing, or reduced-fat—adds about 30 calories
Grilled blackened salmon (deck of cards)
Sautéed spinach (2 golf balls)
White rice (tennis ball)

Approximate serving info (based on *ChangeOne* sizes): Calories 430, fat 16 g, saturated fat 3 g, cholesterol 55 mg, sodium 570 mg, carbohydrate 44 g, fiber 6 g, protein 28 g, calcium 150 mg.

Menu 2
Shrimp cocktail: 4 shrimp and 2 tablespoons cocktail sauce
Green salad dressed with balsamic vinegar and a drizzle of olive oil
Grilled beef tenderloin (deck of cards)
Green beans (2 golf balls)
Steamed asparagus with lemon
Small baked potato (tennis ball)

Approximate serving info (based on *ChangeOne* sizes): Calories 470, fat 9 g, saturated fat 3.5 g, cholesterol 115 mg, sodium 1,020 mg, carbohydrate 60 g, fiber 8 g, protein 37 g, calcium 100 mg.

CHOOSING YOUR MEAL

Appetizers
Seafood appetizers are a popular offering in surf-and-turf restaurants. As long as the seafood isn't fried or swimming in butter or olive oil, it's hard to go wrong with choices like shrimp cocktail, crab legs, or steamed mussels. Green salad is always an option—

BEWARE

- **Béarnaise:** Sauce made with butter and egg yolks.
- **Beurre blanc:** Light-colored butter sauce.
- **Chateaubriand:** Large portion of beef tenderloin, usually for two.
- **Dijonaise:** Dijon mustard and cream sauce.

---

try topping it with shrimp and using cocktail sauce in place of dressing.

Main meals
In most cases you can be fairly confident in the cooking techniques of fish and steak restaurants. Grilling disposes of some fat as the food cooks, and wood or charcoal grilling imparts delicious smoky overtones. But stay alert: The standard 12-ounce tenderloin steak is a full four *ChangeOne* portions, and that's not counting the oversized baked potato with it. Keep in mind that just one tablespoon of melted butter has more than half the calories of the surf and turf entrées below. Here's a list of some popular main dishes, ranked from best to worst on the *ChangeOne* calorie range of about 250 to 300 calories:

Entrée	Serving size
Grilled sea bass	4 ounces (deck of cards)
King crab leg	1
Lobster tail	1
Blackened salmon	3 ounces (deck of cards)
Blue crab cakes	1½
Beef tenderloin	3 ounces
Rack of lamb	2 ounces (deck of cards)

Side dishes
At some restaurants, side dishes come with the entrée. At others you can order them separately. Here are the portion sizes you

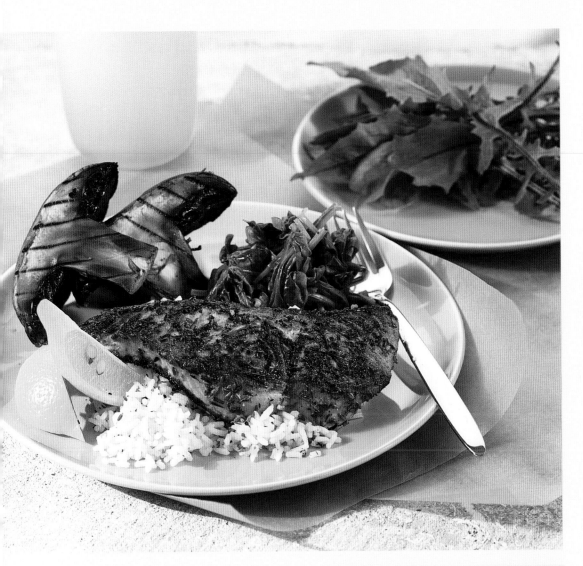

should be aware of for popular selections like grains and potatoes:

Side	Serving size
Baked potato	½ large or 1 small (tennis ball)
Rice pilaf	⅔ cup (tennis ball)
Couscous	1 cup (baseball)
Spaghetti	⅔ cup (tennis ball)
Mashed potatoes	¾ cup
French fries	⅔ cup (½ tennis ball)
Garlic bread	1 slice

TIPS FOR ORDERING

These cooking methods are lean and healthy:

- **Blackened:** Rubbed with black pepper, paprika, and other spices and grilled.
- **Steamed:** Cooked without fat in a seafood steamer.
- **Reduction:** Sauce made by boiling down stock, wine, or balsamic vinegar.
- **Brochette:** Meat, fish, poultry, or vegetables on a skewer.

Take Control of the Table

Be the director of your dining experience right from the start, and you really can have it your way, all the way. Here are four guidelines that will put you in charge:

1 **Ask and you shall receive**
The waitstaff should know how a dish is made, what the ingredients are, and how big the portion size is. So ask, already. Then have it your way. If the burrito looks good except for the fact that it's smothered in sour cream, ask the chef to hold the cream. If you'd like the grilled chicken breast without the skin, say so. If the vegetable side dishes are usually prepared with gobs of butter, request yours lightly sautéed in olive oil or steamed. Pizza tonight? The chef should be more than willing to make yours with half the normal cheese, or none, and an extra topping of vegetables.

2 **Sign up for one course at a time**
One of the pleasures of dining out is taking your time. Or at least it should be. Unfortunately, at too many restaurants waiters snatch up one course and rush in with the next before you've had time to put your fork down. There's a reason. Most restaurants want to turn tables around as quickly as they can to squeeze in as many seatings in an evening as possible. That's their business. Yours is to relax and take the time you need to eat only what you want—and no more. If you're worried about being rushed, order just one course at a time. Start with an appetizer. Once you're done, look back at the menu to consider what you'll have next. A useful rule of thumb: Allot at least 20 minutes per course—the time your body needs to send satiety signals. Do you feel full? You're under no obligation to keep ordering.

3 **Draw the line**
Ask whether the kitchen can prepare half portions. Many restaurants are more than willing to do so. Some even offer half portions on the menu. If the dish you order turns out to be too big, ask the waiter right then and there to divide the portions and set half aside for you to take home. Don't wait until you've started to nibble. Don't depend on

your willpower to eat only half of what's in front of you. If you know in advance that the entrées at a particular restaurant are outsized, ask for a half portion as the meal and request that the other half be brought at the end in a takeout container.

4 Rule the table
When you're dining out, you're in charge—not only of what you eat but of what's on the table. Lots of restaurants start you off with a basket of dinner rolls. If you're hungry when the rolls arrive, you'll automatically gobble up mediocre white-flour bread smeared with butter and loaded with calories without even giving it a second thought. Why waste the calories? Tell the waiter, "No bread, thanks." If you're famished when you sit down, order something more sensible to take the edge off your hunger before you do anything else—a side salad, a vegetable side dish, or a glass of spicy tomato juice, for instance. At the same time, ask for a glass of water. Heck, ask for a whole pitcher. Then you won't have to keep the busboy busy filling your glass. Remember to drink plenty of water with your meal.

And don't forget who's boss. If something arrives at the table that you don't want, politely decline it. No one will mind.

Manage the Menu

Order wisely, and you can put together a meal that's long on flavor and short on calories. Here are five things to consider when you open the menu:

1 Be colorful
Meat and creamy sauces are usually beige, right? Where do most dishes get their brightest colors? From vegetables and fruit, of course. Choose the most colorful dishes on the

(Continued on page 106)

Help!

"I'm used to a glass of wine or beer with dinner. Can I enjoy a drink and still lose weight on ChangeOne?"

Sure. But before you raise your glass, remember one key word: moderation. Alcoholic beverages contain calories—about 120 calories in a glass of wine and 145 in a 12-ounce glass of beer. In fact, the average adult who drinks gets 10 percent of total calories from alcohol, surveys show.

But whether those calories "count" in the same way that food calories count is a subject of debate. Even though drinkers consume more calories than nondrinkers, they aren't more likely to be obese or overweight. What's more, volunteers in controlled studies who are given additional calories in the form of alcohol do not gain weight.

Researchers suspect that alcohol may alter the way the body burns fat, causing it to "waste" calories.

But the new health benefits associated with some alcoholic beverages haven't been enough to convince health experts to advise nondrinkers to start imbibing. The reason: Excessive drinking poses big risks.

Still, if you enjoy a glass of wine or beer with dinner, go on enjoying it. But make sure you have just one.

Diners and Coffee Shops

Americans love diners and coffee shops because they have something for everybody. The catch is that the number of choices can be overwhelming. And the huge portions at many diners give new meaning to the word "abundance." But there is good news: All of those choices make it easy to stick to your *ChangeOne* plan.

MENU 1 (Photo on opposite page)
Small bowl of chicken noodle soup
Green salad with fat-free dressing, or reduced-fat—adds about 30 calories
Hot roast beef sandwich (take home half)
Mashed potatoes (½ tennis ball)
Cooked carrots (2 golf balls)
2 small butter cookies

Approximate serving info (based on *ChangeOne* sizes): Calories 460, fat 16 g, saturated fat 5 g, cholesterol 50 mg, sodium 2,220 mg, carbohydrate 58 g, fiber 8 g, protein 23 g, calcium 150 mg.

MENU 2
Turkey breast (deck of cards)
Turkey gravy (Dixie cup)
Cranberry sauce (2 thumbs)
Candied sweet potatoes (2 golf balls)
Green salad with fat-free dressing, or reduced-fat—adds about 30 calories
1 roll (tennis ball)

Approximate serving info (based on *ChangeOne* sizes): Calories 440, fat 7 g, saturated fat 2 g, cholesterol 80 mg, sodium 1,050 mg, carbohydrate 63 g, fiber 7 g, protein 32 g, calcium 150 mg.

CHOOSING YOUR MEAL

Soups
A typical diner offers two or three different soups each day, usually a broth with pasta or rice, a bean- or pea-based option, a chowder, or French onion soup. Lowest in calories are the broth-based soups like chicken noodle or beef barley. Bean or pea soups have more calories but also are more filling and satisfying. A bowl with bread and a salad is a meal. Highest in calories are soups made with cream, like chowder, or those with cheese.

Appetizers
Most diner appetizers are fried. Be sure to look at other sections of the menu, such as side dishes or breakfast, for surprisingly satisfying appetizers; or play it safe and order a side salad. The list below ranks popular choices by calories and overall nutrition, with calories ranging from about 35 to 65:

Appetizer	Serving size
Grilled vegetables	1 cup (baseball)
Tomato juice	1 cup
Barbecue chicken wing	1
Onion rings	2

Main meals
Here again, portion size is the issue. Also, lots of foods are fried, and meals come in several courses. The three meals at right are all right around the 450-calorie target for dinners:

> ### BEWARE
> - **Complete dinner:** Soup plus salad plus entrée plus sides plus dessert.
> - **Dieter's plate:** Full-fat cottage cheese, fruit, and a burger patty; you could get fewer calories by ordering a regular burger.
> - **Meal salads:** Enough to feed a family, with all the meat and cheese mixed in.
> - **Potato skins:** When they're fried, not baked.

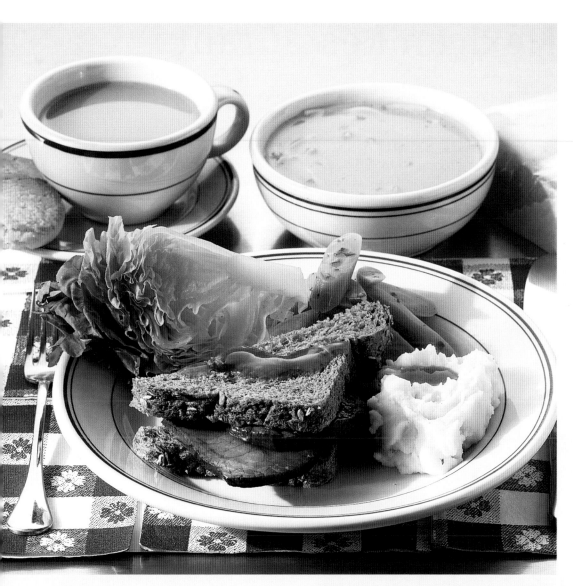

Menu	Serving size
Chicken breast teriyaki	3 ounces (deck of cards)
White rice	1 cup (baseball)
Stir-fried broccoli	1 cup
Meat loaf	3 ounces (deck of cards)
Mashed potatoes	⅓ cup (½ tennis ball)
Green beans	½ cup (2 golf balls)
Dinner roll	1 (tennis ball)
Spinach omelet	2 eggs
Wheat toast	2 slices
Sliced tomatoes	

TIPS FOR ORDERING

Things to look for on the menu:

- **Grilled, broiled, roasted:** When done correctly, fat drips off.
- **Half portion:** Right around the *ChangeOne* recommended portion size.

Mexican Restaurants

There's lots to love about Mexican fare—plenty of beans, fresh fish, grilled vegetables, and salsas. Many popular dishes could feed you and several relatives, however, and they're often drenched in cheese and sour cream. But choose wisely and you can have a delicious Mexican meal that fits nicely into your *ChangeOne* plans.

MENU 1 (Photo on opposite page)
  Cup of gazpacho
  1 chicken fajita with:
  Flour tortilla
  Grilled chicken (deck of cards)
  Grilled onions and peppers
  Guacamole (thumb)
  Unlimited lettuce, tomato, pico de gallo
  (fresh vegetable salsa)

Approximate serving info (based on *ChangeOne* sizes): Calories 430, fat 10 g, saturated fat 2 g, cholesterol 70 mg, sodium 1,310 mg, carbohydrate 47 g, fiber 6 g, protein 40 g, calcium 100 mg.

MENU 2
  Shrimp or fish ceviche
  2 steak soft tacos with:
  2 corn tortillas
  Grilled sirloin steak (deck of cards)
  Grated cheese (palmful)
  Unlimited lettuce, tomato, salsa

Approximate serving info (based on *ChangeOne* sizes): Calories 430, fat 16 g, saturated fat 6 g, cholesterol 155 mg, sodium 590 mg, carbohydrate 33 g, fiber 5 g, protein 40 g, calcium 250 mg.

CHOOSING YOUR MEAL

Soups

Two traditional Mexican soups deliver great taste without many calories. Gazpacho is a cold tomato soup brimming with diced green peppers and cucumber; with all those vegetables, it's wonderfully healthy. Tortilla soup starts with a base of chicken

BEWARE

- **Fish taco:** The fish usually is breaded and fried. See if you can get it with the fish grilled.
- **Tostada or taco salad:** The fried tortilla bowl has more calories than the salad. Order it without the bowl.
- **Frijoles:** High-calorie beans if they've been fried; refried beans are cooked in lard and then mashed.

broth and gets its flavor from lime, cilantro, and pieces of chicken, with crumbled corn tortillas to round out the taste and texture.

Appetizers

Most Mexican appetizers are fried or dripping with cheese. If you must order quesadillas (grilled tortilla cheese sandwiches) or nachos (fried chips with an assortment of toppings), get one order for the whole table. Better yet, try ceviche, a fish or shrimp cocktail marinated in citrus and often accompanied by tomato and avocado.

Main meals

"Grande" is the best way to describe Mexican main courses. To avoid big portions, pick from the à la carte menu and get side orders of beans or rice if you want. One item with soup or a shared appetizer is about the right amount of food. Listed below are several favorites in the 250-300 calorie range when you eat the portion listed:

Entrée	Serving Size
Chicken fajita	Same as Menu 1
Steak soft taco	Same as Menu 2
Burrito	5 ounces (checkbook)
Hard-shell taco	2½ ounces

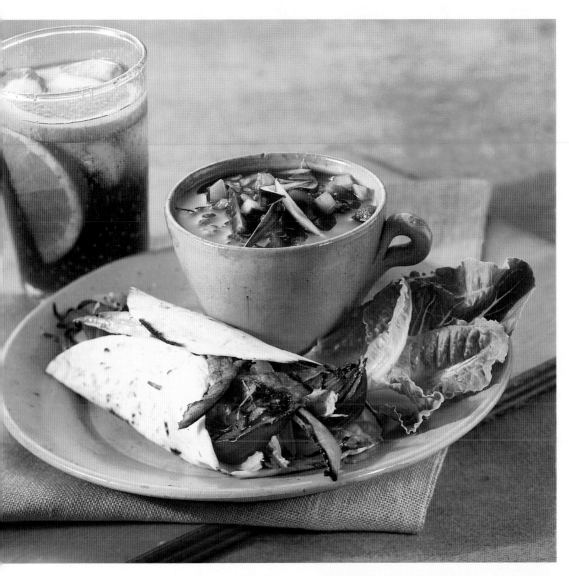

Beef and bean chimichanga	4 ounces (deck of cards)
Beef and cheese chimichanga	4 ounces
Tostada	6 ounces (checkbook)
Chicken taquito	5 ounces
Beef flautas	4 ounces
Cheese quesadilla	4 ounces

TIPS FOR ORDERING

- Ask the waiter to take away the tortilla chips. Better to not be tempted than to try to limit yourself to just a couple.
- Pick just one high-calorie topping— sour cream, grated cheese, or guacamole—and use it sparingly. Guacamole is best, healthwise.
- Make a meal of side orders—for example, black beans, rice, and grilled vegetables topped with salsa.

Help!

I know going out for fast food isn't the smartest thing to do. But sometimes there's no other choice. How do I order and still hold calories down?"

Sure, as long as you can resist the messages to add this and super-size that. Be a contrarian. Choose the smallest sizes. Ditch the secret sauce. Double up on lettuce and tomatoes. Order diet soda or water. Here are 9 meal options to choose from:

- Chicken nuggets (four pieces), sauce (one package), garden salad with fat-free vinaigrette
- Grilled chicken flat bread sandwich (hold the sauce), garden salad with fat-free vinaigrette
- Junior hamburger, garden salad, fat-free French dressing
- Large chili, shredded cheddar cheese (two tablespoons), two saltine crackers
- Plain baked potato, Caesar side salad, fat-free French dressing
- Veggie burger, garden salad, fat-free dressing
- Two beef soft tacos
- Chicken soft taco, pintos, and cheese
- Taco salad with salsa (no shell)

menu, and chances are you'll order the healthiest, lowest-calorie selections. Spicy red salsas, deep purple beets, green salads, yellow corn, bright orange and yellow sweet peppers turn your plate into a rainbow of colors. As long as vegetables arrive without added fat, they're free on *ChangeOne*. Help yourself. And there's another reason for filling your plate with color. Many of the substances that provide fruits and vegetables with their colors are antioxidants—potent disease-fighters that have been shown to lower heart disease and cancer risk.

2 Order appetizers and sides
Another favorite dieting strategy: Forgo the entrée section of the menu and order only from the appetizers and side dishes. With today's oversized restaurant portions, an appetizer or side often makes the perfect meal by itself. Skip things like the deep-fried mozzarella, of course, and make sure your choices include at least two servings of vegetables.

3 Dip into the sauce
Ordering salad dressing on the side and drizzling it on sparingly is one of the oldest diet tricks. Remember that you can order other sauces on the side, too, from gravy to guacamole. Give yourself no more than a tablespoon. And put your fork to good use. Instead of pouring on the sauce or salad dressing, dip the tips of your fork in the dressing and then spear a bite-size portion. You'll make a little bit of a good thing go a long way.

4 Create your own smorgasbord
If you're dining out with friends who share your concern about overdoing it, agree to order and share entrées. If there are four of you, order two or three main dishes. You'll get a chance to sample a wider variety of items and keep portions down to size. Be careful, though: When offered a lot to choose from, some people end up

eating a lot more. Decide in advance to sample only two or three forkfuls of each dish. With lots of dishes on the table, it's especially important to be aware of hunger and satiety signals. Sit back from time to time and think about whether you've had enough. If you have, put your fork down, raise a glass of water, and enjoy the conversation.

5 Be a discerning food critic

Remember the credo of smart dining: If it doesn't taste great, don't eat it. Sure you paid for it, and it's a shame to waste food. But to finish something you don't really like is the true crime. When you're dining out this week, be a tough critic. Pay attention to the first few bites. Decide whether it's good enough to finish, or whether you'd just as soon set aside the calories for something else. If you dine out frequently, consider keeping a diner's diary, with mini reviews and notes on what you had. Use a star system to award top restaurants your own *ChangeOne* rating. You'll find yourself paying closer attention to the food you eat—and enjoying it more.

Weekends and
Holidays

We almost called this chapter "Family and Friends."
Why? Because on weekends and holidays, that's who
you'll be spending your time with, and these people will
have an incredible amount of influence over what you
eat—and how much. In many cases, they'll be instru-
mental in determining your long-term dieting success,
either through their support or lack of it.

Weekends are also when the usual work-week routine
is up for grabs. New temptations arise from every side:
fancy dinners out, hot dogs and French fries at the ball
game, Sunday brunches, and backyard barbecues.

**This week dive into your weekend with gusto.
We're proposing just this one change: Focus
less on food and more on active fun.**

We'll show you that you don't have to hide from
friends, family, or fun to stick to your new eating habits.

Get Together with Family and Friends

By now you know that the real secret to losing weight isn't as complicated as a lot of diet books would have you believe. Like a lot of the volunteers who tested *ChangeOne*, you may have found that making just two or three changes was all you needed in order to start slimming down.

The same principles that have guided you will serve you well when your routine suddenly switches gears on weekends and holidays. Sure, you'll need to be a little creative. But that's not such a bad thing. Learning to be flexible is important. Life, after all, has a way of throwing us a curve now and then. The more confident you feel about adapting your diet to new situations, the better your chances of success. Weekends and holidays are a great way to discover that you can control what you eat in almost any situation.

Why Not Take the Weekend Off?

If you've tried a deprivation-type diet in the past—the kind built around diet shakes or long lists of forbidden foods—you were probably tempted to take a vacation from dieting when weekends and holidays rolled around. But by making a distinction between days when you follow a diet and days when you're on "vacation" from it, you tell yourself that your diet is some kind of unnatural chore. It makes you eat one way to lose weight, but you really want to eat another, very different way in your everyday life. That's the recipe for a diet that will fail. Too many dieters lose weight, then go off their diets and return to the way they used to eat. Almost immediately the pounds begin to pile on again.

ChangeOne isn't about deprivation, as you know by now. It's about good food and a rational way of eating that you can enjoy while you lose weight—and will continue to enjoy and benefit from long after you've lost the pounds. It is a diet you can live with every day.

Check-In

Frustrated that you're not losing weight faster? There's no need to be if you're dropping a pound or two a week. That's a pace that will keep you on track not only to lose weight but keep it off. Wish you were losing that much? Look back at the Fast Track suggestions in the breakfast, lunch, snacks, and dinner sections. Choose two tips from any of those to put into effect this week. Fast Track turned out to be one of the most popular features of *ChangeOne* among previous readers of this book. Many followed the advice in all of them.

That's the key. The more consistently you make smart eating choices, the more quickly they'll become second nature to you. That's why it's so important on weekends and holidays to find ways to use *ChangeOne* strategies even when your normal schedule is thrown up for grabs and you find yourself in situations where plates are piled high and beverages are flowing freely.

The occasional splurge won't make you gain weight; only ongoing excesses do that.

If you're celebrating something special—your birthday, an anniversary, a big wedding, whatever—live it up. But plan ahead. Strike a deal with yourself in advance. In return for getting the chance to indulge a little, agree to skip snacks during the day; set aside 45 minutes for a calorie-burning activity; or put together any combination that lets you, in effect, pay as you go. Keep track of what you eat during the day. Fill in a detailed food diary if you have time.

And remember, one indulgence doesn't mean you've failed. It doesn't even have to bring bad news on the scale. To gain a pound, you have to consume about 3,500 more calories than you burn. That's a lot of calories. Even the biggest holiday feast isn't likely to pack that many. The truth is, a big blowout isn't what typically spells trouble for dieters. The real danger is eating a little too much every day—or every weekend. If you do indulge yourself this weekend, just make a pact to follow the *ChangeOne* meal plans more closely during the coming week and you'll be fine.

When Food Is Love

One big reason weekends and holidays are difficult is that in all the world's cultures, food equals love. Food is a reward. Food is comfort. How do we celebrate Valentine's Day? With chocolate hearts. What do we do for someone's birthday? Bake a cake. How do we mark a wedding? With a feast. The simple act of offering someone food is a way to show love and affection. There's nothing wrong with that. We just need to keep a clear view of why we're eating.

This week and weekend notice the role that food plays for you with your family and friends. If the people who love you press you to eat more than you want or need, look for alternatives. If your mother says, "Eat, eat," to show she cares, say, "No, thanks, Mom. I'm full right now—but let me help you clear the dishes so we can have a chance to talk." If your friends' main device for getting together is dinner out, suggest alternatives that don't have to center on food: cards, bowling, or badminton, for instance, or a hike in a nearby park.

When you do find yourself at the table with friends and family, remember that you don't have to overeat to show you care. Food is only part of what makes sitting down with friends and family a pleasure. We get together to talk and laugh, to catch up on the latest news, to reinforce the ties that

Practicing the Art of Saying, "No, Thanks"

"Have some more," your doting mother-in-law urges you. "You're going to waste away if that's all you eat."

"What?" Aunt Bev says. "You didn't like my casserole? You've always loved my casserole. Come now, just one more little serving. Dessert? But it's a special occasion. You can't say no!"

Of course you can say no—but sometimes only at the risk of hurting someone's feelings. Or so it may seem. But you don't have to let well-meaning urgings to eat cause you to overeat. You can always refuse. And by being diplomatic you won't hurt any feelings in the process. Here's how:

Be up-front. Casually mention to everyone in advance that you're on a diet and watching portion sizes. Make it clear that you don't want to offend anyone but that it's very important for you to keep an eye on how much you eat.

Compliment early and often. If you're oohing and aahing after the first bite, it won't seem as if you disliked the dish when you turn down seconds later.

Pace yourself. If you know Aunt Bev's feelings will be hurt when you don't sample her pecan pie, plan your meal accordingly. Help yourself to smaller portions of the main course so you have a little extra room—and some extra calories to spare—when dessert rolls around.

Say yes to a little. Sometimes it's easier to take a small portion than refuse everything and find yourself staring at an empty plate while everybody enjoys dessert. But be sure that you control the serving size, not Aunt Bev.

Use delaying tactics. You can avoid offending people by saying "Maybe later," or "I'm so full right now I wouldn't be able to enjoy it. Let me wait a little while." Once the plates are cleared away and the festivities move on to the next stage, no one will remember that you didn't have dessert.

Take it home. Another strategy to avoid eating more than you want is simple flattery. When the offer for seconds comes along, rave about how great everything was—and ask if you can take a serving home rather than have seconds now. And taking seconds home doesn't mean you have to eat them. If you don't intend to, make sure you dispose of the leftovers right away. We won't tell.

bind by expressing our feelings for one another. If you're engaged in conversation, no one will notice that you've put your fork down and are sipping from your water glass. Food may nourish our bodies, but it's laughter and expressions of caring, after all, that nourish our souls.

Nurturing Yourself

Family and friends aren't the only people who urge food on us as a reward or show of affection. Some of us do it to ourselves. We eat to reward ourselves or to feel better when we're blue. Especially if you grew up being offered food to feel better, you may have internalized this reflex. Feel bad? Eat. The trouble, of course, is that you'll almost certainly overeat. When you do, you'll feel bad. And what do you do then? Well, eat some more.

How to escape? You may already have found part of the answer in becoming aware of genuine hunger cues and distinguishing them from environmental and emotional triggers to eat. But if you still have trouble resisting the urge to reward yourself with food, make a list of alternatives to eating. What else will make you feel better? If your day is full of stresses, reward yourself with five minutes of quiet time to relax and depressurize. (You'll find more stress-busting strategies in Week 9, "Stress Relief," which begins on page 148.) If you love music, take a few minutes out to play a favorite piece. If you really, really want something to eat, reward yourself with a stick of sugar-free gum, a suggestion we've made before because it really works. Make a habit of it, in fact. Over time, whenever the urge to treat yourself to food arises, you'll think of sugar-free gum.

Have a Plan in Place

Routines may change on weekends and holidays, but that doesn't mean everything has to be thrown up for grabs. Chances are you've already made at least a few plans for this weekend. Before it gets under way, think ahead. Write down a schedule for breakfast, lunch, and dinner, and fill in as many blanks as possible.

Think of it as a reverse food diary. Let's say your weekend plans include a trip to your mother's house to celebrate her

60th birthday with a big family potluck. Your schedule might look something like this:

Saturday
   Breakfast: *ChangeOne* breakfast at home
   Lunch: On the road
   Dinner: Mom's house

Sunday
   Breakfast: Mom's house
   Lunch: Potluck at the park
   Dinner: On the road

Once you've written up a schedule, identify the meals that are likely to pose the toughest challenges and brainstorm ways to prepare in advance to make them easier. In the example above, Saturday breakfast is a breeze, but grabbing lunch on the road could be treacherous, given the long strips of fast-food restaurants between here and Mom's. Family dinners are always a challenge—too much food, too many people urging

Smart Holiday Tricks

When the big winter holidays arrive, there's often no way to avoid being stuck in the house with lots of relatives, friends...and food. Here are some ways to cope:

Be helpful anywhere but in the kitchen. This is a tough one, especially if you're at the in-laws'. But it's easy to nibble when you're surrounded by food in various stages of preparation. Volunteer for other duties: cleaning up, setting the table, being bartender, running errands—anything that doesn't involve food.

Be the activity director. Take the lead in suggesting noneating activities that the family can do together, from playing charades to building a snowman.

Grab a water bottle. When there are lots of high-calorie-beverages around, it helps to have an alternative ready. Keep a glass or bottle of water handy.

Keep "free" snacks and beverages on hand. Satisfy your munchies with very low-calorie treats like carrots, celery, sweet peppers, sliced jicama, and diet drinks. That way you won't have to rely on your willpower to steer clear of all those diet-busting rich foods.

Hang with the kids. If all the adults are circling the food table, spend time with the children. At most ages, kids are more likely than adults to be doing something active. Their energy and playfulness can help distract you from food.

Get lost. If the sight and smell of all that food becomes just too much for you, excuse yourself and get out of the house. Take a stroll or go for a drive.

you to eat. And a potluck on Sunday! Everyone will be bringing family favorites, and the table will be crowded with dishes.

Never fear. There are plenty of ways to plan ahead on a weekend like this. Here are seven ideas to get you started:

1 Do it yourself
The best way to control what you eat is to make it yourself—something we've mentioned a few times so far. If there's not much chance you'll find a decent meal when you're on the road, consider packing your own in advance. You'll save money, frustration, and time. If the weather's good and you can find a nice place to stop, you can turn a bag lunch into a picnic. When the weekend includes a potluck meal, contribute a *ChangeOne* dish. Fix two if you have the time. That way you'll have a choice of dishes you can rely on to be low in calories. Don't forget to bring along sugar-free beverages or sparkling water.

2 Celebrate special occasions with special food
At most big weekend and holiday gatherings, people bring big bowls of store-bought chips and dips along with lovingly prepared homemade delicacies, like Aunt Estella's chicken cacciatore or Grandma Peterson's rhubarb pie. Spend your calories wisely by skipping the run-of-the-mill munchies. Instead, choose from only the special foods that celebrate the occasion.

3 Practice your pace
The big holiday dinner is one time when everyone relaxes and enjoys a leisurely feast. It's a great chance to practice your best tortoise skills. For a long meal, you may have to use every delaying tactic in the book. Drink a sip of water between each bite. Put your fork down frequently. Sit back in your chair and enjoy the conversation for a few minutes without eating anything.

4 Watch the alcohol
Wine, punch, beer, or other alcoholic beverages have a way of flowing freely at holiday meals. Don't let too much alcohol dissolve your best intentions to stick to your diet. Limit yourself to one glass with your meal. The rest of the time have sparkling water or sugar-free soft drinks. Love

Change One success stories

Surpassing Her Goals

Kathy Bennett has been spending a lot of money on clothes lately. Since she started *ChangeOne*, Kathy has gone down three sizes, so she's had to buy a completely new wardrobe.

Not that she's complaining about it. "My original goal was to fit comfortably into my pants, but I eventually lost 30 pounds and over 5 inches from my hips," she says.

And the benefits for Kathy go well beyond pounds lost and brand-new outfits. "My cholesterol count came down from 247 to 183, without any medication," she says. "I also found that I have more energy and less stress, which I'm sure is related to the exercise program suggested by *ChangeOne*."

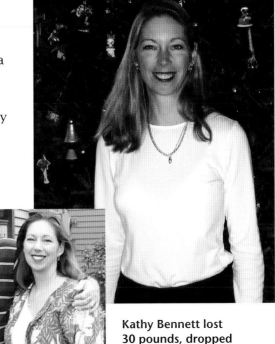

Kathy Bennett lost 30 pounds, dropped three sizes, and lowered her cholesterol 64 points.

Kathy, who has two children, ages 20 and 23, started with ChangeOne because she liked that it was a well-balanced program that allowed her to eat anything, with no prohibited foods.

"I ate everything I loved through my weight-loss process, including penne à la vodka and hot dogs—I just had less of it," she says. "The portion-control tricks are great. The easiest one for me was cutting my meal in half when I went out to dinner—except I ate all the veggies. Because it was so easy, it just became a new way of life for me."

Exercise was also a key to Kathy's success. "I increased my aerobic exercise from once a week to six times per week and used every opportunity to burn calories, including walking up and down 20 flights of stairs on my way to and from the cafeteria every day," she says.

Kathy's family has been extremely helpful with her weight-loss efforts. "My children and my husband were wonderfully supportive through the process, eagerly anticipating my weekly weigh-ins and never once trying to tempt me to eat something off my plan," she says. "It's a real ego boost to have family and friends, even my aerobics instructor, exclaim about how thin I look."

For more ChangeOne *success stories, go to www.changeone.com/successstories*

an icy cold beer on a hot summer weekend? Light beer should be an option, and the offerings in this category are getting better and better.

5 Get out and about

The extra leisure time on weekends offers a great opportunity to plan activities that involve burning more calories. Rally your relatives for hikes, bike rides, walking tours of the city, softball, croquet, a run on the beach, throwing a Frisbee, or just frolicking with the dog. Burn 500 extra calories this weekend, and you can treat yourself to a big piece of Grandma Peterson's rhubarb pie without worrying about upsetting your calorie balance. Activities that the whole family can join in are also great ways to enjoy time together—and they don't center around food.

6 Take time for bedtime

Weekends are a wonderful opportunity to catch up on sleep you may have missed during the week. Lack of sleep can erode your willpower and determination. Obesity experts believe it can even cause you to put on pounds. Get to bed a little early one night this weekend. If that doesn't work, allow yourself to sleep a little later than usual one morning.

7 Fine-tune your expectations

If the coming week is a crowded schedule of holiday parties, be realistic about your goals. Instead of trying to continue losing weight, for instance, relax your goal to simply maintaining your current weight. When the holidays are done, you can start shedding pounds again. Setting standards that are impossible to meet mostly just leads to failure. Unless you have an upcoming modeling session for the cover of a fashion magazine, odds are you don't have to lose a certain amount of weight by a certain date. Remember, this is a weight-loss plan for your entire life. Don't put yourself under needless pressure right from the start. It's far better to take a little while longer to reach your goal than to put yourself under unnecessary stress.

Should You Enlist Family and Friends?

A bit of encouragement, a helping hand, even someone joining you on your walk around the neighborhood can be great morale boosters. So can a shoulder to lean on when things aren't going your way. Help from family and friends also can take the pressure off you and eliminate the unnecessary stresses in your life.

How important are the people around you when it comes to dieting success? At first, behavioral scientists assumed the answer would be "very." The more support dieters had, the assumption went, the better their odds of losing weight and keeping it off. But the results of studies looking at social support and weight loss have been mixed. Some people do better when they have a strong social network. Others do just fine on their own.

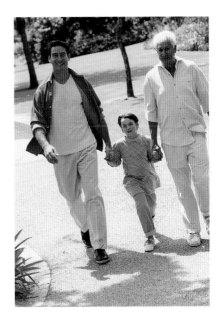

What is consistent among successful dieters is a sense of accountability for their weight loss. A recent study showed that dieters who used a telephone buddy check-in system stayed on track much better than people who had no accountability for their efforts. The bottom line: If you are going to try to lose weight, you will do best if you are serious about it, with goals and rewards. For some of us, having a support team makes a big difference.

Knowing whether you tend to be a team player or a solo flier is the first step in finding the kind of support and encouragement you need to succeed. To find out, answer the questions in the quiz on page 119.

Your Friends in Need

Social support comes in many forms, from the neighbor who joins you on your morning walk to the spouse who decides to do the *ChangeOne* program along with you. The first step in getting the help you need is deciding what you need. Check one or more of the following options:

❑ An activity partner
❑ Someone to talk to when I'm down or discouraged

❏ Someone who can answer specific diet questions
❏ Help in the kitchen
❏ Help around the house
❏ A lunch or dinner companion
❏ Other: _____

Now make a list of possible candidates to fill the positions you've checked. Keep in mind that help and support sometimes come from unexpected places. A colleague at work may be more useful to you than a close family member. A neighbor you meet on one of your walks—someone who's also trying to slim down—may end up offering more help than a close friend.

If you're looking for emotional support, identify someone you're willing to confide in, even if that means admitting weakness or failure. If you're looking for practical help around the house, you probably already know whom to ask. So ask. Be specific about what you need and why you need it. If you're asking someone to do a real favor, think about what you can do for them in return.

Beware of Saboteurs

In a perfect world, family and friends would support you 100 percent. But we live in an imperfect world. Sometimes the people closest to you may be threatened by your efforts to change yourself.

Often it's especially the people closest to you, in fact, who have trouble with your decision to lose weight—a spouse or sibling, for example. If your spouse tends to be a little jealous, your decision to lose weight could be interpreted as a desire to be considered more attractive to other people. If your spouse could stand to lose a little weight, too—but isn't willing to try right now—he or she may resent your determination and success.

There are plenty of reasons that don't take a psychiatrist to figure out, of course. Following a diet requires changes in the kitchen and at the table.

And some family members may not want to be bothered by those changes. They may not like the extra time you spend planning lunches or dinners. They may feel uncomfortable finishing everything on their plate while you eat smaller portions.

Take a moment to think about the people closest to you. Among them, is there anyone who:

Change One quiz
Team Player or Solo Flier?

Some people need the support of people around them. Others do best on their own. To find out for yourself, answer the following:

1. I'm comfortable talking to other people about my weight. △ True ☐ False

2. If things aren't going well for me, I typically turn to family or friends for advice. △ True ☐ False

3. I'm embarrassed talking about my feelings with other people, even people close to me. ☐ True △ False

4. Getting a little pat on the back now and then would help motivate me right now. △ True ☐ False

5. When I set my mind to do something, I don't really need other people to push me. ☐ True △ False

6. I have at least one person in my life with whom I can talk about almost anything. △ True ☐ False

7. I tend to keep my personal feelings to myself. ☐ True △ False

8. The people around me are part of the reason I've had trouble losing weight. ☐ True △ False

9. I've always tended to tackle problems on my own. ☐ True △ False

10. I'm not really sure that the people around me have my best interests in mind. ☐ True △ False

11. Just being able to talk things over with someone when I've got a problem can make things seem better. △ True ☐ False

12. I'm very uneasy about letting people see my weaknesses. ☐ True △ False

13. I've joined groups in the past, and they've really helped me. △ True ☐ False

14. Frankly, I don't trust people to be honest with me or tell me what they're really thinking. ☐ True △ False

Score

Tally up the number of colored shapes you checked—blue triangles or green squares:

△ Blue _____   ☐ Green _____

△ Blue answers indicate team players, people who benefit from the support of others. The more blue triangles you checked, the more likely you are to rely on a strong support network of friends and family. ☐ Green answers indicate the solo fliers—people who typically go it alone. The more green boxes you checked, the more likely you are to depend on yourself.

Most of us are a little bit team player and solo flier, of course. Don't be surprised if your score falls somewhere in the middle. Read on for advice on how to strengthen your social network, along with tips on how you can do a better job of helping yourself.

- Continues to urge food on you even when you say you're not hungry?
- Belittles your efforts to lose weight?
- Throws obstacles in the way of your being more active?
- Seems resentful or threatened by the fact that you've begun to lose weight?
- Expresses anger or frustration when you leave food on your plate?
- Undermines your efforts with negative messages? Perhaps he/she does that with comments like, "I don't know what makes you think you'll be able to lose weight this time," or, "Once the holidays roll around you're going to gain it all back again anyway."

If so, you may be struggling against someone who's trying to sabotage the change you want to make. Often the hardest part in dealing with a saboteur is acknowledging that your personal relationships aren't perfect, and that someone close to you may be standing between you and improvement. It's easier to blame yourself or your lack of willpower. But it's crucially important to recognize when someone is making life harder, rather than easier.

Talk It Out

If you spot a problem like that this week and you think it comes mainly from a lack of communication, ask your problem person for a heart-to-heart talk. Explain why losing weight is so important to you—and why the sincere support and enthusiasm of people around you matter so much. Point out the things that make it hard for you or hurt your feelings.

And be specific about the kind of help you need:

- "I'd rather you didn't offer me seconds. When I say no, I feel as if I'm hurting your feelings. But it's very important to me right now to cut back on the amount I eat."
- "It would help me a lot if we put snack food out of sight in the cupboard, rather than on the counter where I see it all the time. I have a tendency to eat when there's food out."
- "It really hurts my feelings when you say I never stick with things. I'm really trying this time. Your encouragement means a lot to me."

Ask your spouse or friend to talk about his/her feelings. Explore what you can do to make the situation easier. If a loved one feels threatened, make it clear that your love hasn't changed.

Enjoy Yourself

Enjoying yourself should come easy on weekends and holidays. But if you're constantly worried about being tempted by too much food, it's easy to forget that the point of weekends and holidays is to relax and have a good time. So this weekend make sure to do just that. Being physically active on weekends and holidays also adds enjoyment and gives you an opportunity to relax.

Why make a point of enjoying yourself when you're on a diet? Because the more you're able to find pleasure, with and without food, the easier you'll find it to stay with the program and turn healthy eating into a lifelong habit.

How to Be Your Own Best Friend

Whether you're a soloist or a team player, a few strategies can help you get through the inevitable rough patches.

Banish negative thoughts. Most of us have heard the little voice that whispers, "You're never going to make it," or, "You just don't have what it takes." Learn to recognize such negative thoughts and replace them with the kind of positive messages a good friend would offer. "Sure you can do it." "One slip-up is no big deal." "Keep up the good work."

Keep a journal. If that negative voice in your head just won't let up, try carrying a small notebook with you this week and jot down every negative thought that occurs to you. You may be surprised to find that the simple act of writing these thoughts down makes you see how irrational they are. If you can't dismiss them, take a moment to come up with a positive countermessage. "I'm trying to improve myself." "I've stayed with a diet for five weeks, which isn't bad."

"Hey, no one's perfect. I'm doing my best." By keeping a diary, you'll also become aware of the situations and circumstances that trigger negative thoughts. Avoid them if you can.

Reward yourself for a good job. When you reach one of your goals—even if it's something as simple as sticking to *ChangeOne* through a long holiday weekend—give yourself a reward. For a little extra motivation, decide in advance what the reward will be: a new pair of walking shoes, a new music CD, or a trip to the spa.

Learn to laugh at your foibles. Having a sense of humor can go a long way when you're trying to make a big change in your life. Take yourself too seriously, and you'll slip into the kind of all-or-nothing thinking that makes people give up before they've even given themselves a chance to succeed.

Week **7**

Fixing Your
Kitchen

"On days when warmth is the most important need of the human heart," the author E. B. White once wrote, "the kitchen is the place you can find it."

White's words still hold true. Even in today's world of takeout pizzas and microwave meals, the kitchen is still the warm heart of most households.

This week you'll transform the kitchen by tossing out the devilish foods on hand, replacing them with *ChangeOne* choices, and rearranging for easier, healthier cooking.

Why make changes in the kitchen? Because we don't ever want you to think of your kitchen as a place to be avoided. In *ChangeOne*, we want the kitchen to remain a place of warmth, a place that encourages happiness and healthy eating at the same time.

Stocking Up Smartly

Making sure you have plenty of food in your pantry may sound like strange diet advice. After all, who wants a wealth of edible temptations around when you're trying to eat less, not more?

In fact, as many dieters discover, a bare cupboard can actually spell trouble. No matter how scant your provisions are, chances are there's a bag of chips from last week's party or a box of candy left over from Valentine's Day lurking somewhere. And if that's all there is to eat, guess what you're going to grab if you get hungry enough? Exactly.

By keeping plenty of healthy foods around, you'll have plenty of choices, not just for snacks but for every meal of the day. And by organizing your kitchen smartly, you can make sure the best choices are right in front of you when you swing into the kitchen or open the refrigerator door. What's more, a well-stocked, well-organized kitchen can save you time and spare you frustration. With the right selection of essentials on hand, you can put together a simple and delicious meal without having to make a run to the grocery store. Many home chefs are inspired to make interesting dishes simply by opening up the refrigerator, checking out what's there, and conjuring up tasty combinations.

For a detailed analysis of your kitchen and tips on how to make it work better for you, take our "Inspection Time" quiz on page 125.

The first step in designing a diet-friendly kitchen isn't shopping; it's clearing your shelves. So get the garbage bags ready, along with a box for items you can give away. It's time to get rid of food you don't want—and don't need around to tempt you.

Start with the pantry. Ask yourself on each item, "Would I eat this?" If yes, then ask, "Should I eat this?" Keep in mind your family's tastes, of course. But don't

Check-In

Is someone making it harder rather than easier to eat right? If you realized last week that you have a saboteur working against you, consider taking an extra week to resolve the situation as best you can. Keep a record—write down every time someone says something or does something that seems designed to sabotage your efforts. At the end of each day, look over your entries and brainstorm for ways to free yourself. Strategies include avoiding situations that involve food, countering negative messages with positive ones, or simply learning to ignore criticisms or unwanted enticements. Sometimes the best approach is to talk it out. At other times, separating yourself from the source of trouble is a better solution. Use your judgment. Just remember that you're in charge of what you eat—no one else. Be considerate of other people's feelings, but stick to your resolution.

be too generous. If you shouldn't eat it, chances are your loved ones shouldn't, either. Focus in particular on items that have sat around for more than six months.

Move to the refrigerator and freezer next. Clear out those funky old condiment jars, those squishy old peppers, those eight-day-old leftovers.

If it feels good to clear off the shelves, it should. And it'll feel even better when you fill up the space with foods that are healthier, fresher, and more interesting.

Go Shopping

Your next step is making a run to the grocery store to buy essentials. Exactly what those essentials are will depend on your taste, how often you prepare meals at home, and the kinds of foods your family likes. You'll find a master shopping list of kitchen essentials on page 337 to use as your guide. You don't need to stock them all, of course. The more choices you have on hand, though, the easier it will be to put together a *ChangeOne* meal or snack on the spur of the moment.

Before you head for the grocery store this week, keep in mind six essential strategies for smart shopping:

1 **Have a snack before you go.**
You'll get some exercise cruising the aisles and hauling bags, so go ahead and take the hunger edge off before you hit the store. An empty stomach can make you empty-headed. Nothing weakens willpower faster than being hungry. Chances are you've seen shoppers so hungry that they dip into a bag of chips or package of cookies even before they've reached the checkout line. Avoid trouble by shopping after you've eaten a meal. If you find yourself shopping for dinner on an empty stomach, have a *ChangeOne* snack before you start pushing your cart down the aisle.

2 **Start with a list—and stay with it.**
Your local grocery is full of temptations that can be hard to resist. Supermarkets are in the business of selling food, especially items with a big profit margin. The biggest money-makers are often the items that are prominently displayed at eye level or at the ends of aisles. Chances are you'll see row after row of snack foods, cookies, colas, doughnuts, and highly sweetened cereals. Steer your cart

Change One quiz
Inspection Time

How diet-friendly is your kitchen? There's only one way to find out. Put on your kitchen inspector's cap, grab a pencil and a pad of paper, and fill out the following checklist:

1. What are the first three things you see when you open your refrigerator door?
   1. _____
   2. _____
   3. _____

2. What are the first three things you see when you open the freezer?
   1. _____
   2. _____
   3. _____

3. List the three handiest snacks in your kitchen:
   1. _____
   2. _____
   3. _____

4. How many kinds of fresh vegetables does your refrigerator crisper contain?
   ❏ None   ❏ One or two   ❏ Three or more

5. Is there a bowl of fruit on the counter?
   ❏ Yes   ❏ No   ❏ Usually, but not today

6. Do you have the makings of a *ChangeOne* dinner in your cupboard and refrigerator?
   ❏ Yes   ❏ No   ❏ Usually, but not today

7. Where do you keep your grocery list?
   ❏ Posted on the refrigerator door or in another prominent place
   ❏ Tucked away somewhere in the kitchen
   ❏ What list?

8. Rate your collection of storage containers:
   ❏ Plentiful and in a variety of different sizes
   ❏ Enough for a few leftovers
   ❏ What storage containers?

9. How many "too-tempting-to-resist" foods are in your kitchen right now?
   ❏ None   ❏ One or two   ❏ Three or more

10. Which of these is your kitchen lacking?
   ❏ Measuring spoons   ❏ Measuring cups
   ❏ Set of sharp knives   ❏ Microwave
   ❏ Vegetable steamer   ❏ Rice cooker
   ❏ Nonstick frying or sauté pan
   ❏ Set of small bowls and plates

11. Which of the following do you have in your freezer?
   ❏ Skinless, boneless chicken breasts
   ❏ Shrimp or fish fillets
   ❏ Berries or fruit slices
   ❏ Vegetables
   ❏ Frozen yogurt
   ❏ Meal-size containers of homemade chili, soup or stew
   ❏ Homemade soup stock

12. And which of the following can be found in your kitchen?
   ❏ Potato chips
   ❏ Premium ice cream
   ❏ Store-bought cookies
   ❏ Whole milk
   ❏ Doughnuts or cupcakes
   ❏ Salami, bologna, bacon, or breakfast sausage

Turn to next page to tally your score.

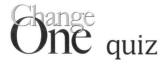 quiz

Score

Assessing your answers:

1, 2, 3. If the first items you see fit on the *ChangeOne* menu, your kitchen's in great shape. If not, your kitchen is working against you. Either get rid of the stuff you'd rather not be tempted by, or tuck it away where you have to work to get it.

4. Vegetables are free, so stock a tempting variety. That will make it easy to throw together a low-calorie meal without running to the store.

5. Put a bowl of fruit out where everyone in the family can see it. That way it will be the first place everyone goes when a snack attack strikes.

6. If you don't have the makings of a *ChangeOne* meal on your pantry shelf, you should. You'll be ready for anything, from a stormy night to a surprise visitor.

7. Invest in an erasable message board that you can mount on the refrigerator. It's a great way to keep a grocery list so that you won't be caught short when you want to cook a quick and simple meal.

8. Keep plenty of storage containers handy. Sure, they're great for leftovers. But you can also use them to divvy up giant food packages from the store into reasonably sized portions when you get home.

9. Why drive yourself crazy keeping foods you can't resist? Toss 'em. Or put them so far out of reach that you'll have to make a big effort to get them. One of our *ChangeOne* volunteers tucked his treat foods behind a couple of rows of wineglasses.

10. For a list of terrific time-saving, diet-friendly kitchen tools, check out page 317.

11. The freezer should be your ally in managing your diet, not an ice-cream shop or frozen-dinner collection. Consider stocking more of these foods for fast, healthy meals and treats.

12. As we've said before, you can't eat what you don't have on hand. Fatty, sugary, low-nutrition foods stop being an issue when there aren't any around to eat. If you must have some every now and then, do it out of the house by buying a single portion.

down almost any aisle, and you'll be surrounded by brightly colored packages specifically designed to lure their way into your cart. "All natural!" "Two for one!" "Giant family-size economy pack!" "Choose me!"

To avoid the hard sell, put together a shopping list in the quiet and comfort of your own kitchen. Build your list around recipes and meal plans. Use the guide to kitchen essentials on page 129, along with our lists of shopping strategies on pages 336-337.

Once you get to the market, stick to your list. Sure, if fresh peaches or ripe tomatoes are in season, help yourself. Don't be afraid to tinker with your meal plan if you find something irresistible in the produce aisle or there's a good bargain at the fish counter. But don't reach for that jumbo-size bag of cheesie-wheezies just because it's on sale this week. If it's not on your list—or your diet—it doesn't belong in your cart. If you don't find what you're looking for at the store, talk to the manager. Most grocery stores are happy to stock what customers want.

Managing Your Food

1. Use opaque storage containers for "treat" foods so you won't be tempted by the sight of the contents.
2. Put notes on food containers to remind yourself of what a sensible portion should be.
3. Decide in advance how much you plan to eat—before you open the container.
4. Attach a list of your favorite *ChangeOne* snacks to the refrigerator door as a reminder.
5. Put a date on leftovers—and a reminder on your calendar of when you plan to eat them.
6. Once a week tour your kitchen, making sure the healthiest foods occupy the most prominent positions.
7. Keep a list of essential items that are running low so that you won't be caught unprepared.

3 **Steer your cart around the perimeter.**
In most grocery stores, the healthiest choices are arranged around the perimeter of the store. That's where you'll find dairy products, the produce section, and the meat and fish counters. Processed foods, including those rows upon rows of brightly colored snack-food packages, are usually in the center of the store. As a general rule, then, the more shopping you do around the perimeter, the less processed food you're likely to run across—and the more food you'll find that fits your *ChangeOne* diet.

4 **Think small.**
Giant food warehouse clubs have risen on the promise of saving money by buying in bulk. There's nothing wrong with saving a few dollars. But if you have a tough time

stopping yourself once a jumbo bag of chips is open, take heed. If you're buying something to eat right away, buy a small package—preferably a single-serving size. If you buy jumbo sizes to save money, divide them into single-serving size, resealable plastic bags or containers right when you return from shopping.

5 **Read the small print.**
With few exceptions, all processed and packaged foods are required to carry detailed food labels that list ingredients and nutritional information. Learning to read a label will help you shop wisely. When your goal is to lose weight, the most important number on the label is calories per serving. Be sure to check how the label describes a serving size. The amount can vary widely even within the same category. Some cereal boxes list ¾ cup as a serving, for example, while others use 1 cup. Some foods may look as if they're low in calories until you discover that a serving size would fit into a thimble.

6 **Keep treats at a distance.**
Don't buy high-calorie items you have trouble resisting once they're under your roof. Do you really want them tempting you all the time? To ensure that treats remain treats, make them part of a special occasion. When the family wants ice cream, for example, go out for it. Don't make it too easy to splurge by keeping a half-gallon in the fridge. Kids clamoring for cookies? Take them down to the java hut or the bakery section of the store and buy a couple of good ones. Decide in advance how much you'll have. One small bite of everybody else's ice cream will let you sample a bunch of flavors and still keep you within the recommended serving size for dessert. A nibble or two on the kids' cookies will satisfy your sweet tooth and keep you on your diet.

Breaking the Chain

The single most important step for many *ChangeOne* participants is learning to shop for food smartly. If you prepare a lot of your meals at home, the decisions you make at the grocery store go a long way toward determining how well you eat.

To understand how important smart shopping is, visualize a chain. Scientists who study behavior talk about chains of

Kitchen Essentials

Use this guide to make sure your kitchen has all the items you'll need for healthy snacking and quick, easy-to-cook meals. Here we list some everyday staples; for a guide to perishables—the fruits, vegetables, dairy products, and meats that you use in *ChangeOne* meals—look at the shopping strategies on pages 336-337.

In the pantry
- Baking powder
- Baking soda
- Cocoa powder, unsweetened
- Cornstarch
- Flours—whole wheat and all-purpose
- Sugars—white and brown
- Vanilla extract
- Vinegars—balsamic, red wine
- Oils—olive, canola, sesame
- Cooking spray
- Peanut butter*
- Broth—chicken or vegetable, canned*
- Soups—mushroom, minestrone, or vegetable, canned*
- Tomatoes, canned*
- Tomato sauce*
- Tuna, canned*
- Herbs, dried
- Italian spices, dried
- Mushrooms, dried

Condiments
- Salt and pepper
- Ketchup*
- Mayonnaise, reduced fat*
- Mustards*—Dijon, yellow
- Soy sauce
- Hot sauce
- Pickles and pickle relish*

- Capers*
- Olives*

Cereals, grains, and beans
- Cereal—ready-to-eat, whole grain
- Oatmeal (rolled oats)
- Couscous
- Legumes (kidney beans, chickpeas, black beans, etc.), canned or dried
- Pasta
- Rice—brown and white

Snacks
- Graham crackers
- Nuts, mixed
- Popcorn kernels
- Whole grain snacks like crackers and pretzels

Fruits and vegetables
- Fruit canned in juice*
- Fruit, assorted fresh
- Raisins
- Garlic, fresh
- Onions
- Potatoes—baking or roasting, and sweet potatoes or yams
- Celery
- Bell peppers, green or red

In the refrigerator
- Butter
- Cheeses for grating, such as Parmesan

- Eggs
- Milk—low-fat or nonfat
- Yogurt, plain—low-fat or nonfat

In the freezer
- Bagels—mini or small (2 ounces)
- Breads—whole wheat and pita
- Berries and other fruit, frozen
- Fruit sorbet or fruit/juice pops
- Beef or chicken bones for homemade stock
- Chicken breasts, individually portioned
- Ground turkey or lean ground beef
- Meatless burgers
- Pizza crust, frozen
- Prepared dinners— reduced-calorie, frozen
- Vegetables, frozen

Miscellaneous
- Carbonated water
- Vegetable juices
- Sugar-free soda
- Iced tea, unsweetened
- Evaporated skim milk, canned
- Herbs, fresh
- Tomato salsa
- Green chiles, canned
- Tortillas—corn and flour, small

*These items may need to be refrigerated after you've opened them.

Help!

"I have three teenage kids, and the kitchen is filled with foods they love—potato chips, soft drinks, ice cream, and all the rest. How can I diet-proof my kitchen against that kind of temptation?"

You can't—not entirely. But you can certainly make your kitchen more comfortable for yourself. If your teenagers are tall enough to reach high, ask them to keep their snack foods on the upper shelves. Assign them a low shelf for soft drinks and other sweetened beverages in the fridge. Insist on reserving the most accessible shelf in the refrigerator for foods that are on your menu. Ask the kids not to leave packages of junk food lying around, and tell them to put all food away in the designated places when they're done eating.

Don't stop there. Try to encourage the rest of the family to follow your example and eat food with fewer empty calories. Sure, it can sometimes seem like an uphill struggle. But many kids these days are surprisingly health-conscious. And since weight problems typically begin early in life, you'll be doing them a favor. Sit down with your kids and explain why losing weight really matters to you. If your children are still young, you can nudge their tastes in the right direction. One *ChangeOne* success story regularly offered his four- and six-year-old children healthy choices, and they now eat whole wheat crackers, broccoli, asparagus, grilled fish, and of course, lots of macaroni and cheese.

behavior—individual decisions that connect like links on a chain. Let's say you give in to temptation one night and eat that whole pint of fudge-brownie ice cream in the fridge. At first that may seem like a single, impulsive act. But in reality, it's the end of a long chain of choices.

Think back to the beginning. That pint of fudge-brownie ice cream didn't get into the freezer on its own, after all. The links in the chain might look something like this:

- You go shopping when you're hungry.
- Rushing out the door, you forget to bring your shopping list with you.
- At the store you see a sign that says: FUDGE-BROWNIE ICE CREAM!—50% OFF! Uh-oh.
- You pop a pint into your cart.
- You pop that same pint into the freezer, telling yourself you'll only have a little, and only on special occasions.
- You're feeling low one night. You know you should get up and out for a walk to feel better, but...
- You're hungry. You open the refrigerator door, but because you haven't gone shopping lately, there's not much there that you want.
- You open the freezer door, and what's this? A pint of fudge-brownie ice cream leaps into your hands.
- You know you should serve up just one small scoop and put the container back, but you're feeling lazy, so you open the lid and grab a spoon.
- You know you should sit down at the counter and eat just a little, savoring every bite. But the TV is on and you wander into the living room. Instead of paying attention to the ice cream, you watch TV while you eat. The next thing you know, the whole pint is gone.

How can you make sure this doesn't happen? Of course, you can break the chain at any one of its links. You can get the ice cream home, realize your mistake, and give it away. Or you can put the spoon down and not dig in. Sure you can, but if you're like most people, the best time to stop the chain is at the store. You don't have to resist eating something you didn't buy. That's something to remember the next time you're tempted by food you know could overwhelm your willpower and set your diet back.

Put Food in Its Place

Once you're back from your shopping spree, it's time to take a serious look at your kitchen. The strategy is simple. Put the healthiest choices in the most prominent spots on kitchen shelves and in the refrigerator. Put "treat" foods—the items you only want to reach now and then—out of sight, even out of reach.

Let's say you like to treat yourself to an oatmeal raisin cookie from time to time. Now imagine that those cookies are stored in a clear glass cookie jar on the counter. Every time you swing into the kitchen for a snack, they're the first option you see. That means every time you enter the room you've got to rely on your willpower to resist turning a special treat into an everyday occurrence.

Why put yourself through that? Imagine, instead, that you keep a bowl of fruit on the counter and a few plastic containers with carrot and celery sticks front and center in the refrigerator. The cookies are safely stored away on the very top shelf of the pantry in a container with a lid that snaps shut—high enough that you need to get the stepladder out when you want them. Suddenly it's easy to grab something low in calories and rich in nutrition—an apple or a handful of carrot sticks. You will need to work to get at those cookies.

By the end of this week, your kitchen will be a place where you can relax, not a place where you have to constantly feel like you're fighting temptations.

How am I
Doing?

"How long does getting thin take?" Winnie the Pooh asks anxiously in A. A. Milne's classic children's book. You may be asking the same question just about now.

You probably have other questions, too. Why do you seem to lose weight some weeks and not others? Are you making reasonable progress toward your goal? What can you do to jumpstart your diet when weight loss stalls?

This week you'll assess how you're doing and find ways to get through trouble spots.

To get you started, take the "Seven Weeks of Progress" quiz, which begins on the following page. You will use its questions throughout this chapter to focus on the best ways to overcome your unique weight-loss challenges.

Change One quiz
Seven Weeks of Progress

Circle the appropriate number in the right-hand column to track your score.

1. How do you feel about your weight-loss progress so far?

Very satisfied	3
Satisfied	2
Disappointed	1

2. How would you rate your energy level since you began *ChangeOne*?

Improved	3
About the same	2
Slumped	1

3. How would you rate your self-confidence while on this program?

Improved	3
About the same	2
Worse	1

4. How many days last week did you closely follow the *ChangeOne* menu for breakfast, lunch, dinner, and snacks?

All or most	3
About half	2
Fewer than half	1

5. How often are you able to stick to sensible portions when you dine out?

All or most of the time	3
About half the time	2
Less than half the time	1

6. Planning is crucial to dieting success; how well are you doing when it comes to planning where and what you'll eat?

Very well	3
Good	2
So-so	1

7. Feeling hungry can whittle away at anyone's willpower; how would you describe your experience on *ChangeOne* so far?

Hunger isn't a problem for me	3
Now and then I get so hungry that I eat more than I should	2
Hunger is a problem for me a lot of the time	1

8. How often do you experience strong cravings for specific foods (chocolate, ice cream, salty snacks, or candy, for instance)?

Never	3
Now and then	2
Frequently	1

9. What phrase best describes your family and close friends?

Behind me 100 percent	3
Somewhat supportive	2
Not very helpful	1

10. How would you rate your overall motivation right now?

Excellent	3
Good	2
Shaky	1

Turn to next page to continue quiz.

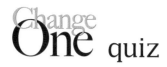 **quiz**

11. Stress can often get in the way when people are trying to change; how are you dealing with it?

Very well	3
Well enough	2
Not very well	1

12. Sometimes it seems there's food everywhere; how would you rate your ability to deal with temptations?

I'm getting better at eating only if I'm hungry	3
I give in to temptation now and then, but not as much as before	2
I still have a very tough time saying no	1

13. Where did you eat in your house during the past week?

Kitchen and dining room only	3
In front of TV or in the bedroom	2
Both in front of TV and in the bedroom	1

14. How many days during the past week did you fit in at least 20 minutes of brisk walking or movement?

All or most	3
About half	2
Fewer than half	1

Score

Add up the combined score of your answers and use the guide below to start evaluating your progress.

A score of 32 to 42: A big gold star for you. But put a check beside any questions that you scored as 1 and read the corresponding numbered tips in the following pages for advice on how to move ahead.

21 to 31: You're doing well, and should be proud of yourself. But the numbers also show that with a little extra help, you could be doing even better. Mark the questions you scored as 1 and read the numbered tips that follow for advice.

14 to 20: Okay, you're having a tough time. Many people do when they first try to lose weight. Read the following advice for doing better, with a particular focus on questions to which you answered with a 1. But first, remember to be kind to yourself! Don't feel bad about your score. Making changes in how you eat can be very hard emotionally. But the long-term benefits are huge. Do all you can to stay motivated and committed, and in time, you will succeed!

Succeeding Your Way

No single approach works for everyone. Even diet experts have been surprised to discover how many ways there are to succeed—or fail—at dieting. Some people like to be told exactly what to eat and then follow a strict plan. Others take a few guiding ideas and handle the rest. Some people need a lot of support from family and friends. Others go it alone.

We've seen the same thing among *ChangeOne* participants. Some began to lose weight with breakfast; others didn't hit their stride until they changed their approach to dinner. There were people who began to lose weight as soon as they changed the way they snacked. Others got the biggest bang for their buck paying attention to what they ate on the weekends. For some, *ChangeOne* was a breeze. For others, it wasn't always easy.

The quiz you just took should help clarify the challenges you've encountered on *ChangeOne*. To help you overcome these challenges, we'll review the quiz questions in detail in this chapter, offering tips and advice as we go to make sure you are getting all you can out of your efforts.

1 Disappointed in your results?
Reassess your goals; renew your commitment.
If you've lost eight pounds or more since you started *ChangeOne*, there's no reason to be disappointed. Experts say a healthy weight-loss plan should average one to three pounds a week. So eight weeks into *ChangeOne* you can expect to have lost anywhere from 8 to 24 pounds. Losing weight more quickly than that means losing muscle tissue along with fat, which could slow your metabolism and make it harder to maintain your weight loss down the road.

If you haven't started seeing the progress you'd like, there may be several reasons. If you've significantly increased the amount of exercise you're doing, you may be losing fat but adding muscle. Nothing wrong with that. In fact, it's the sure-fire way to look firmer and more svelt. But because you're trading fat for muscle, you may not see as much difference on the scale. One sign that you're making progress: your waist size. If it's going down, you're changing for the better.

The most important thing now is not to get discouraged. Make a pact with yourself to use a little extra time and effort this coming month to reach your goal—and make sure the number is realistic. (We'll get into goal-setting in much more detail later in this chapter.)

2 Energy at a low ebb?
Have a snack—and get moving.
While people usually feel much better when losing weight, some people do experience periods of fatigue as well. When you take in fewer calories than you burn, you force your body to turn to the energy it has stored as fat. Falling short on calories can make you feel tired and even grumpy. There's another kind of fatigue: Some people begin to get tired of

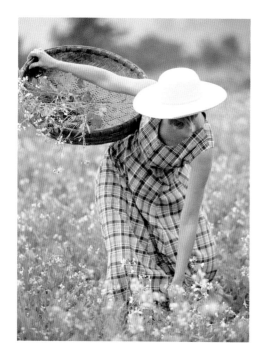

dieting. But you don't have to let an energy drain get in the way of your weight loss.

If you're feeling deep fatigue every day, talk to your doctor. But if you simply have occasional slumps and less energy than you used to, try eating smaller meals and then snack more frequently during the day. Save the piece of fruit from breakfast to eat at mid-morning, or hold off on the sliced vegetables you brought for lunch and have them as soon as you feel hungry in the afternoon. Eating more frequently can steady your blood sugar levels so you won't feel a slump when your energy supplies run low.

Another way to combat fatigue is to fit extra physical activity into your daily schedule. It seems paradoxical to be more active when you have less energy, but research shows that physical activity can actually make people feel more energetic, rather than less. Activity provides a psychological boost that can banish the blues. Getting up and moving also increases your self-confidence. And regular exercise increases stamina, so you'll build reserves of energy for more activity.

3 Need a shot of self-confidence?
Celebrate small victories.
It's easy to lose confidence if you're not reaching your goals and you're not sure why. There's always the temptation to blame yourself. You know how it goes: You tell yourself that

you just don't have the staying power or the willpower to lose weight.

Banish those negative thoughts. You haven't failed just because the pounds are proving more stubborn to shed than you expected. For the moment, focus on your successes.

Here's a trick that worked for many *ChangeOne* participants. Let's say you've managed to lose five pounds so far, which may not sound like a lot. The next time you're at the grocery store, grab a five-pound package of flour, potatoes, whatever. Carry it around the store as you shop. Getting heavy? That's the amount of excess weight you used to carry all the time. Five pounds on the scale may not seem like much; but when you tote it around in your arms and think of it as the fat you've lost, you'll begin to realize the big accomplishment you've achieved already.

Remember, too, that pounds aren't the only measure of success. Make a list of other benefits you've gained by following *ChangeOne*. Maybe your clothes feel a little more comfortable. Maybe you're moving around more easily. Maybe you're simply eating a healthier diet. Whatever your successes are, celebrate them. And remember, if you can make one change, you can make two. If you can make two changes, you can do three. You get the idea.

4 Struggling with a particular meal?
Twice is nice: Go back for seconds.
If you're pleased with your weight-loss progress so far, but you aren't following the *ChangeOne* menu for all your meals, don't worry. Some people find they need to make only one or two small changes—giving up their fast-food habit or switching to sugar-free beverages, for example—to start losing weight.

Pounds not coming off fast enough? Go back to the meal that's giving you trouble and take another week to master it. Set aside enough time so that you can follow that chapter's meal plans to the letter, at least for one week. Try a few suggestions you didn't try the first time around. When you're always too rushed to have breakfast, get everything for the meal ready the night before. If eating too many snacks during the day is your downfall, distract yourself for a few minutes with something other than food—a short walk, an errand, or a chore around the house.

5 Is dining out your downfall?
Zero in on portion control.
If your parents always praised you for being a member of the clean-plate club, you still may have trouble leaving food behind, especially when you've paid good money for it at a restaurant. With today's runaway portion sizes, dining out is a major challenge. Don't let the size of the serving plunked down in front of you determine how much you eat. Keep in mind the *ChangeOne* portion size visuals that we've been using—a baseball or a deck of cards, for example—to remind yourself what reasonable servings of food should look like. Ask the waiter to take away what you don't want and pack it for later. Pay attention to hunger and fullness cues, and eat slowly. For a refresher on navigating restaurants, look back to Week 5, "Dining Out," which begins on page 90.

6 Trouble planning ahead?
Make a list, check it twice.
Knowing where your next meal is coming from is critical to successful dieting. If you're having trouble planning ahead, try this: Set aside 15 minutes the night before or first thing in the morning to make a list of what you'll need to do that day to stick with *ChangeOne*. Your list might include a quick shopping trip to buy what you'll need for dinner, a reminder of when and where you plan to get some exercise during the day, or a note to make a lunch reservation at a restaurant where you know you'll be able to order a sensible meal. Or look for a frozen meal that meets the *ChangeOne* guidelines. Keep several in the freezer. If you're having trouble finding time to pack a lunch, choose a meal that's quicker and easier to prepare: for instance, a macaroni salad you can make in advance and even divide up into single-serving containers.

7 Famished?
Eat more often.
It's fine to be hungry just before your next meal. But if you're getting so famished that you're tempted to give up the whole idea of dieting, it's time for a reassessment. For starters, this week fill out a Hunger Profile form (you'll find it on page 340) for a few days. Keeping tabs on your appetite will zero in on when you typically feel the hungriest during

the day, and what you do about it. Next, begin helping yourself to a snack during those moments when you're feeling especially ravenous. Favor low-calorie, high-fiber snacks that will fill you up without putting you over your calorie target.

If you're still hungry after lunch or dinner, help yourself to an additional serving of vegetables. Keep an eye on your weight. If you continue to lose weight, even if it's a little more slowly than before, that's fine. You're more likely to stick to a diet that doesn't force you to go hungry. If your weight remains steady, that's fine, too. Consider attacking the other side of the calorie equation: Increase your activity level by adding 15 minutes of walking a day to what you already do. And keep in mind that many *ChangeOne* participants report feeling hungry at the beginning of the program. But very quickly their appetites adjusted to *ChangeOne* portion sizes, and they began to feel perfectly satisfied as the weeks progressed—so hang in there.

8 Caving in to cravings?
Forge a new association.

Food cravings aren't hunger pangs. When you're genuinely hungry, you want food, any food. Food cravings are usually for something special—chocolate, potato chips, pizza, whatever. Sometimes food cravings are part of emotional eating. You want chocolate because it makes you feel better when you're feeling low. Food cravings can also be reactions to environmental triggers. You want ice cream after dinner or buttery popcorn when you get to the movie theater simply because all the cues remind you of these foods.

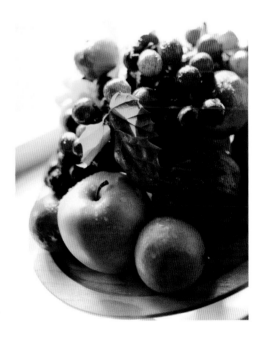

The solution is to teach an old dog a new trick by creating a different, healthier association. Instead of having dessert after dinner this week, get up from the table and go for a stroll. Instead of buttery popcorn at the movies, bring along a *ChangeOne* snack. It won't take long before you associate movie-going with a granola bar or a piece of fruit instead of popcorn. For more on food triggers, emotional eating, and environmental cues, look back to Week 6, "Weekends and Holidays," which begins on page 108.

9 Need a helping hand or a friendly word?
Ask for it.
When the going gets tough, the tough often call on friends and family. If you're not getting the support you need, take this week to explore ways to enlist help or encouragement. The best way to get what you need is by asking for it. Be specific about the kind of help you need. Ask if there's anything you can do in return. Need to cast a wider net? Be creative. If you're looking for an exercise partner, for instance, post a flyer at work or on a neighborhood bulletin board. Wishing you had an eating partner? Consider starting a *ChangeOne* dinner club.

And keep in mind that even though the support of people around you can smooth the way, making a lasting change is ultimately up to you. Even without the active support of family and friends, you can make it on your own.

10 Motivation in need of a tune-up?
Think back to the beginning.
Once the first flush of excitement is over, it can be tough to stay motivated on any diet. Now's the time to remind yourself why you wanted to lose weight in the first place. Write down your three top reasons for starting *ChangeOne*. Below that make a list of the benefits you've noticed so far. These may include the way you feel, the pounds you've managed to lose, the way your clothes fit, or the fact that you're getting more exercise than before. Assign each one a rating of one to three stars, depending on how important it is to you. Post your list somewhere where you'll see it every day (on the refrigerator door, for instance). By reminding yourself of the reasons you started *ChangeOne* and the benefits you've already gained, you'll add oomph to your motivation.

11 Feeling frazzled?
Find a way to let off steam this week.
Being on a diet can be stressful. Add to that the other strains and stresses in your life, and the combination can seem overwhelming. If stress is threatening to derail your efforts to eat a healthier diet, it's time to take action. Next week we'll zero in on ways to deal with stress in much more detail. For this week, think of one change you can make in your life

that will relieve some of the pressure. Ask someone to take on one of your responsibilities at home or the office. Rearrange your schedule to find time to relax. Experiment with different ways to let off steam. Listen to your favorite music, sit quietly and concentrate on your breathing, take up yoga, or go for a walk or a workout. And if exercise is your answer, take heart in the fact that it eases stress and burns extra calories in the bargain.

12 Surrounded by temptations?
Take control of your surroundings.
If your willpower is being tested every time you turn around, take charge of your environment. As we suggested in Week 7, put treats out of sight and make sure that calorie-efficient choices like fruits and vegetables are the centerpiece of your kitchen. At work, don't keep food around your desk or work area. If you find yourself in a situation where you can't remove the temptations, remove yourself—go for a walk, do an errand, or grab a *ChangeOne* snack. Remember, the less you have to rely on sheer willpower to avoid temptation, the more likely you are to reach your goals.

13 Eating all over the house?
Practice the one-room, one-chair rule.
If you eat in practically every room of the house, you're creating associations with food everywhere you go. You'll have no escape from the urge to splurge. Set aside one room and one chair for eating at home. This week make a pact with yourself to go to the designated spot for every meal and snack you eat at home.

14 Sitting on the sidelines?
Get in on the action.
You don't have to start running marathons—all you have to do is find time to walk. This week find a way to add at least 10 minutes of walking during the main part of the day— before breakfast, over the lunch hour, doing errands, or an evening stroll; your eventual goal should be 20 minutes a day. And as we've mentioned above, physical activity can also help you feel more energetic and less stressed.

Goal-Setting, Part II

Back in Week 4 of the *ChangeOne* program, we asked you to sign a goal-setting contract with yourself. It's time to take another look at your contract—pull it out and give it a read. Were you fair with yourself? It's all too easy to have unrealistic expectations when you decide to lose weight—especially when it's the first time you've tried it in earnest. Even people who have dieted in the past tend to set goals that are tough to reach. And when they don't reach them, they give up.

By now you're an expert on what it takes to lose weight. You also know what you're willing and able to do. This is the perfect time to take a clear-eyed, no-nonsense look at what you want to accomplish. In addition, by revisiting your goals and committing yourself to them anew, you'll take a big step toward staying motivated. To get this reevaluation started, fill in the "How Do You Spell Success?" quiz on the next page.

Don't Mistake Success for Failure

Almost anyone who sets out to lose weight on a diet can do it. The crazy thing about many dieters is that when they're doing well, they often don't realize it. *Seriously.* Many people who succeed end up thinking they've failed. That's because they get their minds wrapped around an unattainable goal and never see what they've achieved.

You may guess where we're going with the questions in "How Do You Spell Success?" Most people have several goals in mind when they decide to lose weight. A super ambitious goal is great if it jazzes you up at the start. But if it's too ambitious and you begin to think you'll never reach it, you can begin to feel frustrated, then disillusioned. You may actually succeed in losing a lot of weight and getting all the good stuff that goes with it, but if you didn't reach the mammoth goal, you may consider the diet a failure. Then you might give up, go back to your old patterns of eating, and gain back all the weight you lost.

To test the reality of the typical dieter's expectations, researchers at the weight-loss clinic of the University of Pennsylvania carried out a clever experiment. They asked a group of women at the start of a diet program to describe four different goals.

Change One quiz
How Do You Spell Success?

1. How much did you weigh when you began the *ChangeOne* plan? _____

2. What is your dream weight? _____

3. Let's say you can't reach your dream weight; what's the most you can end up weighing and still be happy with the results? _____

4. If you can't reach that "happy" weight, what weight would you describe as acceptable? _____

5. Let's say that you lose weight, but still don't reach your "acceptable" weight; what ending weight would leave you feeling disappointed? _____

6. Look again at your "dream" weight; what is the number based on?
- ❏ The lowest my weight has been as an adult
- ❏ My ideal weight given my height
- ❏ What I weighed in high school or college
- ❏ The lowest weight I've been able to reach on a diet
- ❏ A healthy weight for me according to my doctor
- ❏ Other _____

7. Numbers on a scale aren't the only way to measure the success of a diet. Besides weight, what other measures are important to you? On a scale of 1 to 5— not important to very important—rate the following items:

Smaller dress or pants size	1 2 3 4 5
How my clothes feel	1 2 3 4 5
How I feel (slimmer, more energetic, more attractive)	1 2 3 4 5
Specific health measures (blood pressure, for example)	1 2 3 4 5
Overall sense of health	1 2 3 4 5

8. If dress or pants size is an important measure of success for you, what goal do you have in mind?
Dress size: _____
Waist size: _____

9. What else do you hope to achieve by dieting? On a scale of 1 to 5—not important to very important—rate the following motivation:

Feeling more self-confident	1 2 3 4 5
Feeling sexier or more attractive	1 2 3 4 5
Being happier about myself and how I look	1 2 3 4 5
Feeling more in control	1 2 3 4 5
Not being embarrassed by my weight	1 2 3 4 5
Feeling fitter	1 2 3 4 5

Score

Congratulations! You got every question correct. There are no wrong answers to the questions we just asked; they are too personal for that. But your answers do say a lot about your expectations. For insights on your comments and some thoughts about whether you are being fair to yourself, read on.

The categories will sound familiar. We borrowed them for the quiz you just completed. The researchers asked the women in the program to specify:

- Their dream weight: The amount they would like to weigh if they could choose their ideal number.
- Their happy weight: A number on the scale that, even if it wasn't perfect, would make them happy.
- Their acceptable weight: The number that they would be

Weight-Loss Goals: Myth vs. Reality

Myth 1: Your ideal weight is what you weighed when you were first married (or graduated from college, or before you had children).

If you're hoping to get back to what you weighed a few years ago, fine. There's a chance you really might get close to that weight again. But if we're talking 15 or 20 years ago, you might want to reconsider. Many people put on weight as they get older. And no matter how hard they try, they have a tough time being as active as they might have been in their early 20s. Don't live in the past. Set a weight-loss goal that's appropriate for the way you live now.

Myth 2: Your ideal weight is the number listed on a standard height-and-weight chart.

Yes, height and weight are often related. Taller people weigh more than shorter ones, all things being equal. But many other factors play a role in determining your weight. For example, your body type: big-boned and solid, small-boned and light, or in between. Your metabolism: whether you naturally burn brightly and move a lot, or take things more slowly. There are other factors as well, like the number of fat cells you have, or how much your parents and other relatives weigh. The numbers listed on a standard height-and-weight chart are just approximations.

Don't let them determine if you've succeeded or failed.

Myth 3: Your ideal weight is the lowest weight you've been able to get to on past diets.

Okay, so you've lost that much before. But the fact that you're dieting again says you gained at least some, or perhaps all, of it back again. If you set a weight-loss goal that's too low to maintain, you'll get caught in yo-yo dieting—losing weight, gaining it back, and trying to lose it again. The best goal is one you can live with.

Myth 4: The less you weigh, the healthier you'll be.

Not true. In fact, many studies show that if you're overweight, losing just 5 percent to 10 percent of your current weight is all you have to do to get the bulk of the health benefits associated with weight loss: lower risks of heart disease, stroke, diabetes, and even some forms of cancer.

Myth 5: If you don't hit your dream weight, you'll never be happy.

You don't believe that, do you? A number is just a number. And if it's a number that leaves you frustrated and stuck in an endless cycle of losing and gaining weight, it's time to replace that number with a more reasonable one.

willing to accept if they couldn't reach either their happy weight or dream weight.

- Their disappointed weight: A number that, even though it was less than what they currently weighed, would leave them feeling disappointed.

The women in the experiment had high hopes. They began the program weighing an average of 218 pounds. Their average "dream weight" goal was 149—a 69-pound loss. Short of that, the women said they'd be happy at an average of 155 pounds. If all else failed, they'd accept a final weight of 163 pounds. And they'd be disappointed if they ended the diet at a weight of 181, an average loss of 37 pounds.

How did they do? The women in the six-month program lost an average of 16 percent of their starting weight, or 35 pounds. Most experts would call that a strong success. The average weight loss at that point in a successful diet program is around 10 percent to 15 percent.

Though the researchers were thrilled, the women were not. On average they had fallen just short of the bottom target—their "disappointed weight"—which would have required them to lose 17 percent of their starting weight. Even the number they described as merely acceptable represented a 25 percent drop. Their dream weight required a 32 percent weight loss, more than double what experts deem a success.

Think about it. These women did great. They lost a significant amount of weight. But without a realistic goal to measure their progress, most of them were likely to consider the diet a failure. That's just crazy.

Divide Big Goals into Milestones

"Uh-oh," you're probably thinking just about now. "So this is where they tell me I can't lose as many pounds as I'd like."

Not for a second. All we want to do is urge you to make sure your first goals are realistic. Especially when you have a lot of weight you'd like to lose, it's helpful to think in terms of gradual milestones, rather than the ultimate weight you want to be. Once you reach your first milestone, you can celebrate your success, take a deep breath, and head on to the next one. The milestone approach helps you gain confidence along the way. It also makes it easy to measure your progress step by step, rather than in a single leap. And that's really what *ChangeOne* is all about.

What's a reasonable first milestone? Many experts say you should first set your sights on losing about 10 percent of your starting weight. To calculate 10 percent, take your weight when you started *ChangeOne* and knock the last number off. If you weighed 222, for instance, 10 percent is about 22 pounds.

Once you reach your first milestone, allow yourself a few weeks to savor the new, slimmer you and to consolidate the changes you've made. Take the time to enjoy all of the other benefits you're likely to experience, from the way you look in the mirror to the way your clothes fit. Then, when you're ready, set the next milestone for weight loss. For many people, weight loss slows as they shed pounds. That's perfectly natural. To avoid becoming discouraged, we recommend setting subsequent milestones at about 5 percent of your starting weight—11 pounds if you started out at 222, for instance.

A Contract with Yourself

Okay, now let's take another look at the *ChangeOne* Contract we asked you to sign at the end of Week 4. Now that you have more experience under your belt—which has moved up a notch or two, we hope—take a look back at your contract. How are you doing? Do the goals you set back then still seem reasonable? Are they the goals that matter most to you?

Write up a revised contract if your earlier goals aren't working for you. This is a contract with yourself, after all. You're doing what you're doing—eating better, being more active, and losing weight—for your own sake, nobody else's. You decide the goals that mean the most and work the best for you. By putting them in writing, you'll be able to keep them in mind—and gauge your progress along the way.

Change One success stories

Looking Good, Feeling Healthy

Concerned about future weight-related health problems, Scott Montgomery had wanted to lose weight for a long time, but he just didn't know how to get started. After reading about *ChangeOne*, he was instantly intrigued and wanted to give it a try.

"It's a very sensible approach to dieting," he says. "So many diets require you to change your eating habits overnight, which is very tough to do. It's a slow change, which is important."

Scott began noticing results immediately. So far, he's lost 70 pounds on *ChangeOne*. "Before, I wore 42-waist pants. Now I wear a 36 and can almost fit into a 34."

He has also made some remarkable health improvements. "I have a lot more energy!" he says. "My blood pressure and cholesterol levels are down. I don't breathe hard when I work out."

Portraits taken just one year apart show how losing 70 pounds had a dramatic effect on Scott Montgomery's appearance.

Scott has enjoyed experimenting with the many different meal and recipe options from *ChangeOne*. He found that eating a healthy breakfast was one of the most important changes he made. "I never ate breakfast, but I never miss it now," he says. "It's important to jump-start your metabolism in the morning."

Exercise has also made a big difference. "Working out helped me drop the weight a lot faster," he says. "But make sure that it's something you enjoy doing and that it burns calories." He also kept track of what he ate, which helped him avoid going off the plan during the day.

Scott is enjoying his healthy life and appreciates the compliments from people who notice his positive changes. "People who haven't seen me for a while just stop and stare," he says. "I have more pride in my appearance."

For more ChangeOne *success stories, go to www.changeone.com/successstories*

Stress Relief

All we're asking you to do this week is relax. That's right, relax. Take a moment or two to shake off the stresses and strains of daily life.

Sound easy? If only it were so. Life can be so hectic these days that taking even a minute off from the pressures of work and family seems impossible. While achieving a stress-free life is unlikely, you can definitely loosen the hold that tension and anxiety often have on you.

That's important, especially when you're trying to lose weight. A rocky period at work or friction at home has knocked many dieters off their program. Stress can rob you of the energy you need to stay focused and motivated. If the pressure gets fierce enough, you may be tempted to say, "Forget it, I just can't do it," and give up your best intentions to stick to a healthier diet.

This week you'll identify the different sources of stress in your life and try out techniques to manage or even eliminate them.

Take the Pressure Off

Like a lot of people, you may find yourself reaching for food when demands get to be too much. That's hardly surprising. Just the act of eating can make you feel better when your nerves are frayed or you're feeling down. Recent studies have shown that eating—especially eating something high in carbo-hydrates—can lower your level of stress hormones and make you feel less frazzled.

In fact, you may feel better after eating because that's exactly what your body was signaling you to do: eat something. Stress itself can trigger hunger, scientists are learning. Here's how it works. Say you're on your way to a very important meeting. You're already running a little late when traffic comes to a sudden halt ahead of you. Instinctively, your body readies itself to do something to deal with the problem. Your brain signals your adrenal glands to churn out a variety of hormones, including the stress hormone cortisol. One of cortisol's jobs is to trigger the release of glucose and fatty acids, in case your muscles need energy.

Back in our hunter-gatherer days, this system made sense. Stress didn't take the form of traffic jams; instead, it was usually a real physical threat—a charging animal perhaps. A fight-or-flight stress response evolved to prepare us within seconds to do battle or run away. These days the challenges we face aren't as straightforward as that. Sure, you might be tempted to stop the car, get out, and run the rest of the way to your very important meeting. If you did, you'd burn off the energy your body had made available. But chances are you sit there and smolder until traffic begins to move again. Afterward, the result of your surge in cortisol is an increase in appetite—your body's way of guaranteeing that you'll replace the energy it released in the form of glucose and fatty acids.

Check-In

At about this point in *ChangeOne*, you're probably having an easier time with some of the changes you've undertaken than with others. No surprise there. Last week you may even have targeted the part that's giving you the toughest time. That's great. But if you get so frustrated that you begin to wonder if it's worth the trouble, ease off. Focus on changes that feel more doable right now. If fitting in activity every day just isn't in the cards, don't worry. Concentrate instead on reining in portions. If paying attention to hunger cues has made a big difference for you, put your energy there and don't worry that you're missing breakfast now and then. Go with your strengths. Target the changes that offer the biggest payoff and concentrate on turning them into easy habits. Go easy on yourself.

A flood of these hormones wouldn't pose much of a problem if it happened only now and then. But a steady tide of tense situations can keep cortisol levels high all day, making you feel hungry almost all the time. As if that's not bad enough, cortisol also triggers enzymes that activate fat cells, priming them to store energy as fat. The most susceptible fat cells are those around your middle, which are particularly sensitive to the effects of cortisol.

You see the problem. Stress makes you hungry. Eating makes you feel better. Stress promotes fat. And you put on weight instead of taking it off. Watching your efforts to lose weight fail can then create even more pressure and tension.

Now is the time to make sure you don't get caught in the spiral of stress and eating.

If stress is getting the better of you, remember that everyone's life has its hassles, small and large. One major difference between people who succeed and those who don't, psychologists say, is how they deal with everyday tribulations.

To see how well you handle stress, take a few minutes to fill out the test on the next page. Your answers will help you analyze how you cope with the challenges of daily life.

Step One:

Solve Problems That *Can* Be Solved

The most direct way to deal with stress is to eliminate the situations that wear you down. Yes, that's easier said than done, but the more irritations and annoyances you can unload, the easier it is to tackle the big issues. You may find there are plenty of petty aggravations you can fix quickly once you start paying attention to them. Every time you feel yourself getting hot, stop and see if you can find a solution. If you find yourself shrieking because you can never seem to find the car keys or your glasses, for instance, establish a place where you put the keys, glasses, cell phone, or whatever, each time you

Help!

"I feel jittery and short-tempered much of the day. I thought it might be too much caffeine—but I have only a couple of cups of coffee in the morning, that's it. What's going on?"

Watch the caffeine you're getting from sources other than coffee. Caffeine is a stimulant, and in some people, it can aggravate stress. Besides coffee, there's also caffeine in teas, colas, chocolate, and some pain relievers. The best way to know if too much caffeine is a problem is to ease back on the amount you consume, but don't go cold-turkey. Caffeine withdrawal can cause headaches and may make you feel even more jittery and short-fused. A better way is to begin mixing regular coffee with decaffeinated coffee. Over a few weeks, gradually add more decaf and less of the high-octane brew. Then, if you decide to give up coffee altogether, you'll have an easier time.

Change One quiz
Stress Test

Read each statement below and check those that apply to you right now:

○ A lot of things in my life seem to be out of control right now.

△ I have several good friends I can call if I need to talk something through.

○ When I'm feeling frazzled, I often have the urge to eat.

△ I'm feeling pretty good about my life right now.

○ I often feel overwhelmed with the thought of everything that has to get done during the day.

△ I feel better once I've made a list of what I have to do.

○ Trying to lose weight has definitely added to the pressures I feel.

○ It's really been frustrating for me to try to find time to be more active.

△ Taking control of my diet has made me feel better about myself.

○ Sometimes I resent all the responsibilities I have.

△ I'm pretty good at taking problems in stride.

○ Lately I notice myself losing my temper when even little things go wrong.

△ Even when things get a little crazy, I still feel as if I'm in control of what's going on in my life.

○ If someone puts me on hold while we're talking and then doesn't come back on the line soon, it really makes me mad—mad enough to hang up sometimes.

○ I don't have much patience for people who make mistakes.

△ Even though my life is pretty crowded, I'm good at keeping my priorities straight.

△ I don't worry much about things I can't control.

○ When I'm under a lot of pressure, I sometimes find myself running in three different directions at once.

○ I frequently wake up in the night feeling anxious about my life.

△ No matter how hectic the day has been, it's easy for me to relax and unwind once I get home.

○ I wish I had more control over what happens in my life.

△ Exercise is a good way for me to let off steam.

○ Social situations often make me nervous.

△ Frankly, I don't tend to sweat the little things—I figure they'll take care of themselves.

Score

What your score means:

How many of each color did you check? If you tallied more blue triangles than red circles, your responses indicate that you've got the pressures of everyday life well in hand. But if the red outnumber the blue, it could spell trouble—stress is hurting your life. If the numbers are about equal—and even if the blue slightly outnumber the red—be aware that a bad day could send you into the red zone. Whatever your score, there are plenty of effective ways to keep cool, calm, and collected. Just read on.

put them down. Post a reminder on the door, if you have to, until you get into the habit.

If getting dinner together makes your blood pressure rise because half the time you don't have what you need on hand, take time on Sunday to stock the pantry for the week. Make double batches of storable dishes to cut your cooking time significantly.

Not all problems are that simple to eliminate, of course. Let's say your boss gives you more work than you can manage. On top of that, you haven't been given the authority you need to do the job. That's a classic high-stress dilemma. What to do about it? The direct solution is to talk to the boss and explain the problem. Frame the talk not as a complaint ("You're overworking me") but as a search for solutions ("It would help me a lot if we could decide on priorities, and if I had your support for making a few key decisions").

Or say your problems are at home—tension in your marriage, for instance, or trouble with one of the children. Talking it through with the person closest to you might help you get to the source of the pressure and relieve it. Yes, it can be hard to ask for help—but it gets easier when you first ask yourself, "What am I getting out of letting things go on the way they are?" You might explain to your spouse or kids why reducing tension in the household is so important to you now: You're trying to make changes that will make your life better. If the problems are more complicated than the family can handle alone, consider enlisting the help of a counselor.

Only you can know which problems you can confront directly and which you may have to learn to live with. Certainly, there are going to be irritations—and worse—that you can't eliminate, at least at the moment. But you can accept them without being overwhelmed by them—and without letting them derail your diet.

Step Two:
Accept the Things You Can't Change

There are people who can shrug off almost any setback. Others get frazzled when even the smallest things don't go right. In either case, the demands may be the same. The difference is in the individual responses. Psychologists don't understand all the reasons why people react so differently to stress. Having a sense of humor seems to help many people. Being able to distract yourself is an added plus. Just having something you really enjoy doing offers a time-out from the pressures of life. Playing a musical instrument, reading a good book, helping out at a local soup kitchen—all of these can take your mind off problems and give you a much-needed vacation from fretting.

Naturally, you can't completely change your personality. But experts say you can change the way you react to hassles and frustrations. On the following pages, we offer seven ways to cool down when your temper flares or the problems in your life feel overwhelming. This week try out several of them. If one doesn't seem to work for you, move on to another. Your goal: to have at least two stress-busting techniques you can turn to when the pressure builds and your nerves begin to feel frazzled. Knowing how to relax and let off steam will help you stay focused and motivated.

Pressure Cookers

For people who compulsively reach for food when tensions reach the boiling point, the simplest solution is the ultimate in common sense: Get away from food. If there are problems at home, don't deal with them in the kitchen. Go to another room of the house to hash them out, and don't take food with you. Under tons of pressure at work? Keep snacks out of easy reach. This week remember our rule: Don't eat to relax. Try one of these techniques first. Then wait 5 or 10 minutes to see if you're still hungry. If so, dig in.

1 **Run away!**
One of the most effective ways to defuse stress is to run away from it—or at least walk briskly. In a 1998 study that asked 38 men and 35 women to keep diaries of activity, mood, and stress, volunteers reported that they felt less anxious on days when they were physically active than on days when they didn't exercise. Even when stressful events occurred, people in the study said they felt less troubled on their physically active days.

Why? Exercise acts as an antidote to life's pressures in several ways. First, it is a simple distraction from problems. Second, it may change the chemistry of stress, blunting the effects of hormones like cortisol. Exercise has also been shown to ease the symptoms of moderate depression. That in turn may help people deal better with daily hassles and aggravations. And then there's the fact that exercise burns calories, an added bonus for dieters. Physical activity makes it easier not only to lose weight but to keep calories in balance once you go off your diet, and that's enough to make anyone feel good.

Virtually any kind of physical activity seems to relieve the effects of stress, although some researchers think that activities that involve repetitive movements—walking, running, cycling, or swimming, for instance—may offer the best defense. Many people consider swimming to be one of the most relaxing exercises, a soothing way to literally go with the flow. Repeating a physical movement over and over again somehow seems to ease mind and body.

Think about some ways to make your workout even more relaxing. If you're a walker, be aware of the way your arms swing from front to back and the rhythm of your gait. Repeat a soothing word or phrase each time you exhale.

If you work out on an exercise cycle or stair machine at a fitness club, you might find yourself parked in front of a bank of television sets. Watching TV can prevent you from getting into the soothing rhythm of your workout. Scientists have found that watching television makes people more jittery, not less. So ignore what's on the screen. Concentrate instead on your breathing and the repetitive movement of your arms and

An Ancient Cure for Frayed Nerves

Looking for a simple way to relax, refresh your energy, become more limber, and strengthen muscles at the same time? Yoga may be just the ticket. Exercise scientists have long known that yoga offers a great way to stretch, increase strength, and improve balance. Now psychologists are discovering it can also ease a troubled mind.

When researchers at the University of Wurzburg in Germany tested 12 women before, during, and after a 60-minute yoga class, they found that the women's heart rates dropped dramatically during the routines. The women also reported feeling less irritable than they did before the class.

Another recent study showed that yoga may well be one of the best stress-easers

around. At Oxford University, a psychologist divided 71 men and women into three groups. One group practiced simple relaxation techniques like deep breathing. The second visualized themselves feeling less tense. The third did a half-hour yoga routine. The relaxers and the visualizers felt sluggish afterward. The people in the yoga group reported feeling more energetic and emotionally content after their class.

How to get started? Several of the stretches you'll find in the Get Stronger chapter are based on yoga positions. If you find that you like doing these stretches, you may want to sign up for a yoga class. Many fitness centers or yoga studios offer them. You'll also find helpful guides in yoga videos or instruction books.

legs. If the gym plays music that gets on your nerves, bring a personal stereo with earphones and your own favorite music, or use noise-blocking earplugs and enjoy a quiet interlude.

2 Do one thing at a time.

Chances are you've heard of Type A behavior—the hard-driven, competitive, take-no-prisoners personality profile once thought to be linked not only to high levels of stress but to greater risk of heart disease. The original term for Type A behavior was the "Hurry Syndrome," because Type A's tend to do everything faster than more relaxed personality types. Type A's feel so rushed, in fact, that they often try to do three things at once. They're the ones you see eating lunch, talking on their cell phones, and driving—all at the same time.

If you find yourself falling into this behavior, make an effort this week to focus on the task at hand. Instead of balancing your checkbook while you're talking on the phone, give the phone call your attention, then return to the checkbook. If you're constantly being interrupted with phone calls while you're trying to work on something, let the answering machine take messages. Call people back when the time is right for you.

In short, do one thing at a time, and you may feel your stress meter begin to tick down.

3 Put out the fire.

Anger can be stressful, especially the "hot-headed" kind that lashes out and doesn't solve the problem that ignited it. But never expressing your anger can be harmful as well.

If you feel your temper about to flare, stop, take a deep breath, and ask yourself three quick questions suggested by Redford Williams, a Duke University researcher who pioneered work in anger control:

Is this really important to me? If the answer is no, leave what sparked your anger behind. If the answer is yes, then ask yourself:

Am I justified in being angry in this situation? Argue the pros and cons, as if you had to make your case in court. If your answer is, "No, I don't really have much to gripe about," you're likely to feel your anger and stress begin to melt away. Of course the answer may be, "Yes, that guy nearly ran me off the road, and he's so busy talking on his cell phone he didn't even notice it!" If so, then ask yourself just one more question:

Is there anything I can really do about it? Honking like crazy isn't going to change anything. It's only likely to make you angrier. So in the case of our driver, the best response is to let it go, take a deep breath, and keep out of the guy's way.

But if your answer to the last question is another yes, then you're in luck. You have the chance to make a real change for the better. Let's say you're angry because one of the kids keeps leaving junk food lying around in the kitchen when you've specifically asked him or her to put it away. Lay down the law. Explain why you don't want junk food lying around. Get mad if you have to, but then let your anger go. If you have trouble doing that, ask yourself the first question again, but with a little twist: "What do I get out of staying angry?" Chances are the answer is "not much," except unpleasant aggravation.

4 Call a friend.
Sure, it sounds a little sappy. But talking to someone else—even just calling someone to say a quick hello—does more than take your mind off your troubles. Swedish researchers recently reported that people with a strong sense of social connection to other people were almost one-third less likely to die after they'd had a heart attack than those who were socially isolated. Part of the reason, the researchers believe, may be the stress-easing effect of close relationships. If you don't have a circle of friends you feel like you can turn to, consider beginning to build one by volunteering for a local charity, joining a club or a church group, or signing up for an exercise class.

5 Talk to yourself.
Sometimes we're our own worst enemies. Instead of easing our pressures, we add to them by thinking in terms of absolutes, using words like "never," "should," or "always." "I should never have done that." "Things always go wrong for me." "I'll never be able to lose weight at this rate." If that sounds like you, be alert to moments when you're being unreasonably hard on yourself and try to lighten up. Counter the negative messages with a steady dose of positive ones.

Don't be embarrassed to say them out loud if you're alone. "Whoa. Easy there. Give it a rest." Replace the harsh absolute

ChangeOne success stories
Dieting Made Easy

With all the success Chris Bellinger has had with *ChangeOne*, she wishes she could take credit for finding the diet. But it was her husband, Bob, who first discovered it.

"He thought the *ChangeOne* diet sounded more like a lifestyle change than just a temporary regimen," she says. "I told him I would give it a try."

As soon as she started, Chris knew *ChangeOne* was different from other diets she had tried. "With other diets, I failed with all of them sooner or later because, even when I lost weight, I inevitably gained it back," she says. "*ChangeOne* is easy to follow and easy to stay with."

Eighteen months after starting *ChangeOne*, Chris is thrilled with her results and knows that this time she will maintain her weight loss. So far, she's lost 140 pounds and lots of inches.

"Before I started, my measurements were bust 54, waist 47, and hips 58. I remember thinking that if I didn't stop gaining, my hips would be the same measurement as my height—I'm 62 inches tall. Today, my measurements are 39, 30, 39!"

Chris's progress has not been only on the scale. Her health has dramatically improved. In fact, her blood pressure has decreased so much that her doctor has taken her off the medication she was using to control it.

There have been other gratifying benefits that she hadn't actually considered, including "fitting into theater seats com-

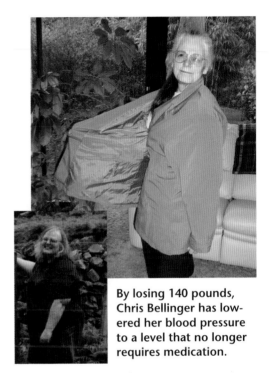

By losing 140 pounds, Chris Bellinger has lowered her blood pressure to a level that no longer requires medication.

fortably, walking up a flight of stairs and not feeling out of breath, going into almost any women's clothing store and being able to try on clothes. Most of all, having more energy—I hadn't appreciated how much effort it takes to carry extra weight around."

And Chris hasn't been alone in her weight-loss journey. Her husband, who followed the diet with her, has lost 45 pounds, and his cholesterol is now in the normal range for the first time in years.

"I am convinced that *ChangeOne* is a permanent lifestyle change rather than temporary weight loss," she says.

For more ChangeOne *success stories, go to www.changeone.com/successstories*

with a more reasonable and forgiving thought: "So it's going to take awhile to lose the weight. So what? No one's pushing me but myself. I'm doing fine." Take the broad view. Things don't always go wrong for you, after all.

The truth is, things occasionally go wrong for everyone. And when they do, everyone has the same challenge: to sort things out and get on with life.

6 Laugh It Off

Laughter actually can be strong medicine, researchers say. The act of laughing eases muscle tension, relieves stress, and has even been shown to lower the risk of stress-related illnesses such as heart disease.

In a study published in 2001, the Center for Preventive Cardiology at the University of Maryland Medical Center

It's a fact: Laughter is measurably good for your health.

tested 300 volunteers for their propensity to laugh at everyday events. Those with a ready laugh were less likely to have heart problems than those who rarely broke a smile, the scientists found. Even among people with elevated blood pressure or cholesterol, the ability to laugh offered protection against heart attacks.

Now it's not always easy to laugh when things go wrong. But if you need a good chortle, try renting a favorite movie comedy, watching your favorite sitcom, or keeping a humorous book handy. Cartoon collections—*Doonesbury,* say, or *The Far Side*—offer plenty of laughs. If you frequently fume in rush-hour traffic, try renting or buying an audio book.

7 Practice Relaxation

Another proven way to ease stress is what Harvard University cardiologist Herbert Benson calls the relaxation response. According to Benson's studies, the method taps an innate mechanism that can be used to counteract the human fight-or-flight response that triggers stress. His research shows that the relaxation technique can lower blood pressure and ease muscle tension. Benson suggests setting aside 20 minutes and following these six simple steps:

- Find a quiet place where you won't be disturbed. Sit in a comfortable position, one that allows you to relax your body. Close your eyes.
- Starting with your feet and moving up, relax each of your muscle groups. End with the muscles of your face. Take a

moment to experience the feeling of being relaxed.

- With your eyes still closed, breathe in and out through your nose, concentrating on each breath.
- As you exhale, begin to silently repeat a short phrase or single word, such as "peace," "calmness," or "easy does it." Choose a word that helps you focus your mind and banish distracting thoughts.
- Continue repeating your soothing word or phrase and concentrating on breathing. The experts usually recommend doing this exercise for 10 to 15 minutes. Don't set an alarm, though, or you'll constantly be thinking about it. Have a watch or clock handy and open your eyes now and then to check the time. And don't be discouraged from doing the relaxation routine if you don't have a full 15 minutes. Even a few minutes will help.
- Sit quietly for a few more minutes, first with your eyes closed and then with them open. Savor the way your body and mind feel.

Sound easy? In fact, most of us have a hard time letting our minds go quiet and our bodies relax. You may need to practice relaxing a few times before you master the art. But with some practice, you'll find that you can slip quickly into relaxation and away from stress.

Making the Change

Choose at least three of the strategies in this chapter and try them this week. You probably already have an intuitive sense of which ones are best suited to your temperament. But don't be afraid to try at least one that sounds a little far out. You may be surprised at how effective it can be.

Whatever you choose, don't put added pressure on yourself by thinking you have to squeeze yet one more change into an already crowded schedule. Most of these stress-busting techniques take no time at all. Even those that do, like practicing the relaxation response or exercising, are well worth the extra time. By taking a few minutes to relax, you may find that you're more focused and productive when you get back to work. Certainly, you'll feel calmer. And that's a change that will help you stay in charge of your diet and your life.

Superfoods

Yes, we know what we told you: On *ChangeOne,* you get to eat the foods you want—and we're not backing off from that promise! But we have a feeling that after reading the next few pages, you'll be eager to put these weight-loss superfoods on the menu.

Thanks to two decades of research, we now know that many delicious foods have an uncanny talent for helping people lose weight. The *real* weight-loss superfoods? Grilled salmon. Nuts. Fast-food chicken. (No kidding!) Crunchy salads and hearty soups. A bowl of cereal with fresh fruit. And that's just a sampling.

So this week, you'll enjoy adding a *ChangeOne* superfood to at least one meal each day.

Over time, you'll learn how to make them your *automatic* choices when you are hungry, stressed out, pressed for time, or find yourself in a situation that could encourage overeating.

Change One quiz

What's Your Superfood IQ?

We've studied the research, consulted the experts, and come up with 10 foods that have the most significant weight-loss benefits. They're not always what you might think, so see if you can identify our superfood picks in this rather challenging quiz.

1. For weight loss and health, research shows that the best drink to have frequently is:

a. Milk   b. Fruit juice
c. Water   d. Coffee

2. Which of the following breakfast foods was proven in a recent study to keep dieters feeling fuller longer?

a. Eggs   b. Wheat toast
c. Oatmeal   d. Cornflakes

3. Which snack helped dieters who ate it daily lose 18 percent more weight than those who skipped it?

a. Pretzels   b. Chocolate
c. Almonds   d. Popsicles

4. A recent study showed that starting lunch with this item reduced calorie consumption at the meal by an average of 100 calories. Which item is it?

a. A bowl of soup   b. A glass of water
c. A piece of fruit   d. A garden salad

5. Another study showed that dieters who ate this food four or more times a week ended up losing more weight than those who didn't eat it. Which food is it?

a. Soup   b. Shrimp
c. Chocolate   d. An apple

6. Yet another study showed that women who frequently consumed this common breakfast food weighed 9 pounds less on average than those who generally didn't eat it. Which is it?

a. Grapefruit   b. Orange juice
c. A banana   d. Cereal

7. Which of the following common entrée choices has the fewest calories per ounce?

a. Shrimp   b. Lean pork
c. Chicken breast   d. Salmon

8. Which of these protein superstars is so versatile that it plays a starring role in *every* popular weight-loss plan?

a. Tofu   b. Pinto Beans
c. Chicken   d. Lean beef

9. This low-calorie food is eaten for breakfast and dessert; added to sauces, dips, and spreads; and even mixed into drinks. Plus, it contains nutrients that may speed up weight loss. Which is it?

a. Ricotta cheese   b. Yogurt
c. Peanut butter   d. Apricot jam

10. In the USDA's list of the 20 foods that have the most fiber per ounce, 15 are in the same category. What is this superfiber food family?

a. Cereals   b. Squashes
c. Beans   d. Root vegetables

Score

Welcome to the *ChangeOne* superfoods list! Each of the questions above corresponds to the superfood of the same number on the following pages. Be prepared for some surprises!

Food to the Rescue

Our superfood all-stars are a lot like superheroes: Each has a unique power. In this case, those powers help you lose pounds and keep them off. Some superfoods trick your tummy into telling your brain that you're already full. Others are rich and satisfying to eat, yet their calories don't seem to end up as fat on your hips. Some reset your appetite so you'll want to eat less at your next meal without even thinking about it. Others fine-tune your metabolism so your body burns calories effectively throughout the day.

To earn their places on our exclusive list, though, these edibles had to do even more. Each offers special health benefits, such as protecting against heart attack and diabetes, boosting immunity, lifting your energy level, or guarding your vision, for example. In summary, here's what we looked for.

- **Easier weight loss.** We scoured medical research to find out if any foods can truly help you lose more weight. Sure, there are lots of products that claim to melt pounds, but could any healthy foods make the same claim? What we found surprised us: A snack food long seen as decadent—nuts—actually seems to help people shed pounds. Nuts don't melt fat, of course, but they may help by making you feel so full that you simply eat less later on. Their tough cell walls may also block fat absorption, researchers suspect.
- **More satisfaction.** Nothing torpedoes a new weight-loss plan quicker than cravings. You know how that goes: You eat a Spartan breakfast and a sensible lunch, and at 3 P.M. your body seems to propel you, as if in a dream, to the cafeteria for a doughnut and a soda. That's the power of a craving—most often triggered by a slump in blood sugar. We've found the foods that keep blood sugar low and steady—thanks to fiber and protein—freeing you from the roller coaster of up-and-down blood sugar levels and a surge of food cravings.
- **Better metabolic burn.** Lots of research suggests that some foods, such as green tea and hot red pepper, turn up your body's fat-burning ability, but those effects are small or short-lived. We've found something better: low-glycemic eating. Low-glycemic foods not only keep blood

sugar low, they also keep your metabolism higher while you're on a weight-loss program, according to amazing research from Children's Hospital in Boston. You can actually burn 80 calories more each day when you eat these foods as compared with eating a typical low-fat diet. The result: more weight loss, fewer cravings, and more energy.

- **Easier calorie reduction.** We also wanted to help you eliminate unnecessary calories from your daily eating plan without sacrificing pleasure or nutrition. We found the ultimate weapons—a first-course strategy proven to cut mealtime calories and an age-old beverage that could save you hundreds of calories a day. And, we promise, there's no need to ever feel hungry.

Ready to dive in? For each of our fabulous 10, you'll discover their full range of benefits, some ideas for getting more into your diet, and guidelines on how much to eat for optimal effect.

SUPER FOOD Water

Good old H_2O has all the right stuff: zero calories, low cost, and convenience (just turn on the tap or grab the bottled version, available virtually everywhere). Sipping this precious fluid instead of one soft drink per day can save you a whopping 1,400 calories in a week—and could help you lose 21 pounds in a year, say nutrition experts from the University of North Carolina.

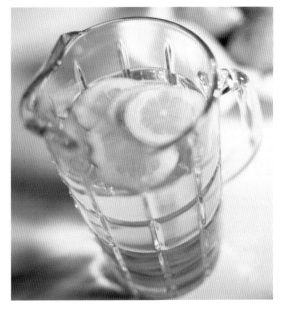

That's why water is the official *ChangeOne* beverage—we recommend it as your drink of choice at meals and between meals, too. (Read on for ways to add flavor without adding sugar and calories.)

What about recent reports that Americans are overly worried about water and dehydration? Well, sure, you don't see people falling over in the streets from thirst, but that's a silly way to look at it, isn't it? The truth is, only a third of us are getting enough for optimal health and weight. And while foods, especially fruits and veggies, do contribute to your daily fluid quota (as do tea and coffee), nothing keeps you hydrated as well as a refreshing, cool glass of water. Unfortunately, though, we need to explode two myths right now: Water *won't* flush fat out of your fat cells, and it *won't* raise your metabolism enough to burn significant calories, even if it's icy cold.

Hold the Salt

Carbonated water goes by many names, including club soda, seltzer, soda water, and effervescent water. While the names are often used interchangeably, the drinks aren't all the same. In particular, some types of carbonated water have salt added to them. Check the bottle's label and skip those! Too much salt in your diet can cause several health problems, including high blood pressure.

Water's real weight-loss power? Keeping you hydrated, which can help you avoid overeating caused by "stealth thirst"—unrecognized signals of early dehydration. It can help you feel full. It's the perfect substitute for snacks eaten out of habit, boredom, or anxiety. And it can help you cut hundreds of calories a day if you substitute it for sweetened soft drinks.

Health bonus: Drinking more than five glasses a day cut heart attack risk by 41 percent in women and 54 percent in men in a study at California's Loma Linda University. Researchers think staying hydrated may cut the risk of developing heart-threatening blood clots.

Keep it interesting: Sip club soda with a splash of orange or grape juice; add a slice of lemon, lime, or even cucumber to ice-cold water; or make iced (or hot) herbal or green tea.

Get this much: How much do you need each day? About 1 ounce of water for every 2 pounds of body weight. This is just enough to replace fluid lost naturally through breathing, sweating, and trips to the bathroom. If you weigh 160 pounds, that's 80 ounces. How many glasses is that? It depends on your glass! A teacup or small juice glass often holds just 6 ounces; a large drinking glass could hold 24 ounces. Our suggestion: Find out how much liquid your everyday glasses hold (surprisingly, few people know), then figure out how many glasses you need to drink. Probably, it'll be between 6 and 10.

Important note for exercisers: Drink an extra cup or two of water before you get started and again afterward—and sip a half-cup every 15 to 20 minutes during your workout.

SUPER FOOD Eggs

Satiety—that satisfied, filled-up feeling that makes snacking and overeating the furthest thing from your mind—may be as close as the dozen eggs nestled in a carton in your fridge. In a recent study, women who ate two eggs, toast, and jelly for breakfast reported feeling fuller longer than those who started the day with yogurt and a bagel slathered with cream cheese.

The egg eaters went on to eat 29 percent fewer calories at lunch and nearly 400 fewer calories for the entire day. (The bagel group had 2,035 calories each, while the egg group ate 1,761 apiece.) And how's this for staying power: They even ate less the following day, according to researchers from the Rochester Center for Obesity Research in Michigan. "Eggs have a 50 percent greater satiety index than breakfast cereal or bread," the researchers concluded.

Why? Ah—there's the mystery. It could be the balance of protein and fat or some other combination of nutrients in eggs. Experts aren't certain. They do know that eggs ranked in the same "super-satisfying" category as cheese, meat, and fish in a study of the "fullness factor" of foods conducted at the University of Sydney in Australia.

Health bonus: Egg yolks are rich in lutein, an antioxidant that protects the eyes against age-related macular degeneration, a leading cause of blindness.

Keep it interesting: Store extra hard-boiled eggs in the fridge (they'll keep for up to five days), then slice some into your lunch or dinner salad to create a fast main course or chop and mix with low-fat mayo and a little relish for egg salad (add a sprinkle of curry powder for an exotic change of pace). Make a two-egg omelet with a dusting of grated cheese and some roasted veggies for lunch or dinner.

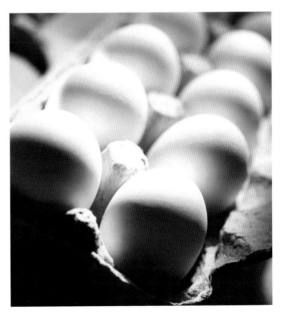

Get this much: If you're not at risk for heart disease, it's okay to have one egg a day—a total of seven per week, says the American Heart Association.

SUPER FOOD Nuts

At last, there's no reason to feel guilty about thoroughly enjoying a handful of nuts. Once a forbidden food, these little nuggets are packed with good fats, protein, fiber, and a variety of important vitamins and minerals. We've known this for a while, but the "new" news is that a growing stack of studies shows that nuts can help you lose weight, too.

In one eye-opening study at Purdue University in Indiana, people who snacked daily on oily, salty cocktail peanuts for eight weeks didn't gain weight. Why? Scientists suspect that those who munched nuts were so satisfied by the fat, protein, and fiber that they ate less at meals and other snack times without even knowing it. There were even signs that the nuts boosted metabolism ever so slightly. And in another amazing study, dieters who added almonds to their daily menus lost 18 percent more weight than those who didn't, according to researchers from the City of Hope National Medical Center in

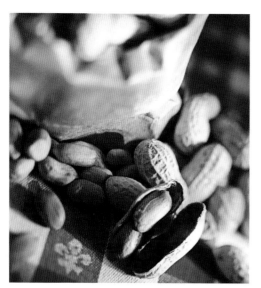

California. The magic? Almonds, like other nuts, make you feel full. And, researchers say, it's possible that their tough cell walls prevent digestion and absorption of their fat.

Health bonus: Good fats in nuts can prevent blood clots, promote a healthy heartbeat, and lower blood pressure.

Keep it interesting: Pack nuts in single-serving portions in small zipper-lock bags as soon as you buy them. Buy several varieties and combine them. That way, you'll get a wider variety of beneficial nutrients and fats.

Get this much: As we mentioned earlier in this book, eating nuts requires a little planning—otherwise, this weight-loss strategy becomes a calorie binge. If you snack on nuts or plan to add some to a salad, we suggest counting out your allotment, then putting the container away before munching. A palmful of nuts provides about 200 calories; a 100-calorie serving equals about 8 walnut halves, 15 almonds, 10 to 12 cashews, 10 pecans, 5 or 6 macadamia nuts, 12 hazelnuts, or 1 tablespoon of peanut butter.

ChangeOne success stories

Leading the Way, One Step at a Time

Susan Miller joined ChangeOne.com with hopes of losing some weight. "I needed to change how I ate, and I really liked the concept of changing only one thing at a time," she says.

A busy mother of four kids under age 11, Susan loved that she could be on *ChangeOne* without preparing special foods or reforming her entire diet overnight. "I like that there's a clear understanding of how much I can eat, and I learned to do this with the foods I normally eat," says the 36-year-old. "I was able to do it at my own pace and be successful in baby steps."

Now 43 pounds lighter and 28 inches smaller overall, Susan is thrilled with her progress. And she's using her success and enthusiasm for the program to help and inspire others. Fellow ChangeOne.com members have grown accustomed to seeing frequent motivational and inspirational messages from Susan on the site's message boards. "I've made many wonderful friends," she says.

Susan particularly enjoys posting hints and tips for people just starting *ChangeOne*, encouraging them to get started and stick with it. "I've seen women from all walks of life be successful at this—if we can, you can, too!" she tells them.

Susan has passed healthy *ChangeOne* tips on to her kids, too. "I've learned

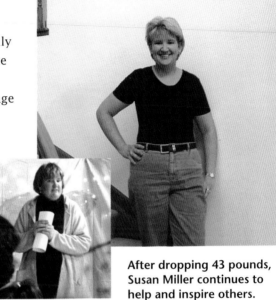

After dropping 43 pounds, Susan Miller continues to help and inspire others.

correct portion size, which I can now teach to my children."

Susan is also a lot more active than she used to be. "I am willing to try new things since I don't feel 'conspicuous' anymore," she says.

Another bonus is the frequent compliments she gets from friends and family. "They're thrilled for me!" she says. "It's very fun to see someone I haven't seen for months and hear comments on how good I'm looking."

Susan continues to lose weight, and she plans to stick with her new healthy habits. "I really love *ChangeOne*," she says. "It's not a diet—it's a way to relearn how to eat."

For more ChangeOne *success stories, go to www.changeone.com/successstories*

SUPER FOOD Salad

Rock-'n'-roll stars and politicians are usually grabbing head-lines—but mixed greens? Recently, a salad got top billing in national newspapers and on network news shows when researchers revealed that eating a veggie medley topped with

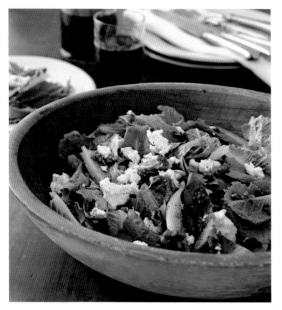

fat-free Italian dressing helped dieters eat 100 fewer calories at lunch than they did when they skipped this produce-rich first course.

The secret? Salads made with ingredients such as lettuce, carrots, tomatoes, and peppers are big in size (and flavor) but low in calories, due in part to their high fiber and water content. Dieters in the study filled up on 3 cups of salad—nearly a day's worth of nutritious vegetables—without consuming more than a few dozen precious calories. Just as important, the salad influenced how much they ate for the rest of their meal. Crunchy vegetables are satisfying to munch, and their chunky shapes and sizes stretch your tummy so that receptors on the stomach lining send "all full" messages back to your brain.

For added benefits, sprinkle your salad with vinegar. Arizona State University nutritionists found that this condiment can cut blood sugar by up to 30 percent after a meal—an effect that could reduce cravings later in the day.

Health bonus: Eating more veggies will increase your daily intake of fiber and antioxidants, cutting your risk of heart disease, diabetes, and even some cancers.

Keep it interesting: As a base for your salad, try baby spinach, radicchio, mixed field greens, or spicy arugula or other interesting lettuces from the supermarket produce section. Each has a unique character.

Get this much: We suggest starting lunch or dinner every day with a high-volume, low-cal salad, especially if you tend to overeat. Start with a generous bed of lettuce, top with chopped tomatoes, grated or sliced carrots, cucumber rounds, and cut-up green or red peppers, and add any of these:

shredded zucchini, sliced raw mushrooms, onions, fresh herbs
(basil is heavenly), celery, fennel, or shredded cabbage. Top
with fat-free dressing or about one capful of low-fat dressing.

SUPER FOOD Soup

When you're craving comfort food but want to avoid fat and
calorie minefields such as macaroni and cheese or lasagna,
simply start with soup. Hot, hearty, and a pleasure to eat,
soup's a proven weight-loss star that fills you up so you eat
fewer calories during the rest of the meal. In University of
Pennsylvania study of 500 dieters, those who ate soup at least
four times a week lost more weight than those who ate it less
often. Pennsylvania State University researchers found that
eating a 200-calorie bowl of soup before lunch was more satisfying than having the same number of calories from cheese
and crackers—and helped dieters eat less during their meals.
Why? Think quantity: The cheese and crackers appetizer was
less than 2 ounces; the soup was a satisfying 20 ounces.

Soup is a great alternative to salad as a first course during
cold weather, it makes a satisfying snack, and it's the perfect
calorie-control secret weapon when
dining out. Just look for broth-based
soups made without cream and with little
butter or fat. At home, start from scratch
or use fat-free, reduced-sodium broth.
Add fresh or frozen veggies to first-
course soups. For a main course, pump
up the nutrition and calories with lean
meat, beans, and even whole grain
noodles, barley, or lentils. For a low-cal
"cream" soup, puree the liquid and half of
the cooked veggies in a blender, then add
to the rest of the vegetables. Top with
plain yogurt instead of sour cream.

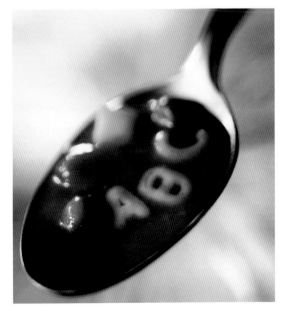

Health bonus: Extra fluid, plus veggies that help protect your heart and cut
the risk of cancer.

Keep it interesting: Add extra frozen vegetables to canned
chicken vegetable soup; toss fresh or dried herbs into soup to
intensify the flavor (try dill in chicken soup, rosemary in

white bean soup, and cilantro in black bean soup); keep low-sodium broths and canned beans on hand as the base for quick, healthy lunch or dinner soups. Serve with a salad.

Get this much: We suggest having soup on days when you don't feel like starting lunch or dinner with a salad. Strive for at least four bowls per week.

SUPER FOOD Cereal

Healthy, filling, and ready to eat, high-fiber cereal is the perfect weight-loss food any time of day. Studies show it can rein in your appetite and work as a clever, low-calorie "meal replacement" at lunch or dinner.

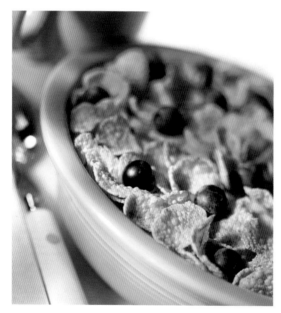

Instead of thinking of that cereal in the pantry as breakfast food, see it in a new light: as a snack, quick lunch, or even the centerpiece of a healthy dinner. In a Purdue University study of 109 overweight women and men, those who ate cereal with fruit and fat-free milk for breakfast and either lunch or dinner cut 640 calories from their daily intake. Meanwhile, a recent survey found that women who had cereal several times a week weighed 9 pounds less than those who generally bypassed it.

The key is picking the right cereal—one with at least 3 grams of fiber per serving. More is even better: Some cereals pack 6 to 11 grams per serving. When 60 women and men had high-fiber oatmeal for breakfast instead of low-fiber cornflakes, they ate 30 percent fewer calories at lunch, reported researchers from the New York Obesity Research Center at St. Luke's–Roosevelt Hospital. The appetite-control factor seems to be all that satisfying fiber, which helps you stay full.

It's also important to look for cereals with low sugar content. That way, you'll control calories and stay off the blood-sugar roller coaster that leads to midmorning hunger pangs and food cravings. (A British study found recently that eating sugary cereal actually led to overeating at lunch.)

Health bonus: A Harvard study found that participants who ate whole-grain cereals every day were 17 percent less likely to die over the next several years from any cause, and 20 percent less likely to die from cardiovascular disease, than those who "rarely or never" ate those cereals.

Keep it interesting: Mix it up—the smart way. *ChangeOne* suggests setting aside an extra 5 to 10 minutes on your next shopping trip to explore the cereal aisle. Take your reading glasses so you can compare the fiber and sugar content of various brands. (You'll find this important data on the Nutrition Facts label on the side or back of the box.) And remember to look up high and down low; the healthy cereals are often relegated to inconvenient spots on the shelves.

Get this much: Make cereal your breakfast default—have a bowl any morning you don't have time or the inclination to prepare fancier fare. If controlling portions is a challenge at lunch or dinner, we recommend having cereal once in a while instead. Set a goal of eating at least five bowls of high-fiber cereal a week.

SUPER FOOD   Seafood

Shrimp grilled with pineapple and red peppers. Poached oysters on a bed of freshly sautéed spinach. A gorgeous salmon fillet dressed up with yogurt-dill sauce. If there's a glamour food on your list of sensible, weight-pampering edibles, it should be seafood.

Low in calories, high in mouthwatering flavor, loaded with satisfying protein, and packed with nutrients (including zinc and omega-3 fatty acids), seafood can control your appetite without padding your middle or clogging your arteries with bad fats. Even better, seafood can feel like a splurge—a lifesaver when you're faced with some of the toughest challenges to sensible eating, such as navigating a party buffet or ordering at a restaurant. So get the shrimp—4 ounces has just 120 calories. Or go for the salmon: A 3-ounce

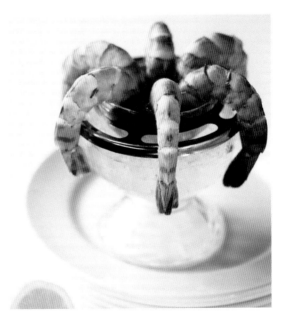

piece has just 200 calories and more than a half day's quota of omega-3 fatty acids. Go ahead, enjoy the broiled scallops! Four ounces has just 151 calories and delivers omega-3's and lots of vitamin B_{12}.

Want an example of proof that seafood's a smart choice? In a four-month-long Australian study, fish was shown to help volunteers lose weight and reduce their risks of heart disease and diabetes.

Health bonus: The good fats in seafood protect your heart by helping blood flow smoothly. B vitamins help lower levels of homocysteine, a compound in the blood associated with clogged arteries and heart attack, and may also protect against colon cancer.

Keep it interesting: Check out the single-serving foil packs of salmon and shrimp in the canned fish section of your supermarket. And don't overlook canned salmon—it's an inexpensive, widely available form of wild salmon that's great in a quiche. Or mix it with low-fat mayo to make salmon salad. Other ways to expand your seafood habit include having a bowl of Manhattan clam chowder (the red, brothy type) once or twice a week, a grilled fish fillet every Tuesday evening (we particularly like tilapia), and an occasional bowl of pasta topped with bay scallops sautéed with vegetables, olive oil, and wine.

Get this much: Try for at least two fish meals per week. That should be easy: a tuna sandwich for lunch one day, sautéed shrimp for dinner another day, and you're there.

SUPER FOOD Chicken

This all-American favorite earned a gold star as a *ChangeOne* superfood for purely pragmatic reasons: There's no high-protein, low-fat weight-loss food that's more convenient.

True, chicken earns top marks in almost every weight-loss plan in existence—low carb or high carb, low fat or high protein—and it's no wonder. A roasted, skinless breast weighs in with just 120 to 140 calories and is packed with all the satisfaction of protein and less than half the fat of a trimmed, Choice-grade T-bone steak. How satisfying is chicken? When French researchers gave either a high-protein chicken snack or a high-carb rice pudding snack to a group of volunteers, the carb group got hungry as quickly as another group of volunteers who had no snack. But the chicken snackers reported feeling full for nearly an hour longer than all the others.

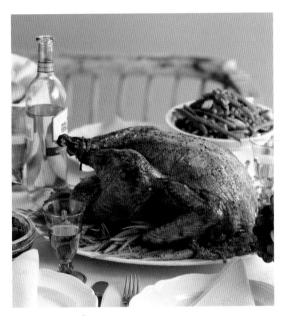

We believe that any protein-rich, low-fat food will help you stay satisfied longer, but here's why we love chicken: You can find it, ready to eat, virtually everywhere. Need a snack on the road? Pull up to the drive-through window for a grilled chicken sandwich, no sauce. Toss the bun and eat the chicken for a hunger-stopping 160-calorie snack. Need a quick dinner? Go for grilled chicken (on a bun or, even better, on a salad) at your local fast-food joint. Planning menus for a busy week? Grab precooked chicken breast slices or quick-cooking boneless, skinless breasts at the supermarket. And stock up on those little 3-ounce cans of white-meat chicken, which is great on bread, in a salad, or in soup.

One warning, which you already know: Avoid eating the skin, which is absolutely loaded with calories.

Health bonus: Chicken is packed with B vitamins, important for energy production and heart health.

Keep it interesting: Chicken's mild flavor makes it a blank canvas for culinary adventure: Top with chopped cilantro, a squirt of lime juice, and a dollop of fat-free sour cream; barbecue in teriyaki sauce; cube and mix with chopped garlic, basil, and balsamic vinegar or with tarragon, grapes, and low-fat mayo. Yum!

Get this much: Hungry? Think chicken. There's no reason not to have it several times a week.

SUPER FOOD Yogurt

Most dairy products can help you slim down faster if you're on a low-calorie program like *ChangeOne*. But only one can be part of breakfast or dessert, a vegetable dip or a base for a sauce, or the main ingredient in a summertime drink. We're talking about versatile, hardworking yogurt—and it's better than ever.

Yogurt is a powerhouse full of calcium and protein, factors that may help explain studies showing that dairy foods can

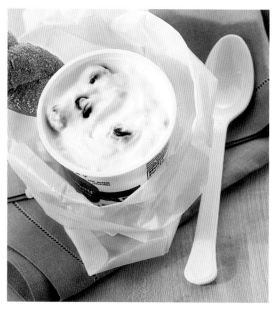

turbo-charge your weight-loss efforts. But unlike milk or cheese, yogurt's smooth, pudding-like consistency allows it to go places other dairy products fear to tread. You can blend fat-free yogurt with fruit and ice for a low-cal smoothie; freeze it in the carton, then whirl it in a food processor with fresh or frozen fruit for an intensely flavored dessert; or mix it with herbs and lemon juice to make a dressing or dip. You can also drain out the liquid to create a cheese-like spread that's great on bagels.

Buy yogurt plain rather than flavored and in large containers rather than in small cups. Flavored yogurts are very high in sugar and calories; buying plain yogurt and adding a teaspoon of fruit jam—and perhaps some nuts, raisins, or cereal—is almost always healthier.

Health bonus: Look for yogurt that contains live, active cultures. These probiotics—the name scientists use for beneficial bacteria—can help digestion and may fight infection.

Keep it interesting: Build a healthy parfait: Layer yogurt, fresh fruit, and granola in wine glasses or dessert cups for a pretty dessert. Or add a fruity liqueur, such as Amaretto or Chambord, to yogurt for a simple yet wonderful sauce for cakes or fresh fruit.

Have this much: Work yogurt into your meals several times a week. Have some every day if you don't like milk or are lactose intolerant. (Enzymes in yogurt convert milk sugars into a digestible form that's perfect for you.)

SUPER FOOD Beans

Whether black or pinto, kidney or cannellini, beans may seem too starchy, simply too heavy in carbohydrates to get top billing as superfoods. But look again: These morsels have what weight-loss experts call satiety power. Thanks to their unique blend of fiber and protein, beans keep your blood sugar low and steady. Eating beans will help you feel full longer and sidestep blood sugar swings that lead to ravenous slipups at the soda machine or snack bar.

In fact, no other natural, ready-to-eat food has more fiber than beans. They pack the top of the USDA's list of fiber all-stars. (Fifteen of the 20 top fiber sources on the chart are beans!) The lowdown: A cup of black beans, kidney beans, peas (actually members of the bean, or legume, family), or even beans and franks delivers 15 to 17 grams of fiber—half of your daily needs. And all that fiber, plus protein, means that beans are ranked low on the glycemic index (GI)—a measure of a food's impact on blood sugar.

Low-GI foods are weight-loss good guys because they raise blood sugar levels only slightly. A growing number of studies show that building your meals around low-glycemic choices can help you lose weight faster and more easily—without feeling so tired or hungry. That means you'll be more likely to stick with your plan longer and have the energy to get up and get active—another key component of success on the *ChangeOne* plan.

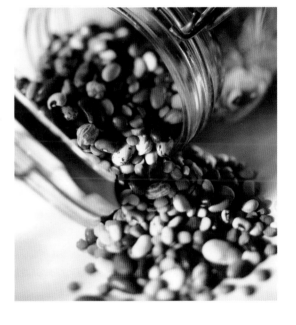

Health bonus: Beans contain two kinds of fiber: insoluble, which helps your gastrointestinal system eliminate waste products more quickly, and soluble, which forms a gel in your intestines that helps lower levels of "bad" LDL cholesterol by whisking cholesterol out of your body. Research shows that eating a cup of beans per day can reduce cholesterol by up to 10 percent in just six weeks.

Keep it interesting: Use beans in place of meat in soups and on salads. Toss together a quick lunch salad with rinsed, canned beans (½ cup is enough), fat-free dressing, and chopped veggies. Experiment with bean salads—as simple as white beans with olive oil, red wine vinegar, and parsley, or as bold as black beans with southwestern spices and chiles.

Get this much: Have beans five times a week.

Keeping
on Track

By now you're hitting your stride. You're dropping pounds, and the success feels great.

Still, as almost any successful dieter will tell you, it's essential to monitor your progress. The pressures that surround us to eat, eat, eat, don't go away. Portion sizes have a way of creeping up. Plans to go for a walk or hit the gym can fall by the wayside. And the pounds have a way of sneaking back.

This week you'll devise your own "first-alert" program to sound an alarm if you begin to get off track.

We're not suggesting that you measure every bowl of cereal or pasta serving for the rest of your life. But staying alert to how you're feeling, what you're doing, and how much you're eating will have a huge payoff in terms of weight, health, and self-confidence.

Schedule a
Regular Checkup

With the end of the 12-week program just around the corner, it's time to take a moment to appreciate how far you've come. If you're like many *ChangeOne* participants, you may have already reached your target weight. Now it's time to make the transition from a diet that contains fewer calories than you need to one that balances your calorie intake with the number that you expend.

If you began *ChangeOne* hoping to lose a significant amount of weight, you may still have some pounds to go. There's nothing wrong with that. Slow and steady is the best kind of progress to make.

Wherever you are on the path to your desired weight, start planning now for the future. Almost any diet program will help you lose weight during the first few months. That's the easy part. If you've dieted before, you know that the real trick is maintaining weight loss—which requires turning the healthy changes you've already made into lifelong habits.

Sadly, that's where most diet plans falter. We've already mentioned one pitfall: Call it the on-off trap. People go on a diet to lose weight and go off it once they've shed the pounds. And unfortunately, that means going right back to the way they ate before. You know how the story ends. Before long the numbers on the scale are right back where they started.

There's another pitfall, and one that's probably more common. As people near their desired weight, they begin to ease up a little. They stop paying as much attention to portion sizes. They splurge a little more often on rich desserts. They grab an extra snack. Nothing dramatic. But if they're not watching, all those little nibbles can add up to a pound here and a pound there. Before they know it, they've gained back a chunk of the weight they lost.

Regaining a few pounds shouldn't be a big deal. You already know what it takes to lose those pounds, right? But losing ground spells real trouble, for several reasons. If you begin to gain weight back again, it's natural to assume that the diet isn't working and to abandon it completely. Worse, it's easy to begin to blame yourself and replay all kinds of negative messages in your head: "I'm a failure." "I'll never be able to lose the weight and keep it off." "I'm destined to be fat." Losing weight only to gain it back can also make you reluctant to try again. And when you do, you might feel discouraged from the start.

Thanks to the careful work you've already put in, this is far less likely to happen to you than it is for people on faddish diets. You've learned that eating should be a pleasure, not something that you have to fear. You've seen that you can lose weight and keep it off while eating regular food that you actually like to eat. You've also discovered on *ChangeOne* that you can eat sensible portions without feeling hungry. Along the way, you've seen which changes have made the biggest difference for you.

Now all it takes to ensure that weight creep doesn't happen is to keep a watchful eye not only on your weight but also on how your clothes fit, how you feel, how much you exercise, and what's on the menu.

The *ChangeOne* First-Alert Program

Starting this week, take a few minutes once a week to do a quick self checkup. Record your weight. Estimate about how much physical activity you were able to get. Rate your overall mood. And jot down any issues or problems you may be dealing with. That's it. To make your weekly checkups even easier, we've included a *ChangeOne* Progress Log on page 343, which will allow you to track four weeks of checkups. At the end of those four weeks, chart how your weight has changed on the simple graph at the bottom of the form.

We're not suggesting you fill out weight-monitoring forms for the rest of your life. But we do recommend logging your progress for the next two months. If your weight is holding steady and you're comfortable with how things are going, tuck the form away in a drawer and get on with your life. Celebrate your success. Forget about dieting for a while.

But don't forget to pay attention. Weigh yourself once a week. Keep track of how your clothes feel or where you notch your belt. Be alert to your moods. If you notice a change for the worse—if your favorite trousers start feeling a wee bit snug or you're going through a rocky period at home—grab a copy of the progress report and start filling it in weekly again.

Remember, most people's weight goes up or down a little, week by week. You probably already know how much yours normally varies. If the scale creeps up more than five pounds from your desired weight, it's time to take action. Don't panic—you haven't failed. And don't give up. You already know exactly what it takes to lose weight. You've done it before, and you can do it again.

Tally Your Activity

Keeping track of exercise isn't as easy as watching pounds on the scale. True, if you follow the *ChangeOne* fitness plan in the coming pages, you'll be exercising each and everyday for short but effective bursts, making monitoring as easy as saying, "I did it" or "I didn't." But if your exercise consists of doing everyday physical activities—taking the stairs, walking from the far end of the parking lot, doing a circuit around the block during commercial breaks—keeping track can be trickier.

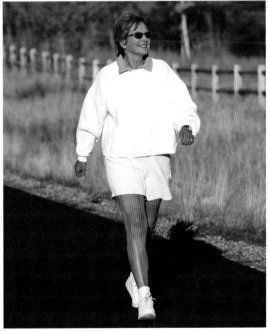

One approach is to fill out an activity log, tallying up the time you spend every day. (Remember, we've included one for you on page 342.) Your goal should be to add at least 30 minutes of moderately intense activity daily.

Another strategy, which many people come to love, is using a step-counter, also called a pedometer. Step-counters are devices about the size of a pager that can be attached to your belt or waist-band. By way of a mechanical pendulum that moves back and forth with each step you take, the device automatically records your every step.

The simplest devices, the ones that just count steps, are the best buys. Pedometers that compute the distance you've covered aren't very accurate; models that claim to tell you how many calories you've burned are even more unreliable, since they can't distinguish between a leisurely stroll and a heart-thumping run. A basic step-counter will run about $25 and can be found at most sporting goods stores.

For the first few days, wear the counter but go about your usual day. At the end of each day, jot down how many steps you took. This number will serve as your baseline. Then set your first goal to increase the amount of walking you do. Without doing anything but going about your daily business, you're likely to take about 3,000 steps. Doing roughly 15 minutes' worth of walking, stair climbing, and other everyday activities will add about 2,000 steps. The optimum goal for weight maintenance is around 10,000 to 12,000 steps a day.

The easiest way to monitor your activity level? Wear a step-counter.

Okay, so you're not there yet—don't worry. Scale up your weekly goals gradually. Start by shooting for 7,000 steps one week, for example, and the next week increase your goal to 9,000 steps. Like many people, you may find that using a step-counter will give you a little push when you need it. From time to time each day, check to see how many steps you've taken. If you're barely up to 2,000 steps when lunchtime rolls around, consider a brisk walk after you eat. If you're done with dinner and are still short on steps, turn off the television and take a hike.

If you decide to use a step-counter, include the average number of steps you take on your four-week progress log. That way you can track your increasing activity at a glance.

Monitor Your Moods

While you're keeping tabs on your weight, how your clothes fit, and how much exercise you get, also be alert to how you feel—happy, sad, enthusiastic, busy, bored, gung-ho, whatever. You'll find a place on the progress log to record what your overall moods were like during the previous week.

Staying in touch with the way you feel is important for several reasons you probably already recognize. For a lot of people, stress, boredom, loneliness, or feeling blue are triggers for eating. If you're among those emotional eaters, keeping tabs on your mental state will help you begin to see patterns. You may see that the times your weight tends to creep back up again are times when you're bored.

The solution could be as simple as making a list of three things to do when you're feeling that way that don't involve eating. Let's say that stress at work is your downfall; every time you start checking the "stressed out" box on your progress report, you can almost be sure your weight will start to climb. Simply recognizing that pattern can help you change it—by finding healthier ways to deal with stress than eating, for instance, or by increasing your exercise time.

Remember the First-Alert Plan

Like many people, you may discover that paying attention to your moods allows you to notice early warning signs of trouble. You realize that you're beginning to feel worn down by stress before you become completely frazzled. You notice the first signs of feeling blue.

That awareness can help you remedy the situation before you find yourself in a deep slump. Get together with friends. Schedule something you really love. Set aside extra time for exercise, which is a proven mood-booster. Turn your attention back to healthy eating as a way to avoid overeating when you're feeling discouraged or down.

The truth is, everyone feels down now and then. Sometimes there's a perfectly good reason for it. Money problems, relationship difficulties, a bad day at work. But some people find their moods dragged down again and again when there's no good reason except a feeling of low self-esteem. Given the emphasis our society places on being thin, it's not surprising that many people who struggle with their weight end up having a negative image of their bodies. The problem is compounded by a tendency on the part of many people to think that being overweight is the result of a lack of willpower. It's not that at all. It's the result of a complicated mix of factors, from genes and family eating patterns to body type and psychology.

So here's another reason for monitoring your moods: If your mental state tends to turn sour because of low self-esteem, take time to remind yourself of how far you've come in making healthful changes. Remember that not all of us are magazine cover models. Healthy bodies vary tremendously in terms of size and shape. Don't get into the trap of wanting the "perfect" body. Concentrate instead on achieving a healthy, reasonable weight for who you are.

Of course, that's easier said than done. Sometimes feelings of low self-esteem reach all the way back to childhood, making them very hard to change on your own. Feeling sad or hopeless can be no more than just a passing emotion for some people, but for others, it can be a symptom of clinical depression. If you find yourself struggling without success against feelings of sadness, hopelessness, or low self-esteem, talk to your doctor. There is a proven link between depression and weight gain. And treating depression, studies show, can have the additional effect of helping people get down to a normal weight.

Taking Action

If you notice your weight beginning to climb—or your clothes or belt beginning to feel tight—search for the reason. You may know exactly why you're gaining weight. Stress at work, per-haps, or long stretch of holiday party-going. Maybe you've just stopped being as strict as you were before about keeping portions under control. The notes you've jotted down should tell you a lot. To do more in-depth troubleshooting, fill in the diagnostic checklist below.

Once you've zeroed in on the specific problem, take action. Don't try to address all your issues at once. That's

Diagnostic Checklist

When the first-alert warning bell rings, use this checklist to identify the sources of trouble. ☺ A smile means you're doing just fine. ☺ A neutral expression means you're holding your own. ☹ A frown—well, you know what that means. After you're done, look over the categories that scored a frown. These are the areas to focus your troubleshooting efforts.

	☺	☺	☹	For Help
Breakfast				Page 22
Lunch				Page 36
Snacks				Page 52
Dinner				Page 76
Dining out				Page 90
Stress				Page 148
Resisting pressures to eat				Page 110
Environmental triggers				Page 56
Emotional eating				Page 60
Self-esteem				Page 181
Stopping when I'm satisfied				Page 78
Motivation				Page 140

what *ChangeOne* is all about, after all: focusing on one change at a time.

Having trouble with a specific meal? Check back to the first four weeks of *ChangeOne* for advice on how to take control of breakfast, lunch, dinner, or snacks. Eating when you're not really hungry? Make a conscious effort to stop and ask yourself whether you're actually responding to an emotional or environmental cue. If you're not truly hungry, distract yourself by doing something else—take a walk, do a chore, brush your teeth, or grab a stick of sugar-free gum. Feeling just plain overwhelmed? Your best bet may be that tried-and-true jump-start for any weight-loss plan: the food diary. Keep one for a week. Even if you make no other change, chances are you'll see progress on the scale.

Keeping track is so important that we urge you to set aside a particular time each week to conduct your *ChangeOne* checkup. Many prefer to do theirs on Sunday evenings. Use whatever day and time works best for you. Just try to stick to it. Put a reminder on your calendar. Post your weekly checkup form on the refrigerator or beside your desk—wherever it's easy to find. If you have a tendency to misplace pieces of paper, record your weight and activity level in a couple of places—a notebook or your computer, for instance. That way you'll have a backup. And if all is going well, then you'll have several reminders to tell yourself, "Congratulations! Be proud!" By learning the *ChangeOne* way to lose weight, you have changed yourself in untold wonderful ways.

ChangeOne...
for Life!

It's celebration time. Put down the book for a moment, take a deep breath, and let out a victory yell.

You've reached Week 12, the end of the formal *ChangeOne* program. Over the past three months you've done something remarkable. You've redirected your life. You've changed the way you eat. More important than that, you've proved to yourself that you are in control. You've learned that small steps in the right direction can add up to a giant leap forward.

So in this final week, have fun. We want you to be playful with food. At least twice, try a new combination or flavor you've never had before.

Why? Because the enemy of weight loss is boredom. Eat the same way all the time, under tight restrictions, and you'll soon rebel. And if *ChangeOne* is about anything, it's about a love and respect for good food.

Reward Yourself

Give yourself a big pat on the back, but don't stop there. Reward yourself with something special. Make it a complete extravagance, if you want—a weekend getaway or a night on the town. Or choose something that reinforces your changes, your results, and the new you: running shoes, a new bike, a gift certificate for yoga classes, or an enticing cookbook.

Why make a big deal about rewarding yourself? Because too often we tend to be aware of when we've fallen short and take our progress for granted. Even people who have lost weight and made healthy changes in the way they live may think they've failed—unless they celebrate their successes.

Acknowledging a job well done also serves as a way to mark those milestones we talked about before—the small steps you take that add up to a giant leap forward. Unless you celebrate them, you may not even be aware of how far you've come. And when we say celebrate your victories, we mean all of them. Some of your successes are easy to recognize. Eating a healthier breakfast, for instance. Or taming runaway snacks. But other positive changes may be more subtle, though more important: discovering that you can decide on a plan of action and stick to it; gaining self-confidence; banishing a negative voice that used to echo in your head; learning that you can slip for a day or two and get yourself back on track.

Small steps? Sure. But each one of them makes an important difference. This week take a little time out to think about the obvious and not so obvious ways you've changed over the last 12 weeks. Give yourself kudos for every positive step you've taken.

Aren't the people around us supposed to give us a big pat on the back when we've done something wonderful? Sure they are. And maybe you're lucky enough to have someone who does give you accolades for what you've accomplished. Still, it's important to give yourself a job-well-done, too. As helpful as other people can be, changing for the better is up to you and you alone. You have to be your own best friend. By giving yourself rewards, you also reinforce positive self-messages—a powerful antidote against those discouraging words that can sometimes repeat in your ears.

Trust Your Instincts

Yes, you'll celebrate your success this week. But—and no surprise here—we've included a lesson for the long haul. Relax. It's a lesson you'll love.

First, a question: What's the toughest challenge dieters face when it comes to keeping the weight off? When we asked some *ChangeOne* participants as they were beginning the program, many of them listed things like "snacks," "hunger," and "a sweet tooth." Most people starting a diet figure the hardest part will be resisting temptation. In fact, as we mentioned at the start, the biggest pitfall dieters face over the long haul is something much more basic: boredom.

People often give up on a diet because it gets tiresome. They grow weary of tracking calories or consulting long lists of foods they should or shouldn't eat. They rebel against the rules that most diets include.

We've made sure *ChangeOne* doesn't include a lot of strict rules, banned foods, complex theories, and other guidelines that tie you up. A healthy diet, after all, is about eating sensible servings of tasty and (mostly) nutritious food. You can eat just about anything, but if your choice is rich in calories, you'll have to watch portions. It's that simple.

But even with the varied *ChangeOne* menu, you could be feeling a little restless. So this week you'll shake things up. Fix something you haven't eaten before. Get creative in the kitchen and concoct a dish of your own. Treat yourself to a fancy meal at a restaurant you've been anxious to try. Forget the *ChangeOne* meal plans for a whole day. Heck, take the whole week off, if you want. Imagine that you're taking the training wheels off and going for a solo spin after 12 weeks of learning how to keep your balance. This week let the *ChangeOne* principles guide you as you venture out on your own.

To get started, turn the page for a party of festive ideas; then go to page 190 for more eating adventures.

Try Something New

How you'll shake things up this week is up to you. If you've been sitting down to cereal every morning, see how a yogurt

(Continued on page 190)

An Appetizer Dinner

Appetizers let you enjoy a diversity of flavors, textures, and cuisines. Plus, it's a playful and social way to eat. Here's just one approach.

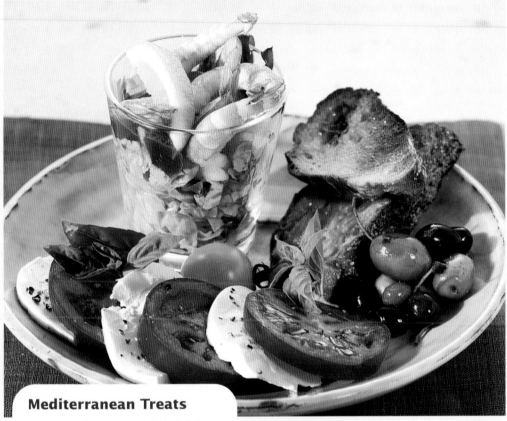

Mediterranean Treats

14-ounce shrimp cocktail (4-6 shrimp, plus cocktail sauce)

1 ounce fresh mozzarella (coaster) atop tomato salad with slivered basil and balsamic vinegar

10 herbed olives

1 slice crusty bread

Calories 430, fat 13 g, saturated fat 4 g, cholesterol 190 mg, sodium 1,350 mg, carbohydrate 46 g, fiber 5 g, protein 33 g, calcium 250 mg.

VARIATIONS

For balance and calorie control, pick one item from some or all of the following:

Protein foods: Ceviche, ½ cup; Thai satay (grilled chicken or beef strips), 2 skewers; smoked salmon, 2 ounces; prosciutto, 3 thin slices; steamed mussels, 1 cup (out of shell).

Vegetables: Unlimited, as long as they are not prepared with added fat. As an option, you can top them with 1½ ounces fresh mozzarella, 1 ounce cheese slivers, or 1 tablespoon peanut butter, but keep the add-ons to reasonable portions.

Nibbles: 10 olives, handful of nuts.

Bread: 1 slice, your choice of flavor, or try a medium-sized hard roll.

Taco Party

Tacos migrated from Mexico to become one of the most popular dishes in the United States. But why eat fatty restaurant tacos? It's more fun to make tacos at home. Set out a self-serve buffet of tortillas, chopped vegetables, low-fat cheese, and grilled or sautéed meats or beans, as shown. A serving is two tacos, based on our taco-building approach.

HOW TO BUILD A TACO:

1. Put corn or small flour tortilla on plate.

2. Top with ¼ cup (golf ball) of either lean ground beef, ground turkey, shredded turkey, meatless crumbles, or fat-free refried beans.

3. Add 2 tablespoons (2 thumbs) shredded reduced-fat jack or cheddar cheese, guacamole, and/or sliced olives (total of 2 tablespoons).

4. Cover with vegetables and sauce—chopped tomatoes, shredded lettuce, diced red and green peppers, minced red onion, diced or sliced jalapeño peppers, chopped green chiles, salsa.

5. Fold over and eat.

For corn tortilla and ground beef: Calories 430, fat 22 g, saturated fat 10 g, cholesterol 80 mg, sodium 670 mg, carbohydrate 33 g, fiber 5 g, protein 27 g, calcium 300 mg.

TIPS ON CHEESE

Mexican *queso fresco* is a soft white cheese with a mild flavor, similar to Monterey jack cheese. Check the label to make sure yours is made from pasteurized milk, which limits the chances of bacterial contamination. Other popular taco cheeses include pepper jack and cheddar. Look for grated reduced-fat varieties to save a few calories, or shred your own using a grater with fine holes. Chill the cheese well before grating to help prevent it from falling apart.

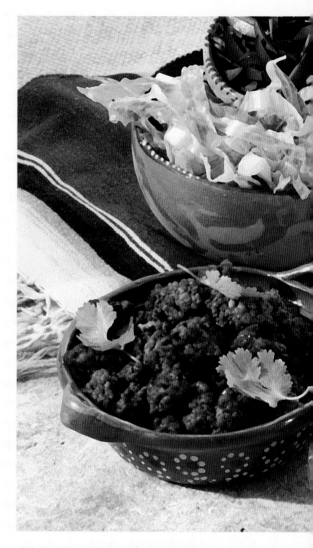

ABOUT REFRIED BEANS

Traditional Mexican refried beans, *frijoles refritos,* are made by sautéing diced onion and sometimes garlic in lard, then adding and mashing pinto or other types of beans. Make your own lower-fat, lower-calorie version by cooking onion in a nonstick skillet with a teaspoon or so of olive oil and a splash of chicken or vegetable broth until the onion is soft. Add a can of pinto beans plus a teaspoon of ground cumin and mash the beans as they cook in the skillet. Or you might find fat-free canned refried beans in the specialty foods section of your grocery store.

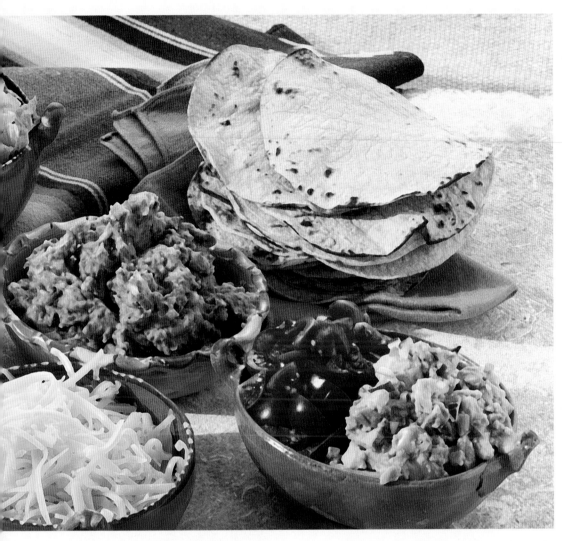

TIPS ON TORTILLAS

- Corn tortillas have fewer calories than flour tortillas because they aren't made with added fat. And corn tortillas can deliver another bonus: When they're made with lime, a calcium compound, they dish up a decent amount of this important mineral.
- Colored corn tortillas are made from corn kernels that grow in a rainbow of colors, most commonly blue and red. They are just as nutritious as regular corn tortillas. Some say that blue corn tortillas have a stronger corn flavor. In any case, they add to the festivity of a taco party.
- Crisp tortillas usually are fried, and that gives them about double the calorie count of a soft tortilla.

HEALTH TIP

Keep your total portion of cheese, chopped olives, and guacamole to no more than 4 tablespoons. While they add great flavor and texture to tacos, all are high in fat and calories.

parfait grabs you. If you've been packing a sandwich, take yourself out for lunch this week. If you've been following the *ChangeOne* dinner meal plans scrupulously, pull a couple of cookbooks down from your kitchen shelf and try out a few new recipes. Do a *ChangeOne* makeover of an old family standard. Throw a big dinner party. Take the family out for a lavish meal. Splurge on a dessert you haven't had for a while. Visit the local farmers' market or produce stand and take home something you've never tasted before.

Losing weight should never get in the way of enjoying new and interesting foods.

Giving yourself a little freedom doesn't mean putting your progress at risk. Last week you set up a first-alert system that will warn you if you get off track. Trust it. And trust your instincts to guide you. Gaining the confidence to make healthy choices is one of the measures of lasting success.

Not sure how to add excitement to the menu this week? Here are a few suggestions:

Make your own salad bar

For a family dinner one night this week, put together a salad bar and invite the crew to create their own salads. Include at least two vegetables that aren't usually on the menu—jicama, beets, radicchio, edamame, or artichoke hearts, for instance. Warm up a loaf of whole wheat or whole grain bread. For dessert, serve up a selection of colorful sorbets topped with berries.

Throw a taco party

As you've seen, tacos are a terrific way to serve up lots of vegetables—tomatoes, lettuce, grilled sweet peppers, and onions. Put all the ingredients out on the counter and let everyone make their own. Mix things up by using black beans instead of refried beans, help yourself to as much salsa as you want, don't forget to dab on some guacamole, and go easy on—or skip—the sour cream.

Slim down an old family friend

Choose a favorite casserole, pasta, or other dish and give it a boost by adding a serving of vegetables. Broccoli is terrific in tuna casserole. Garbanzo beans (also called chickpeas) make a great addition to spaghetti with tomato sauce. Green peppers can liven up, and lighten up, a bowl of chili. If fish sticks are a family favorite, serve them with a special salsa for added zest.

If you'd like, use a calorie-counter to tally up the precise calories in your makeover meal.

Order a feast of appetizers and sides

Choose a restaurant with a wide range of appetizers and vegetable sides and have a feast. Share the dishes with your dinner companions, and you can order practically every small dish on the menu without having to worry about portion sizes. Start with only as many dishes as there are people at the table. If you're still hungry, order more. Steer clear of fried foods, of course, and include plenty of vegetables.

Go fish

Chances are your local fish market features at least a few kinds of fish you haven't tried. Be adventurous and cook up something new for you—orange roughy, giant prawns, or mahi mahi, for instance. Choose a recipe that involves baking or grilling, not frying. There are many low-calorie ways to give fish a burst of exotic flavor. Many markets now offer spices that create the "blackened" flavor of traditional Cajun cooking, for instance. Spicy salsas or a scattering of capers are also terrific on fish.

Bake bread

As a special treat, take the time this weekend to bake your own loaf of bread. If you don't have a bread machine, consider investing in one. They simplify bread-making. Pop the ingredients in, head out on a couple of errands, and by the time you're back, the house will be filled with the aroma of fresh baked bread. Choose recipes that include whole wheat flour and, even better, whole grains like oats.

Have a pizza extravaganza

Most markets sell do-it-yourself pizza crusts that make preparing a homemade pizza fast and easy. Get a group together for a pizza party. Include at

Pasta Shapes and Sauces

Yes, everyone knows spaghetti goes with tomato-based sauce, but what about the rest of those noodles? In general, the lighter and more delicate the pasta, the lighter its sauce should be. Thicker or textured pastas go best with heavier and chunkier sauces. Here's a pairing of pasta shapes and sauces:

- Angel hair (thin spaghetti): light sauces.
- Conchiglie (shells): cheese-flavored sauces, and also good in soups.
- Farfalle (bow ties): chunky sauces.
- Fettuccine (ribbon): creamy sauces, tomato-based sauces.
- Fusilli (twisted spaghetti), ravioli (stuffed pillows), rotelle (spirals): chunky, tomato-based sauces.
- Macaroni (elbows), ziti and penne (hollow tubes): meat sauces.
- Tortellini (small stuffed dumplings): tomato-based sauces.

least two vegetable toppings. Use shredded cheese rather than slices, and you'll get more coverage with less cheese. Try smoked mozzarella instead of plain for more flavor.

Make a new acquaintance

It's easy to get into a rut, especially when you go shopping. This week look a little more closely at things you've been skipping in the produce section and take home a vegetable you haven't tried before. Many markets carry once exotic leafy greens like arugula, watercress, radicchio, and chard. Never tried jicama? Roasted fennel? A fresh artichoke? Then you're missing out on some of the world's great taste treats. This week add a new vegetable to your repertoire.

Create your own signature pasta

No other dish is as versatile as Italian pasta. Pasta itself comes in a wide range of shapes and colors, from familiar fettuccine to fun shapes like wagon wheels, bow ties, shells, corkscrews, tubes, and ears. And the ingredients that show up in pasta are virtually limitless—from shrimp or chicken to savory olives, artichokes, basil, diced ripe tomatoes, fava beans, tuna, capers, mushrooms, cauliflower, broccoli, Parmesan cheese...You get the idea. Put on your chef's hat this week, and create your own pasta masterpiece.

Travel the world

America's melting pot has created a rich variety of ethnic cuisines unmatched almost anywhere in the world, from Italian and French to Indian and Moroccan restaurants. This week sample a cuisine you haven't tried before, or at least one you don't eat very often. If you're an avid home cook, try preparing something from a cuisine you've never explored before. Check your library or local bookstore for a cookbook

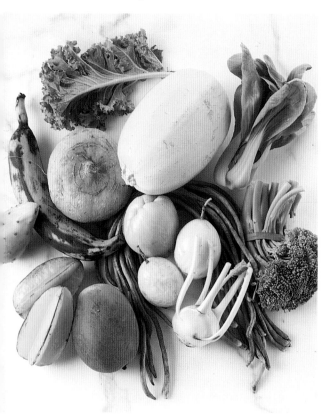

Colorful fruits and vegetables add pleasure to your plate. Clockwise from top: kale, spaghetti squash, bok choy, broccolini, long beans—wrapped around (from top to bottom): chayote, two passion fruit, and kohlrabi—mango, two starfruit, plantain, prickly pear, and kabocha squash.

that specializes in a particular ethnic cuisine. Chances are you'll discover a world of new ingredients and tastes.

Find a New Move

While you're shaking things up this week in the food department, do the same with exercise. The goal is simple: Find something fun to do this week that you haven't done before, something that involves being active. Take the plunge at the local pool. Go for a hike in a nearby park. Take the kids canoeing. Go power-walking at the local mall. If you haven't given the *ChangeOne* strengthening routines on pages 240-263 a try, do it this week.

And don't hide behind the excuse that you don't like being active. Don't tell us that you don't like strolling in a beautiful park, playing catch with the kids, walking past the shop windows downtown, or riding a bike around the neighborhood. Those are the kinds of activities that make life worth living.

Strike a Balance

ChangeOne is based on the simple principle that to lose weight, you have to take in fewer calories than you burn. To maintain your weight, you have to balance calories in and calories out.

That notion of striking a balance is a powerful one and worth keeping in mind as you move forward. As far as diet goes, there are many ways to build that healthy balance. One is to watch every bite you eat. Another, more relaxed way is to be aware of what you eat throughout the day, balancing a little indulgence here with a little restraint there.

If you treat yourself to a sumptuous brunch with friends, for instance, go light on supper and try to fit in extra exercise.

If there's a big birthday dinner planned in the evening, go easy on snacks and have a simple lunch.

As you've probably learned by now, one day of overdoing it on food doesn't mean the end of your diet. Cut back on portion sizes for the next day or two, and you'll be able to regain your balance. Even a week of overdoing it won't bring your diet crashing down. Naturally, people worry about the big holidays at the end of the year, when every occasion seems to center around food. The reality is you can enjoy yourself over the holidays without much danger of putting on a lot of weight.

It used to be held as a gospel truth that people typically gain about five pounds during the holidays. Not true, according to recent research from the National Institutes of Health, which tracked 200 men and women from late September through early March using weight and other health measurements. The average weight gain was about one pound. And it turns out that extra pound may have had less to do with eating than with exercise. People who said they weren't physically active during the roughly six months of the study typically gained about 1.5 pounds; those who stayed active through the cold winter months actually lost weight.

No, we're not advising you to throw caution to the wind when holidays or special occasions roll around. It's still important to make smart choices. Our point is that even a couple of weeks of eating more than usual aren't enough to topple your healthy diet. Become extra active, and you can counterbalance the extra food you eat. Even if you do gain weight, it's not likely to be that much. When you return to healthier habits as the holidays end, you'll regain your balance and steadily lose any weight you might have added.

Keep Your Perspective

There's one more way in which keeping your balance is important as you set off from here. You've already heard about the pitfalls of all-or-nothing thinking. It's the tendency to think that a diet is working as long as you're losing weight and that it has failed the moment you hit a plateau or gain a pound or two. It's the tendency of some people to think, the moment they slip up, "I'm a failure." All-or-nothing thinking doesn't acknowledge anything in between and is nothing more than a skewed perspective.

One thing we hope the *ChangeOne* approach has given you is a more balanced perspective on what it takes to lose weight and keep it off. It's not an all-or-nothing proposition. It's about the choices you make every day. If you go overboard on portions one day, you have the next to restore your balance. If your weight plateaus for a while, so be it. You haven't failed. The diet hasn't failed. You can give yourself a little time-out and then

One More Week at a Time

One of the things that has amazed us most as *ChangeOne* has grown has been the interest among participants for more weekly tasks. Many of us are successful at making one small change at a time and see no reason to stop after 12 weeks!

At changeone.com, members have the option of making one change per week for an entire year, and a surprising number of people do so. If you are the type who likes the discipline and rewards of weekly assignments, here are five more to try.

Conquer your cravings: This week, don't just resist your cravings, but figure out why you have them and try to deal with their root causes. Remember: Hunger doesn't have food preferences; if you are craving a particular flavor or food, it's your mind talking, not your stomach!

Eat by color: This week, make sure that you eat three different colors at every meal, and that a day doesn't go by in which you don't eat some red (peppers, tomatoes, apples) and orange (carrots, oranges, cantaloupe), plus plenty of green. There's no better indication that you are eating healthily than having a diversity of color on your plate. The brighter, the better, assuming it's natural coloring!

Get on your feet: Exercise is great, but that doesn't permit you to be sedentary the rest of the time. This week, stand as much as you can—when you are on the phone, reading the newspaper, peeling onions. Get used to being up and moving, rather than sitting.

Laugh it off: With a positive attitude, you can conquer anything! And what better indicator of your attitude than the amount of laughter in your day? This week, monitor your laughing and pursue lots more of it. If you don't have 10 or 15 good laughs in a day, you've got some unserious work to do!

Master your liquids: For the first few days of the week, log everything you drink in a day. Then review it for two things—are you drinking enough, and are you drinking the right stuff? A healthy day of drink would include at least eight glasses of water, a glass of milk, a glass of wine, perhaps a juice in the morning, and one or two cups of tea or coffee. Soda should be treated like candy—a sweet treat that falls in the snack or dessert category.

make another change or two when you feel ready. If you gain a few pounds when things at work or home are stressful, no big deal. You know what it takes to lose it again. The only way to fail is to decide that you've failed—and to give up.

Keep that in mind as you relax a little this week and move into the weeks beyond, and you'll be just fine. You've got what it takes to do almost anything you want. Just take it one step at a time. Keep your spirits up and your resolution firm. Stay positive. Have as much fun as you can. If you hit a rocky stretch, go easy on yourself. Set your sights on a new goal. Figure out the best ways to get there. And go for it!

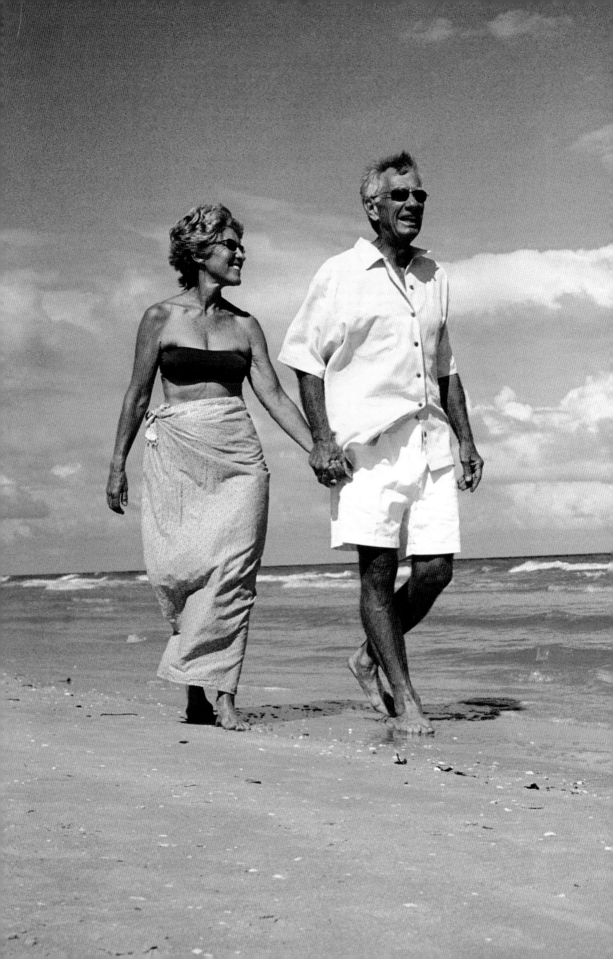

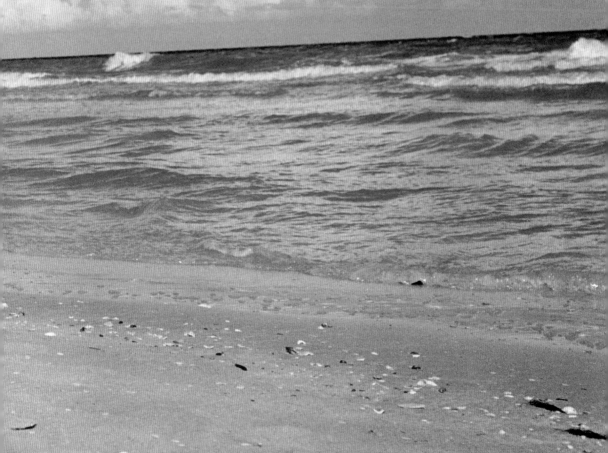

Part 2

Change
One

Fitness

The Truth About
Fitness

Consider the strange history of Product X. By all rights, it should be a huge success: Everybody needs it, and most have tried it—over and over again. Yet 8 in 10 people say that they simply can't use Product X, no matter how hard they try.

In the business world, X's spectacular failure would be blamed on the product, not the customers. But what if we told you that Product X is actually *exercise*? Surprised? Don't be. We firmly believe that a big reason 80 percent of us have given up on exercise is the sweaty, competitive, numbers-driven, "no pain, no gain," testosterone-pumped definition of exercise that the fitness industry has pushed upon us.

It doesn't have to be that way. In this chapter, you'll learn to forget about athletes, supermodels, sports drink commercials, and national health-club chains.

The *ChangeOne* approach to fitness is 100 percent natural, fun, and easy. Try it, and you'll never look at exercise the same way again.

Traditional Fitness: For Jocks Only

There's a good reason why most exercise routines—and most gyms—make you feel as if you've suddenly, inexplicably signed up for high school football or time-traveled back to phys ed class with your school's most notorious drill sergeant as a teacher. The fact is, most exercise programs are based on the old sports-team model of getting into shape: Lots of grunting and perspiration...lifting heavy weights until your muscles shake...pushing your body hard and then even harder... constantly measuring results and striving for improvements that can be expressed in numbers...workouts that involve counting repetitions and watching the clock and constantly checking your heart rate...competition, with others and yourself...odd clothing you'd never wear on the street...routines that must be performed in special places—certainly not at home with the kids, with a friend, or while you do the dishes! Anything less, this model asserts, just isn't fitness.

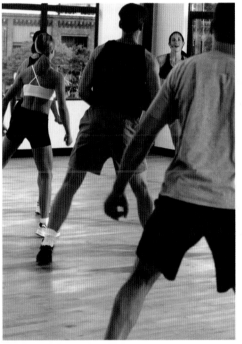

This approach may assure victory on the gridiron for Homecoming Day—and it's a good fit for a small percentage of athletically inclined women and men. But for most of us, it's beyond useless. It hurts. It's boring. It's time-consuming. It's punishing. Whatever the reason, it's just the wrong approach.

But if you want to exercise—to lose weight, get healthier, boost your energy, or for any other reason—it has long been the only "official" way. Even the government has gotten in on it, putting forth an official, national standard for fitness based entirely on formal exercise sessions and all types of measurements and exertion thresholds.

So you try it. You sweat and grunt—and eventually, you stop. And you probably feel pretty guilty about it, too.

You're not alone. At least two million Americans join health clubs each January (more than at any other time of year except perhaps in the month or two before swimsuit season). But

Casual Wins

If your workplace allows you to come to work dressed casually, take advantage of it—you just might lose more weight. When University of Wisconsin researchers checked the activity levels of 53 women and men who wore pedometers to work, they found that the number of steps they took—and calories they burned—increased significantly on casual days.

Study participants took an average of 491 (or 8 percent) more steps on casual days. Over the course of a year, that could translate into burning an extra 6,250 calories—and help you lose (or offset the gain of) nearly 2 pounds.

only one in five keeps going to the gym for more than a month or two. (There go hundreds of dollars, lost to an unused gym membership!)

What's more, just 20 percent of Americans are physically active on a regular basis, leaving 80 percent of us at home on the couch, despite the fact that we know darned well that activity is crucial to weight loss and better health. So why aren't we out there exercising? A recent poll by the President's Council on Physical Fitness and Sports found that 40 percent of Americans say they don't have enough time, 20 percent say they get enough exercise at work or at home (we think those people are on to something!), 15 percent can't exercise due to health problems, 12 percent say exercise is boring, 10 percent believe they're too old, 9 percent think exercise isn't necessary, and 7 percent are too tired.

The usual reaction from fitness experts? Get over it! Get out there! Go! Go! Go!

So you go, go, go for a while...and stop again. And maybe you start feeling as if *you* have failed at fitness—as if maybe you *don't* have a natural-born right to a toned, healthy, happy body. Which, of course, you do. Because the truth is, fitness has failed *you*.

Natural Exercise

ChangeOne says it's time not for a new gung-ho attitude but for a completely new definition of fitness.

Stroll into a summer morning, alive with birdsong and the scents of blooming flowers. Slowly strengthen and stretch your muscles until you feel as lithe as a Siamese cat. Park as far from the supermarket as possible and smile as you walk to get your cart—you've just added some secret, calorie-burning activity to your day. Swim, sail, garden, or play with the kids this weekend, secure in the knowledge that simply enjoying yourself under the blue dome of the sky is good for your mind, body, and spirit.

Your Fitness Attitude

How do you define fitness, and is that definition helping or hurting you? To find out, answer these questions as honestly as you can and keep a record of your answers.

1. If there were a gym within a short walking distance from where I live, I would:
- a. Still not join; I just don't like gyms.
- b. Probably join, but not use it much. Who has time?
- c. Be there all the time.

2. I find that doing the same exercise routine over and over again is:
- a. Boring, of course.
- b. Okay for a short time, but then I try to vary things.
- c. The proper approach; practice makes perfect, after all.

3. In high school, gym was:
- a. My least favorite class.
- b. Occasionally fun, particularly when we were doing a sport or activity I liked.
- c. One of the classes I most looked forward to.

4. I have played on this many organized sports teams in my life:
- a. Very few, if any, unless you count neighborhood kickball games.
- b. A fair number over the years, but never very competitively.
- c. Loads, and some were highly competitive.

5. My favorite vigorous activity is:
- a. Gardening or fixing up my house.
- b. Hiking, cruising on a bike, or some other outdoor pastime.
- c. Running, working out with weights, or playing a high-intensity sport.

6. My attitude toward sweating is:
- a. It's a miserable feeling that I try to avoid.
- b. I don't mind it on occasion when I'm outdoors and in the right clothes.
- c. I love it—it means I'm being active, healthy, and alive.

7. We keep the following in our home for strengthening exercises:
- a. Nothing really, unless you count a lawn mower or hammer.
- b. A few dumbbells or other basic exercise tools.
- c. A weight-lifting bench, a barbell set, and more.

8. When I see world-class weightlifters competing on television, I think:
- a. What a waste of a person's life.
- b. Definitely not for me, but I respect their achievements.
- c. If only I could get to the gym more...

9. When I'm on a bicycle, I like to:
- a. Chitchat, look at the world around me, and make frequent stops.
- b. Have a mildly strenuous but mostly pleasant ride to a nearby destination.
- c. Put my head down and go, go, go.

10. When I see a TV commercial for a sports drink that features overachieving athletes, I think:
- a. This is gross!
- b. Clever marketing, but not for me.
- c. I've gotta try that!

Turn to next page to continue quiz.

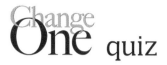

11. My idea of a good time in a swimming pool is:

a. Dozing while lying on a float.

b. Playing games in the shallow end with the kids.

c. Swimming laps, having races, and making up competitions.

12. I know the following statistics about my fitness level:

a. Not a thing, but ask me about the Yankees.

b. I know my basic medical numbers—my weight, pulse rate, Body Mass Index—but not much else.

c. A lot; I monitor things like my daily step count, heart rate, maximum weight levels I can lift, and more.

Score

Give yourself 1 point for (a.) answers, 2 points for (b.) answers, and 3 points for (c.) answers. Tally up your score and check below to find out where your fitness attitude falls.

12-15: Anti-exercise. Not only don't you exercise much, you also have a negative attitude about fitness. You sorely need a new, more positive mind-set. The *ChangeOne* approach is perfect for you, since it will slowly get you moving in easy, fun ways that won't intrude much on your everyday life.

16-22: Apathetic. You aren't anti-exercise, but you probably don't think about it much and don't worry about getting it into your life. *ChangeOne* will help you see why exercise is important to health and weight and show you that getting the amount you need won't require much effort at all.

23-28: Healthy. You understand the benefits of active living and probably enjoy the outdoors, but you aren't committed to formal exercise regimens. *ChangeOne* is great for you in that it will inject a little routine into your efforts, making sure you get all the fun and movement you need on a daily basis for health and weight loss.

29-36: Athletic. You are quite comfortable in the world of exercise and sports and enjoy the rigors and benefits of formal workout routines. *ChangeOne* is still very useful to you, though, because it will broaden your perspective on fitness and show you how to integrate movement into your entire day.

Welcome to *ChangeOne* Fitness! We feel that physical activity is far too important to leave to traditional sports-based workouts alone. We have a new, more natural way to help you get the benefits of physical activity, without the need to work out like a jock.

But first, let us not deny that exercise is crucial for health—and a healthy weight. After all, activity is *the* most effective way to boost your metabolism (so your body burns more calories all day and night, even while you sleep). Regular exercise turns flabby fat into sleek and shapely muscle. It burns calories, helping you lose weight and keep it off. It boosts energy, increases your overall attitude, and, when done right, is a whole lot more fun than watching weeknight television.

ChangeOne Fitness lets you get all the benefits of exercise in just a half hour a day, plus about 2 hours of fun time on the weekend. The components of our plan:

A brisk daily walk: Your target is 20 minutes a day—long enough to kick your body's fat-burning power into action, yet short enough to fit into your lunch break or to be an after-dinner activity. This is the fat-blasting part of the plan.

More daily activity: You'll discover dozens of ways to add extra steps and movements to your day—from parking at the far end of the company lot to washing the dishes by hand—and see how they can add up to a significant calorie burn. This part of the plan helps you replace activity that's slowly been erased from daily life over the past 50 years—one of the reasons Americans weigh more now than in the past.

Outdoor fun: Clear your Saturday morning or Sunday afternoon schedule; we want to see you having fun in nature for 2 hours a week. Get the kids outdoors for touch football; rake leaves, then have a fall barbecue; take a hike; go to the beach. What you choose is up to you. We just know that moving and having fun out in sunshine, fresh air, and natural surroundings is happiness defined. You'll feel more alive—and ready to get out there again soon!

Muscles Aren't Fat!

Lots of fitness experts warn that if you stop exercising, your muscles will "become" fat. That's not true. Inactivity allows muscles to shrink, leaving room for larger fat deposits, but the cellular makeup of the muscles themselves doesn't change. Good news: Experts say you don't have to join a gym to hold on to precious muscle. Vigorous everyday activities, from walking Fido to sweeping the porch to cutting the lawn with a push mower instead of a tractor, is usually enough to maintain muscle density.

Strengthening and stretching: Just *10 minutes a day* will help you build sleek, high-metabolism muscle. You'll lose fat faster, keep it off more easily, and get strong and confident. And—ahh!—our stretches will pamper your body, relieving aches and pains and helping to build flexibility. This component helps protect and rebuild muscle lost to aging and to reduced-calorie eating, and it can help keep you from getting stuck on a weight-loss plateau.

Sound too good to be true? Too easy to work? In fact, a growing stack of research proves that this smart plan works *better* for most of us than heavy-duty workouts.

Smarter Fitness

Don't be cowed by the snobbery of the weight room or the über-confidence of the regulars in that fancy-footwork aerobics class. You can take the *ChangeOne* Fitness plan seriously—we do!—because it's amazingly effective. Research proves the benefits:

■ *Slow and steady means better results:* Moderation burns more calories, say researchers at Maastricht University in the Netherlands. When they compared the fitness levels of people who participated in moderate physical activity, such as walking and biking, with those who exercised vigorously, they found that those who exercised vigorously for short periods of time made up for their efforts by spending more time being inactive the rest of the day. In contrast, the moderate exercisers tended to be more active overall.

■ *A lean, sexy figure:* You'll replace fat with muscle in just 10 minutes a day. Don't worry about bulking up: You won't. In fact, it'll be the opposite. Muscle tissue takes up much less space than fat tissue, and our exercises are gentle in nature, meaning they create lean, not bulky, muscles.

■ *An energy boost:* We're bowled over by the number of studies showing that simple, easy activities supercharge your energy level. For example, one study found that a 10-minute

Be a Better Lover

One of the most exciting, though least discussed, benefits of physical activity is that it pays big dividends in bed. Studies show that exercise can:

- Help you feel more sexually desirable and experience greater levels of satisfaction.
- Cut the risk of impotence.
- Boost circulation for better potency and orgasms.
- Cut stress and boost your spirits so you'll be in the mood.

ChangeOne versus Traditional Exercise Programs

Here's how *ChangeOne* helps you overcome the most daunting exercise roadblocks and how traditional exercise programs handle the same issues.

ROADBLOCK: I don't have time.
Traditional approach: Make time! Fitness is important!
ChangeOne **approach:** Do everyday activities and super-short routines.

ROADBLOCK: It hurts!
Traditional approach: No pain, no gain.
ChangeOne **approach:** You may feel a little sore, but fitness should *never* hurt.

ROADBLOCK: I'm too tired.
Traditional approach: Do it anyway.
ChangeOne **approach:** Just do a little—you'll be energized!

ROADBLOCK: It's boring.
Traditional approach: Keep doing the same routines; just change the exercises.
ChangeOne **approach:** Choose activities you like.

ROADBLOCK: I'm not in the mood.
Traditional approach: Do it anyway.
ChangeOne **approach:** Not ready for your walk? Garden instead!

---

walk gives you more energy than eating a chocolate bar, because exercise increases levels of an energy-boosting hormone. Other studies show that people who begin exercise programs greatly increase their physical activity around the clock and also are more likely to take up new hobbies and pursuits.

■ *Efficient weight loss:* Combining *ChangeOne* Fitness with our diet plan guarantees faster, easier weight loss. The proof? When 24 overweight women walked three times a week and followed a reduced-calorie diet similar to *ChangeOne*, they lost 8 percent of their body weight—and their body fat fell by an amazing 15 percent, meaning they had replaced flabby fat with lean, calorie-burning muscle. Wow!

■ *Staying skinny for life:* By increasing the amount of muscle in your body, our 10-minutes-a-day strengthening plan also revs up your metabolism. That means your body burns more calories around the clock, no matter what you are doing!

■ *More calorie burn without exercising:* Fifty years ago, Americans burned about 700 more calories per day than we do today—not by running marathons but via a host of daily activities that we've engineered out of our lives, from rolling down car windows by hand to washing the dishes. We'll show you how to put activity back into your days—a move that burns hundreds of calories more than you could in a formal exercise program. In fact, adding "lifestyle activity" keeps weight off more successfully than formal exercise classes, say University of Pennsylvania researchers who compared the body weights of women in a step aerobics class with those who simply fit more activity into each day.

■ *Natural happiness:* We often spend 20 to 23 hours per day being inactive—in the car, at work, watching TV, eating meals, sleeping. We'll show you how to get outdoors, have fun, and once again feel the happiness that comes from time spent in fresh air and sunshine amid flowers and trees.

■ *A graceful, ache-free body:* Each of our strengthening routines ends with a couple of refreshing stretches. These are more than feel-good moves (although stretching can help you relax, physically and mentally). Stretching makes muscles more flexible and increases your range of motion.

Getting Started

As you can see, *ChangeOne* Fitness isn't about formal exercise sessions a few times a week. It's a lifestyle, meaning it's part of each and every day. It's choosing to stand rather than sit and to walk rather than stand. It's about bounding up stairs with energy rather than taking the elevator and leaning sleepily against the mirrored walls inside. It's starting the morning with a 10-minute, in-your-pajamas workout that revs you up for the rest of the day rather than staring blankly at the morning news while the coffee brews. It's about getting outdoors in the evening rather than watching nature shows on TV. None of that requires workout clothes, a gym membership, a personal trainer, or sports drinks.

And like the *ChangeOne* approach to eating, this change in your fitness personality is best achieved one small step at a time. We haven't broken down this section into a 12-week plan, because one such program is enough to follow. But you know what to do—first, focus on walking. Once that becomes a regular habit, try to increase your time outdoors. When that's working, take on the daily 10-minute workout. Along the way, whenever you have a chance to be up and moving, do so!

Most people think that exercise makes you tired, but the opposite is true—the more you get, the *less* tired you feel. If you've been reading the *ChangeOne* success stories, you've probably noticed how almost every person has mentioned that the combination of more exercise and less weight has made them more energized—so stop using "I don't have the energy" as an excuse for not getting up and moving. The moment you can overcome the urge to sit, you will begin a wonderful journey back to the energy and weight you so desire.

One caveat: If you're over age 40 and have had a sedentary lifestyle, or you have a chronic health condition, talk with your doctor before starting the *ChangeOne* program. She may want to check you out to make sure everything is in working order. She will probably advise you to go easy but definitely to start exercising. That's because easy fitness can help a wide range of conditions.

Read through the chapters ahead and get started! *ChangeOne* Fitness, you'll discover, will bring a surprising amount of fun and relaxation into your life. And your weight-loss efforts will go so much easier!

Get Ready for
Action

A mystic once said that every journey begins with a single step. This is literally true with *ChangeOne* Fitness, which begins with nothing more complicated than walking. But before you take that first step toward fitness, take the *ChangeOne* quiz on the next page.

We'll show you how to use your answers to create an active lifestyle that you'll love, full of pleasure, energy, and easy moves guaranteed to get results.

As you start your *ChangeOne* Fitness journey, you may remember past exercise attempts that fizzled, plans that sounded great but just didn't fit into your life, activities that seemed promising but were in reality no fun at all. This journey will be different—we promise—because you'll tailor it to suit your fitness level, your personality, and even your secret hopes and dreams.

Change One quiz
What's Your Starting Point?

1. **On a typical Saturday afternoon, I'm:**
   a. Watching the game on TV or otherwise deepening the depression in my chair.
   b. Working in the yard, playing golf, or doing something else active.
   c. Watching the kids' soccer or baseball game or driving around to do my errands.

2. **If I walked briskly for 15 minutes, I would feel:**
   a. Invigorated and ready for another lap.
   b. A little pooped, but still able to hold a conversation.
   c. Like someone knocked the wind out of me.

3. **I would rate my strength as:**
   a. Not what it used to be; the grocery bags seem to weigh a ton, and I think twice before picking up children.
   b. Pretty darn good; I could lift a bag of potting soil or carry luggage.
   c. Embarrassing; when I get out of a chair, I have to push off using the armrests.

4. **My attitude about exercise is:**
   a. Ugh! I get flashbacks to junior high gym class.
   b. It's a waste of closet space; my house is jammed with dusty exercise bikes, treadmills, and thigh slimmers.
   c. Once I get going, I know it will feel good.

5. **I enjoy physical activity most when it's:**
   a. Playful; if I'm feeling the wind in my hair, moving to my favorite tunes or throwing a ball with my kids, I'm happy.
   b. Practical; if it gets the house cleaned, or the car washed, I'll do it.
   c. Barely noticeable; I'd rather sneak it in while socializing or watching TV.

   d. Competitive; nothing motivates me like winning.

6. **When I was a kid, I loved:**
   a. Competition; whether it was backyard baseball, kickball, or touch football, I was in on the action.
   b. Adventure; I liked to explore, climb trees, swim, skate, and walk on stilts.
   c. Fantasy and fairy wings; I loved to dance, create, and pretend.

7. **My average day is:**
   a. Fairly leisurely, with plenty of holes in my schedule.
   b. Sometimes hectic, but I can usually break for lunch.
   c. Crazy; once the day gets going, there's no time to stop.

8. **My biggest fear about exercising is:**
   a. It will tire me out.
   b. I'll get big and bulky.
   c. I won't be able to do it.

9. **My top secret wish about exercising is:**
   a. That I'll be able to eat everything I want.
   b. That I'll spot-reduce my tummy, waist, hips, or thighs.
   c. That I'll look and feel like I did 10 years ago.

Score

As we're sure you figured out, there are no right or wrong answers. But to help interpret your answers, the rest of this chapter offers advice and guidance based on each of these nine questions. Armed with this information, you'll be in a much better position to get moving, *ChangeOne* style.

Set Aside Your Doubts

What is stopping you from starting up a daily walk? From turning off the TV and going outside? From trying a little stretching? Sure, some of it is lack of knowledge—you want to know the right way to exercise—but for most of us, the obstacles are things like lack of time, or fear, or ingrained habits and daily patterns that don't include exercise. The following tips will help convince you that it's time to reject all those internal arguments against exercise and finally get started.

1 Weekends too busy for fun?
Fix your schedule—and your attitude.
More everyday movement, more outdoor fun—those are the simple tenets behind *ChangeOne* Fitness. Saturdays are the perfect times to be outside, having a good time. So make a commitment to it: From 10 A.M. to noon, it's fun time. Or 3 to 5 P.M.; whenever works. If you spend your Saturdays doing errands and chores, learn to get these tasks done on weekday evenings. If you're a sports watcher, either learn to record broadcasts to watch later or set a goal: For each hour spent watching a game, you spend an hour outside being active. If you're at a child's sporting event or practice, get up, walk around, and be playful while you cheer. Your kids are having fun on this beautiful Saturday and so should you! You'll find more ideas for getting active throughout the following chapters.

2 Not ready for vigorous walking?
Start slow and smart.
The key to successful exercise, for *every* fitness level, is to exert yourself based entirely on your current capabilities, and from there, progress *slowly* but steadily. If you plunge into some crazy exercise regimen, the odds are high that you'll throw in the towel in no time. Remember, exercise is never an all-or-nothing proposition. With *ChangeOne* Fitness, it's simply about adding more movement to the life you're already leading.

Whether you are an experienced, super-fit walker or a first-time fitness walker coming off a long period of sedentary living, your exertion level is the same: Walk at a speed and for a distance at which you feel you are breathing a little heavily, but you can still hold a conversation. Whether you reach that point during a slow 10-minute stroll or an arm-churning, hour-long power walk, it's the right pace for *you*.

From there, slowly build up the length and intensity of your activities. If you're already fit, look for small ways to take things up a notch. This approach isn't wimpy—it's super-smart. In a recent study of 78 inactive people, those who set small, doable exercise targets (in this case, adding just a bit more walking to their days) were three times more likely to stick with it than superambitious types who started with Everest-size goals.

You probably don't need to check with your doctor before beginning our gentle fitness program. However, if you take medication for high blood pressure or a heart condition; feel extremely breathless or dizzy after a little activity; develop pain or pressure in your chest, neck, shoulder, or arm after exercising; or have a bone or joint problem or a chronic medical condition such as diabetes, do consult your doctor first.

3 Consider yourself too stiff or weak for muscle-strengthening exercises?
Start easy and give it a few weeks.

As we keep saying, *ChangeOne* Fitness isn't about achieving someone else's idea of acceptable strength. You are accountable only to *you*. Don't be hard on yourself if you have fallen out of shape—as we said in the last chapter, 80 percent of Americans are in the same position, thanks in good part to a fitness industry gone haywire. Just start easy and progress slowly.

Remember too that muscle strength and flexibility naturally diminish as we get older. When we don't exercise, the results start to show themselves in everyday ways: big and little aches, trouble bending and stretching, a harder time picking up a full bag of groceries or a gallon of milk. *ChangeOne* Fitness will help you gradually reverse that decline with our daily 10-minute stretching and strengthening program. After a few weeks, you'll begin to discover a sleeker, fitter, stronger you, minus the aches and pains. The bonus: More muscle mass means your body burns more calories 24/7, so it will become easier to lose weight and keep it off. But reject the old philosophy of "no pain, no gain." If an exercise hurts, skip it. If you're very sore afterward, take it easier next time.

4 Had too many bad experiences with fitness?
Think enjoyment, not punishment.
Forget about that whistle-blowing gym teacher, those get-fit-quick gimmicks, and those overexuberant aerobics classes you tried years ago. *ChangeOne* Fitness is based on a new definition of exercise: fitting fun, pleasure, and natural movement into every day. Translation: Gardening, playing with the kids, walking the dog, and catching up with a friend as you stroll through a gorgeous summer morning all count! And we promise, you'll never have to wear skin tight Spandex or do jumping jacks.

Why our way works: You'll get hooked on enjoying movement, and you'll see results. In a four-year study of 124 overweight women and men, National Institutes of Health researchers discovered that people who tried fitting short periods of exercise into their days or getting a half hour of "lifestyle activity" such as gardening, heavy cleaning, or walking the dog daily lost as much weight as those who signed up for a traditional aerobics class—and they were more likely to still be fit a year later.

5 Have unique exercise likes and dislikes?
Work with your personality.
Just as our tastes in spouses, friends, and spaghetti sauces aren't all the same, neither are our activity likes and dislikes. With *ChangeOne* Fitness, the idea is to move your body more, no matter how. If you enjoy group fitness classes, go for it. If the idea of bouncing or bending in front of 12 other people mortifies you, get on your bike instead. Need to see concrete results to feel good? You'll discover how to turn everyday chores into calorie-burning mini-routines. Like to do good in the world? Find ways to add a higher pur-pose to your activities, such as walking to raise money for your favorite charity.

If you're a true TV addict, get your exercise by dusting off that treadmill-turned-clothes-hanger and walking while you watch, or do the 10-minute exercise routines starting on page 240. (We still want you to turn off the tube once in a while and get outside, though.) Always have a phone to your ear? Get a cell phone with a headset and move while you gab. The point is that fitness shouldn't be work, but it should work for you.

6 Forgotten the pleasures of active fun?
Return to your childhood.
The key to succeeding in business is also the key to succeeding at exercise: Do what you love. If you're not sure what that is anymore, then try doing what you *used to* love as a child. That could mean bike rides, basketball, dancing, tennis, or merely walking in the woods. Recapturing childhood joy adds excitement and "can't wait to do it again" enthusiasm to your new active lifestyle. If you loved the competition and camaraderie of team sports, look for an amateur league to join. Are you an explorer at heart? Discover new worlds by joining a local kayaking or canoeing club or planning an adventure vacation with a hiking or walking group. Have the soul of an artist? Express yourself by learning how to rumba or belly dance. The bottom line: Get in touch with what makes you tick, and you'll never run out of batteries.

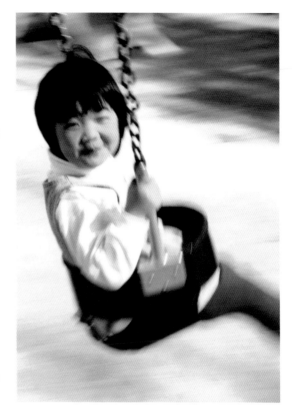

7 Don't have time in your day for exercise?
Start by finding just a few minutes here and there.
Fitness, particularly the *ChangeOne* Fitness approach, can work with *any* schedule. If you're the type who can take a break, relax for a few minutes, and then get back to work, you may find that short bursts of activity are perfect for you. (How about a brisk stroll around the office parking lot?) If there's no time to stop once you get going, fit in a 20-minute walk in the morning, before the craziness begins. You'll be energized for the day and have a sense of accomplishment before you've even turned on your computer or started your first task. And if the day just never stops, consider using that lovely, golden hour after dinner for a stroll around the neighborhood—imagine you're taking an old-fashioned Italian *passeggiata,* or evening stroll—or an hour of gardening.

Still struggling? Then you need to analyze your time more carefully. What is it that's taking up 16 hours of waking time a day? Is there TV time that can be sacrificed or half of a lunch or dinner hour? Can you hold one-on-one discussions at work while walking? Is there a way to alter your commute times so you aren't in the car during peak driving hours? All you need to start is 10 minutes a day for our strengthening and stretching program, along with moments here and there for brisk walking. Make it a priority, and you will succeed in finding the time.

8 Intimidated by the prospect of daily exercise?
We understand, but you can overcome it.
When the American Council on Exercise asked 1,500 certified personal trainers to name the top fitness myths, three answers to question 8 topped the list. Afraid you'll be tired? The truth is, activity boosts energy in several ways. It cuts stress, improves sleep, and helps your body better use the oxygen, blood sugar, and fat it burns for energy. Will you bulk up? Only if you embark on a Schwarzenegger-style bodybuilding routine. (And if that's what you want, you're reading the wrong book!) Afraid you won't be able to keep up or won't have the time? *ChangeOne* Fitness is meant to work with your schedule, your personality, and your fitness level. You'll never ever feel as if you can't do it. That's a promise.

9 Worried that you might fail?
Right-size your expectations.
It's better to have modest hopes and be pleasantly surprised by your progress than to have wild expectations and lose heart when they don't pan out. Unless you run marathons, you won't be able to eat with wild abandon—but you *will* be able to indulge occasionally without seeing the results on your butt, belly, or thighs. That's because exercising burns more calories than sitting still, and it increases your metabolism slightly.

Can a fitness routine magically shrink one body part? Probably not. Expect to look sleeker all over as you firm up your flab and trim body fat. Doing extra tummy, hip, or leg exercises could make muscles in those areas tighter more quickly, but it can't banish fat selectively.

If your big hope is to look and feel younger, you're in luck. Exercise literally turns back the clock. In one amazing study at the University of Texas Southwestern Medical Center at Dallas, five out-of-shape, middle-aged guys who exercised for just six months became as fit as they'd been in their twenties. Who wouldn't want to feel like a 20-something again?

Exercising Her Way to Success

Although she wasn't an avid exerciser before she started *ChangeOne*, Donna Westog has made physical activity part of her daily routine. The results have been spectacular.

"The weight just fell off me," she says. Already down 46½ pounds, she's well on her way to her goal of 125 pounds.

Being active has made a huge difference for Donna. "If you expect to lose weight and become healthier—get moving! I make sure I get some form of exercise or physical activity in daily. Since I began *ChangeOne*, I've only missed a total of seven days."

Donna's latest toy is a new treadmill. "I just love it!" she says. "I still walk outside whenever possible, but with the treadmill, I am now working toward running and am training to run a 5K. This is something I never, ever dreamed of doing before *ChangeOne*. I have a marathon-running brother who is hoping someday I'll join him. We'll see!"

The portion-control tips have also been extremely helpful to Donna. "I have discovered how much food I *don't* have to give up as long as I am watchful of portions," she says.

Donna confesses that she can't take all the credit for her success with *ChangeOne*. She gets a lot of advice and

Donna Westog lost more than 46 pounds by getting some form of physical activity every day.

encouragement from friends on the ChangeOne.com message boards. "I never could have gotten this far without their support," she says.

She advises people on *ChangeOne* to be patient. "Just change one thing at a time, and you will become a healthier person—and thinner, too! Your extra weight did *not* come on overnight—don't expect it to come off that quickly. So many think that the pounds will magically disappear! It takes a ton of hard work and discipline, but this plan is so great."

For more ChangeOne *success stories, go to www.changeone.com/successstories*

9 Tips for Fitness Success

For every 10 people who begin a fitness program, as many as 7 will drop out in less than six months. Here are ways to help you from contributing to the dropout statistics.

Start Slowly

1 The *ChangeOne* philosophy is the same whether you apply it to healthy eating or to fitness: Make just one small change at a time! That's the best way to guarantee that the changes you make will become permanent. So while we hope you ultimately adopt all of the *ChangeOne* Fitness tenets, focus on only one at a time. Even then, start slowly. Remember: You are making changes that should last the rest of your life. Don't rush them.

Avoid Boredom

2 It's among the top reasons people drop out of exercise regimens; after all, who wants to be bored? Take it upon yourself to keep things fresh. Vary your walking route or work in new activities to keep your routine fun and different. Do your usual walk in reverse, go biking next week instead of walking, stop and investigate outdoor places and activities that have always piqued your interest.

Surround Yourself with Support

3 Some people can stay more committed if they have a regular fitness partner. In one study that tracked 309 people for two years, those who had a support group lost 30 percent more weight than those who dieted alone. If you can find someone who shares your enthusiasm and exercises at the same pace and for the same length of time as you do, you'll be more likely to stick with your plan—and have fun along the way. And remember: Think beyond just close friends, coworkers, and family members. An online group, a hiking club, or a gym or exercise class may offer just the support you're looking for. Most important, end up with an arrangement that helps you succeed. If you're a loner, having a partner could hurt, but having someone cheering you on might help. Be true to your personality.

Dress for Success

4 There's no reason to spend money on specialized workout clothes for the *ChangeOne* Fitness program. Comfortable pants or shorts and a top made from breathable material such as cotton will do just fine. In fact, you don't even need to change your clothes for most *ChangeOne* Fitness activities. But if you do, make sure they are clothes you love to be in. Clothing should motivate you, not embarrass or irritate you.

Fuel Up

5 Nothing takes the pleasure out of an activity more than running out of energy. Too little water or too little food beforehand can make that happen, so be sure you're hydrated and not hungry before you start out. If you think you'll be exerting yourself, have a large glass of water and a healthy snack 30 minutes before starting. If you're active for more than 30 minutes, be sure to drink more water every 15 to 20 minutes.

Adopt a New Attitude

6 Be a little selfish about your exercise time: Schedule it, commit to it, and protect it by gently reminding intruders—including your spouse and children—that sorry, but you're busy doing something important and that exercise is a priority you'll be sticking with. Do the same at work. Don't let peer pressure force you to eat lunch with the usual gang when you've planned to be outside walking. And don't feel guilty! In fact, be proud of your new priorities. You may not realize it, but you're being a role model for your friends and family, and perhaps some of them will soon follow in your footsteps.

Celebrate Fitness Success

7 Sure, you're paying attention to your weight-loss achievements. Ultimately, that's what *ChangeOne* is for. But as you progress down the fitness path, you're probably going to want to monitor progress directly related to the exercise. Consider keeping an exercise journal to note your personal observations, and think about monitoring your energy levels, body measurements, sleep patterns, or sports performance—anything that would improve as a direct result of your new exercise patterns. When you show improvement, as you inevitably will, reward yourself!

Work With—Not Against—Your Body

9 Elsewhere in this chapter, we talk about respecting your personal likes and dislikes when it comes to choosing activities. You also need to respect your unique physical limitations. For example, if a physical condition makes it difficult for you to walk, there are many other wonderful ways to keep moving for 20 minutes, whether swimming or using a rowing machine or merely doing calisthenics in a chair. Similarly, chronic conditions such as arthritis or back pain can limit your mobility. Respect that, and find movements you *can* do and enjoy. What's crucial is that you don't use physical limitations as an excuse not to get moving.

Just as important, play to your physical strengths. If you have strong legs, resume a hiking or biking regimen. If you have strong arms, there are plenty of sports, such as tennis and softball, that are great for you. Are you naturally graceful? Sign up for a dance class. With *ChangeOne,* it's not the specific activity that matters; just that you are active. Improvise as necessary for your unique needs.

Stay Motivated

8 Goals, treats, inspiration, fun, and lots of positive self-coaching can help you stick with your new fitness plan. There are many ways to do this: Get a portable music player and load it with upbeat music so you can have fun listening whenever you're on the go; create an inspiration wall from a bulletin board or poster board to display logs of your improving health statistics, photos of you as you slim down, and other motivating photos or quotes; constantly keep up the positive self-talk ("I can do it!") and ban negative self-talk ("I can't do it"); and give yourself nice rewards (a book, a movie, earrings) for reaching small thresholds, such as five consecutive days of walking or getting through the entire strengthening sequence for the first time.

Get Walking

Stride along on a sunny morning alive with birdsong. Take a lap around the mall before hitting the clearance sales. Walk to the neighborhood mailbox instead of leaving your letter in your own box. Opportunities to walk are endless, and that's exactly the point.

Walking is the most natural, intuitive, and practical form of exercise. Besides getting you from point A to point B, it burns calories, boosts energy, improves mood, wards off food cravings, and helps keep you slim. That's why foot power is at the heart of *ChangeOne* Fitness.

Our goals for you? Fit more calorie-blasting steps into your daily routine, and take a dedicated 20-minute brisk walk every day.

In this chapter, we'll prove to you that this simple strategy (no gym memberships, no equipment, no fancy moves, no huge time commitment required) is the most powerful way to lose weight and feel great—for life.

Change One quiz
What's Your Walking Quotient?

1. My thinking about walking is:

    a. It's a slow but cheap mode of transportation. Period.

    b. It's probably good for you, but certainly not serious exercise.

    c. It's a legitimate form of exercise I should do more of.

    d. It's not only great exercise but also a wonderful source of relaxation and pleasure.

2. If the weather's nice, I might walk for this long:

    a. 1 minute—the time it takes to get from my car to the supermarket entrance.

    b. 5 minutes—the time it takes to find a nice bench in the park.

    c. 20 minutes—a relaxed stroll in the sun is a rare but pleasant treat.

    d. 30 minutes or more—I jump at every chance to be outside and moving.

3. My usual walking shoes are:

    a. Fuzzy slippers or old socks; that's all you need for strolling around the house.

    b. My everyday work shoes; who has time to change shoes for a little walking?

    c. Sandals, clogs, or flip-flops; feet like sunshine, too.

    d. Dedicated sneakers or hiking shoes; *sturdy* and *supportive* are the operative words.

4. My favorite parking spot at the mall is:

    a. I don't know; I shop online.

    b. Right up front; I'll circle the lot endlessly until a primo spot opens up.

    c. Relatively near; I don't obsess over getting close and don't mind a little extra walking.

    d. The farthest lot; this gives me a chance to get in one more brisk stroll.

5. I stash my walking shoes:

    a. Umm, don't you walk in *all* your shoes?

    b. When last glimpsed, my circa-1998 Keds were buried at the back of my closet.

    c. Relatively new, well-fitting sneakers are prominently arrayed with my other shoes.

    d. I keep dedicated walking shoes in the car, at work, and by the front door.

Score

We were pretty obvious with this one—for each question, the answers go from worst to best. Here are some of the underlying messages of each question.

1. Walking is for real. As you'll read shortly, study after study shows the substantial, measurable benefits of regular walking to your health, weight, and mental state.

2. Walking is a pleasure. It's a simple, convenient, fun way to add exercise to your life and an effective way to lose weight.

3. If the sneaker fits, wear it. Your feet were made for walking, and your shoes should be, too. Studies show you're likely to walk more during the day if you're wearing comfortable shoes.

4. We're talking about a lifestyle, not fitness quotas. *ChangeOne* Fitness is a philosophy as much as a plan. Any chance you see to fit a few more steps into your day—such as parking your car in Siberia—you should grab.

5. Ready, set, go. You'll know you're in the *ChangeOne* Fitness mind-set when you're ready to walk, stroll, or play outside at a moment's notice.

Walking Your Way to Weight Loss

A growing stack of research shows that if you want to lose weight, combining a sensible eating plan with exercise such as walking is far smarter than just cutting calories. It also tames the dreaded "jiggles," helping you look and feel firmer.

One example of the power of this strategy: In a recent University of Maryland study, researchers asked 24 over-weight, inactive women to begin walking three times a week (one day on a treadmill in the lab for 30 to 45 minutes, and two days on their own for any length of time they wanted) and to cut 250 calories per day from their diets, following an eating plan based closely on the nutritional guidelines of *ChangeOne.* After six months, the volunteers had lost 8 percent of their body weight—about a 14-pound reduction for a 180-pound woman. Nice, but get this: Total body fat fell by 15 percent, meaning each woman shaved off about 27 pounds of fat and replaced half of it with muscle. And they all felt stronger because their aerobic capacity—a measure of the lungs' ability to take in oxygen—increased by 8 percent. The bottom line? Thanks to the diet-plus-walking strategy, these women were slimmer, fitter, and had more stamina.

The benefits of walking are many. It can help you:

Burn fat. Blasting fat requires using your body's biggest muscle groups—those in your buttocks and legs—rhythmically, briskly, and consistently for at least 20 minutes at a time. (That's exactly why we ask you to dedicate yourself to a brisk 20-minute walk every day.) During an aerobic workout such as walking, your muscle cells first burn sugar stored as a fuel called glycogen; after about 15 minutes, your cells turn to fat as their primary power source.

Trim stubborn belly fat. Walkers lost significant abdominal fat—the stubborn fat that can be toughest to lose (and the kind that raises your risk of diabetes and heart disease) in one Tufts University study.

Make your "skinny jeans" your everyday jeans, for good. Adding just 2,000 steps a day to your regular activities—that's just 15 minutes of walking—

Help!

My knees and shins hurt after a walk. What can I do?

First, make sure you've picked a walking surface that's kind to your body, one that's firm but not too hard. Avoid concrete, the hardest walking surface of them all. Best are grass, wood-chip paths, dirt paths, a cinder track, or a regular running track. Next, be sure you're also doing the *ChangeOne* strengthening/stretching program to build the muscles around your knees. Increase your time and speed gradually. And be sure your walking shoes have flexible soles.

could mean you'll *never* gain another pound, say top weight-loss experts from the Center for Human Nutrition at the University of Colorado Health Sciences Center.

Have energy to burn. California State University researchers found that the more people walked, the more energetic they felt. Even better: Just a short walk is all it takes! In a 1997 study, scientists found that a brisk 10-minute walk gave people more energy than eating a chocolate bar. Why? Exercise boosts a hormone that increases energy.

Turn on your happy switch. Can you walk your way to happiness? Absolutely. In fact, Duke University psychologists have found that walking relieves mild-to-moderate depression better than drugs.

Brisk Walking Basics

If you're new to walking or haven't hit the pavement for a while, or if your doctor—or your body—tells you to start slowly, we recommend beginning with baby steps. Walk for just 10 minutes at a comfortable pace and gradually, over the next few weeks, build up to the full 20 minutes. *Then* pick up the pace. If you already walk regularly or are reasonably fit, go for 20 minutes most days a week right away. (Of course, if you fall in love with walking, there's no harm in going longer!)

Perfect timing. We recommend walking in the early morning, before your day gets going. This strategy guarantees that you'll fit your walk in and will add a relaxed, energetic glow to everything else you do. If midday or evening's better for you, or if your best time changes from day to day, that's fine, too. Just try to identify your walk time the night before so you can build it into your day. Keep walking shoes and socks in your office or your car (or on your feet) so you can get out when the getting's good.

Best places. Feed your soul, feast your eyes, and breathe clean, sweet air by choosing the prettiest streets in your neighborhood or the nicest nearby parks or trails. Avoid walking along busy highways or in parking lots. It's no fun being assaulted by traffic noise and breathing bus fumes.

Walk this way. Everybody knows how to walk, right? Yes...and no. Just as we don't always sit the right way, we don't always walk the right way. When they're walking for

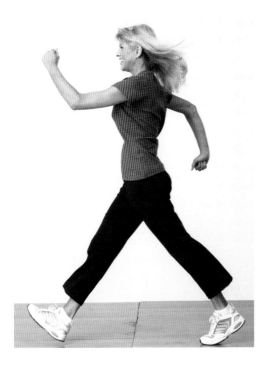

fitness, people sometimes do funny things. They flap their elbows as if they were doing the chicken dance or march along stiff-armed; they take super-elongated strides or lean forward as if heading into a hurricane.

The best walking style is natural and free, but not lazy. Stand up straight, tuck in your tummy, relax your shoulders, and look forward, keeping your gaze about 20 feet ahead rather than down in front of you. (Of course, if you're walking on an uneven surface, do look down!)

The right pace? Simply aim to walk briskly—at the speed you'd reach if you were about 10 minutes late for an appointment. You should be breathing a little hard but still be able to carry on a conversation in full sentences. This easy "talk test" works as well as a heart monitor for making sure you get to, and stay in, the best calorie-burning, fitness-building zone. If you're breathing normally, pick up the pace a bit.

Boost the calorie burn. Once you're comfortable with your 20-minute brisk walk, you can burn even more calories by adding a few fast-paced intervals. Here's how. Walk at your usual speed for 3 to 5 minutes, then walk even more briskly for 1 to 2 minutes. To pick up the pace, take short, quick steps. (Most people try to walk faster by elongating their strides, but this actually slows you down and can lead to joint and shin injuries.) Bend your arms at 90 degrees and pump them quickly. After your fast-walking interval, settle back into your usual brisk pace for 3 to 4 minutes, then pick up the pace again for 1 to 2 minutes. Do this several times during your walk. Boosting the intensity intermittently can increase the calorie burn by 60 percent.

Stepping Up Your Steps

Researchers estimate that today, Americans burn half as many calories a day as we did a half century ago—in part, because we don't walk to the store, the bus stop, school, the movies, or during chores as our parents did. In addition to a dedicated

20-minute walk every day, we want you to buck fattening, 21st-century sitting disease by adding steps back into your life.

Extra steps really can add up. "Wherever I go, I park my car as far away from the entrance as possible," one *ChangeOne* participant says. "The steps add up eventually. I know at work, I add 250 steps to my day just by parking in the farthest space." How can you fit more steps into your day?

Volunteer on the homefront. Have an outdoor mailbox? Walk to the mailbox to get the mail instead of popping out of the car. Instead of sending your husband or kids to bring up the laundry, let the dog in, or get the newspaper, see these chores as an opportunity for a brief burst of exercise—and some extra steps. Love TV? March in place during a half-hour sitcom, use your treadmill, or walk around the house during commercials. On the phone? Don't chat from the easy chair. Take calls on a cordless phone or cell phone and walk while you talk.

Make Every Step Count

Can a little plastic gadget that costs under $30 help you walk more and lose weight? Count on it. Pedometers are scarcely larger than a book of matches and clip unobtrusively to your belt or waistband. They count each step you take, and some also track miles and calories burned. For many people, simply knowing that the number on the readout is increasing with every step inspires them to take more. "The pedometer is a wonderful, motivational tool. I love mine," says one *ChangeOne* participant.

Experts recommend shooting for an ultimate goal of 10,000 steps a day for weight loss and fitness. We recommend a more modest goal of adding 5,000 steps (including those you accumulate on your daily 20-minute walk) to what you're doing now.

Those 5,000 steps add up to a real weight-loss advantage, reported researchers in a recent University of Pennsylvania study of 179 women and men.

They all followed a *ChangeOne*-type diet, and for 40 weeks, they either went to the gym four times a week, did calisthenics at home, or simply tried to increase their daily steps by 5,000. At the end, the steppers lost as much weight as the others and kept it off just as easily.

How to get there: First, wear your pedometer on a typical day *before* you begin the walking program and note how many steps you walk. Watch that number increase as you begin the *ChangeOne* Fitness walking plan. Basic, everyday activities such as taking out the trash and picking up the mail use about 100 steps per minute. So does strolling at a lively yet relaxed pace while shopping at the supermarket or mall. Hustling to a meeting or appointment tallies about 130 steps per minute. Walking a mile requires about 2,000 steps. We estimate the *ChangeOne* 20-minute fitness walk will add 2,500 steps to your day.

Step it up at work. Get off the bus a stop or two early and walk the rest of the way. Choose the farthest entrance from your work space, then park as far away from it as possible. Take a walking break every half hour at work and head to the water cooler or bathroom farthest from your office. Go to a coworker's desk when you have a question instead of always using e-mail or the phone; you may find that you even improve your working relationships.

Get out of the car, up from your seat, or off the bleachers. Running errands? See which ones you can do by walking from home. For others, park in a central location and walk to as many stores as possible. Circle the field during kids' sporting events. Take a walk instead of waiting in the car or the hall during play practices, piano lessons, and so on. Stuck at the airport? Take a good walk around the terminal and skip the moving sidewalks.

Keep It Interesting

Stay motivated, enjoy your walks more, and walk in all weather with these tips.

Pair up with a buddy. Sometimes the pull of inertia is irresistible, but if you have a walking date to keep, you're much more likely to make it past the threshold of your front door. If you don't have a friend who wants to walk with you, find a walking partner by asking around your neighborhood or at work (for lunchtime walks) or by posting a notice at your church, gym, or community center.

Get a gadget. Invest in an iPod or a Walkman-style cassette or CD player with earphones and walk to your favorite tunes. Upbeat songs can help you maintain a faster pace. Or catch up on your reading with books on tape. Another idea: Equip your cell phone with a headset, hit the road, and dial Mom, Sis, or your best friend for an uninterrupted chat.

Outsmart the seasons. If the mail carrier can deliver mail in any weather, you can walk in any weather, as long as you're dressed for it. But if you live in a climate that's often too hot or too cold for comfort, consider investing in a treadmill. A word of advice: Try before you buy. Features to think about include the deck size (a longer walking surface feels less cramped than a short one, but be sure your chosen machine will fit the space available in your home), shock absorption (thicker belts, floating decks, and special shock absorbers decrease the wear and tear on your legs and feet but also raise the price), and the range of speeds and incline levels. (Most walkers will be fine with a top speed of 5 to 6 miles per hour, but consider a wide incline range so you can vary your walks and add a bigger challenge.)

Try an indoor track—with cash registers. Many malls open early for walkers. You could also easily walk for 20 minutes in a big buying-club store or at a Walmart or Kmart. "I began walking five times a week at the local mall about three months ago," reports one mall-walker on the *ChangeOne* plan. "I walk along the interior walls and through one or two of the larger stores. I wasn't going to look at the scale that often, but when my coworkers kept asking me if I was losing weight, I checked, and I'd lost the first 10 pounds easily—plus some inches, as my pants had become baggy."

Be inspired. Once a week, find and walk in a special new spot—a lovely neighborhood across town, a pretty hiking trail, a riverside towpath. Feel at one with nature and yourself by focusing on your breathing and your steps. Or repeat a soothing word or phrase as you walk. Soak up the year-round beauty of nature and enjoy it even more with inspirational quotes from a book we like, *With Beauty Before Me: An Inspirational Guide for Nature Walks,* by Joseph Cornell. (One idea from the author: Pretend you're seeing everything around you for the very first time.) Check the newspaper for local nature hikes and walking tours of local homes, gardens, and historic spots, too.

Give back. Plan to participate in a fund-raising charity walk a few months from now. Many are 5K's—5 kilometers, or 3 miles, long. You'll stay motivated as you "train" on your daily walks and help support a worthy cause such as breast cancer research or preventing birth defects.

ChangeOne Shoe Tips

The only equipment you really need is a good pair of walking shoes. Finding them is a cinch—just be sure they're comfortable. You shouldn't need to "break them in." When shopping for shoes:

- Wear the socks you plan to walk in, not thicker or thinner ones.
- Look for flat shoes (your heel and the ball of your foot should be at about the same level) with lots of toe room.
- Do the twist test. A good walking shoe should be flexible enough to accommodate your foot's natural heel-to-toe roll. If the shoe doesn't bend at the ball of the foot, and you can't twist the sole from side to side, it's too stiff.
- Reserve these shoes for walking to preserve their useful life. Experts recommend replacing walking shoes every 500 miles—about every 10 months on the *ChangeOne* Fitness program.

Get
Outdoors

"The world is mud-luscious and puddle-wonderful," wrote the poet e. e. cummings. If you can't remember the last time you splashed in—or at least walked around—a fine, fat mud puddle, you've come to the right chapter.

In these pages, you'll be inspired to reconnect with the outdoors and with your own sense of playfulness and fun. The payoffs? Energy, happiness, and a return to the calorie-burning activities of your youth.

And if life doesn't afford you much time for outdoor fun, we'll show you how yard work and even home maintenance projects can count toward your *ChangeOne* Fitness goal of spending at least 2 hours a week outdoors. Why 2 hours? We want you to break away from indoor disease—the sitting, snacking, sedentary lifestyle that packs on pounds, zaps energy levels, and leaves you choosing between an endless round of chores and watching endless TV sitcoms and reality shows. It's time to live a little—and we think getting outside is an essential component of a happy, healthy life.

Outsmart Indoor Disease

If you're plopped on a bed, couch, or chair right now, surrounded by four walls and a ceiling, you're taking part in America's number 1 *anti*-activity-indoor disease. It's the top reason more and more of us are overweight and under-energetic. This housebound, car-bound, office-bound lifestyle claims *at least* 20 to 23 hours out of the days of most adults in the United States. Shocked? Check this sobering arithmetic: Add up 2 hours for cooking and eating meals, 1 to 2 hours sitting in the car, bus, or train while commuting, 7 to 9 hours on the job (or working at home), 3 hours of watching TV, and 7 hours of snoozing. Not much time left for activity, much less for going outside, is there?

The *ChangeOne* response? Turn off the TV, push the footstool away from the sofa, lace up your shoes, and get outdoors for a minimum of 2 hours of fun a week. What you do once you land on the other side of the front door is up to you. Follow your bliss. Of course, ahead in this chapter, you'll find dozens of ideas for backyard fun, practical house and garden projects, and short jaunts and longer trips in the wide, beautiful, natural world. But we believe that even enjoying your morning coffee or an after-work glass of iced tea on the patio counts, because the more you get outside, the more likely it is that you'll stay and stay—strolling across the lawn to check out the first purple crocuses or the last summer tomato, walking next door to chat with a neighbor, or playing catch with the kids or fetch with Fido. (Or finally tacking up that sagging bit of gutter on the garage...)

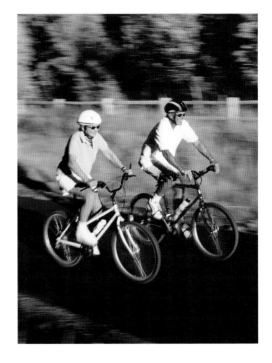

Your mission is simple: Just get outdoors and trust that nature will take its course. We bet your personal happiness index will go up, stress and fatigue will begin to melt away, and you'll find yourself inventing excuses to get back out there in the sunshine and fresh air again real soon. Even better, you may find that the more time you spend outside, the faster the pounds will fall away.

Personal Benefits

Need hard facts about the benefits of living outside the big box called home? You'll:

Cash in on extracurricular weight loss. A half hour of TV watching burns a piddling 37 calories. In contrast, 30 minutes spent painting the house will work off 200 calories; gardening uses 189; a fast-paced touch football game works off 320; washing the car uses up 178; and mowing the lawn uses 189 calories—if you rake afterward, you'll sweat off 199. In winter, shoveling snow burns 236 and stacking firewood burns another 241.

Multiply your happiness. Looking at flowers eases depression, say Rutgers University psychologists who tested the moods of 100 women and men in the presence and absence of colorful flowers. Meanwhile, exposure to sunlight lifted depression in a University of San Diego study. No surprise there—most of us have heard (and know instinctively) that sunlight has the power to lift winter depression. Yet the researchers also found that we don't always act on what we know. When they issued sunlight meters to study volunteers to measure their exposure to sunlight over two days, they found that most got just an hour of exposure, and some had none at all.

Feel pleasure, have fun. Kick off your shoes, taste a sun-ripened strawberry, smell the fall leaves. Every little kid delays coming indoors as long as possible after a day in the open air, and that kid is still inside you. Nature is gloriously romantic. The poet Kahlil Gibran said, "Forget not that the earth delights to feel your bare feet and the winds long to play with your hair." Or, as one *ChangeOne* participant told us, "Whenever I garden, I forget time, aches, or even to eat! I would sooner be outside, even pulling weeds, than doing most anything else!"

Spend kid-approved quality time with the family. In one eye-opening survey of 500 families by the Boys & Girls Clubs of America, kids confided that they spend hardly any meaningful time with their parents—by which they meant doing something fun together. (Parents thought they spent lots of quality time teaching their kids how to do things.) We think getting outdoors together will bring you closer to your children or grandchildren and create a lasting, deeper bond.

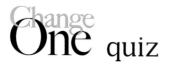
One quiz

Are You an Indoor or Outdoor Person?

Answer each of the following true-or-false questions as honestly as you can.

1. I can swim and like to do so.
   ☐ True ☐ False

2. If I were invited to play in an easygoing softball game, I'd probably say yes.
   ☐ True ☐ False

3. Sunsets, wildflowers, and mountaintop views make me very, very happy.
   ☐ True ☐ False

4. I'd rather grow my own tomatoes than buy them.
   ☐ True ☐ False

5. I understand why people are attracted to the game of golf.
   ☐ True ☐ False

6. When I see a well-equipped playground, the kid inside me wants to stop and play.
   ☐ True ☐ False

7. I'd rather read a book in a hammock than on a sofa.
   ☐ True ☐ False

8. I'd rather take an evening stroll than watch the evening news.
   ☐ True ☐ False

9. At least one pair of shoes in my closet has dried mud caked to the bottom.
   ☐ True ☐ False

10. I have my own bicycle, and it's ready for riding.
    ☐ True ☐ False

11. I can identify at least three constellations in the night sky.
    ☐ True ☐ False

12. I can identify at least five different types of birds where I live.
    ☐ True ☐ False

Score

Tally up your "true" answers. Here's how to rate your score.

9-12: You are clearly a person who loves the outdoors! Now that you know that being outdoors is part of the active, healthy-weight lifestyle, you should be motivated to get out even more often.

5-8: You enjoy the outdoors, but being outside probably isn't an integral part of your life. Find outdoor activities you particularly enjoy and pursue them as much as you can. In time, you'll broaden your activities and become far more passionate about your time in the fresh air.

1-4: Modern living has clearly gotten the best of you. The time has come to reconnect with your childhood spirit and to relearn the joys of cool breezes, soft grass, and outdoor play. Try to do your walks outdoors, and slowly find interests that get you out of the living room, out of the stores, out of the car, and into nature.

Build self-esteem. People who spend lots of time outdoors tend to be doers, not watchers. Not only are they physically stronger than their sedentary counterparts, they also often have lots of self-confidence as well. They are often leaner and healthier, thanks to all the activity they do, and they frequently have more positive attitudes about life as well. Sure, we admit these are stereotypes, and there are plenty of exceptions. But think about people you know who are passionate about the outdoors. Are we very far from the truth?

Get Ready

As a kid, your wardrobe was probably sharply divided between "good" clothes, "school" clothes, and grungy, the-dirtier-the-better "play" clothes. We'd like you to revive the play clothes category so you're prepared, at a moment's notice, to get out in the sunshine (or moonlight). Here's how.

- Gather into one drawer or onto one shelf your oldest, machine-washable T-shirts (long- and short-sleeved), shorts, and jeans; a warm sweatshirt; comfy socks that can get dirty; and for women, a supportive bra you won't mind sweating in.
- Keep outdoor shoes and a brimmed hat by the front door. Store sunscreen and a bug repellent. If you don't like chemical repellents, try one with picaridin or oil of lemon eucalyptus. According to the Centers for Disease Control and Prevention, they're just as good as DEET for repelling mosquitoes.
- Put on your outdoor clothes when you get home from work or first thing on weekend mornings when you don't have to go anyplace.
- Resurrect the toy box. Stock it with things you might enjoy playing with, such as Wiffle golf balls and a 9-iron, a Frisbee, a jump rope, a fishing pole (practice casting into a bucket), a bocce set, horseshoes, or even a paint set. If you have children, grandchildren, or neighborhood kids who visit, include a kickball or soccer ball, chalk for drawing hopscotch squares in the driveway, and maybe even a hula hoop. You'll always be ready to play at a moment's notice.

Plan It, Then Do It

If your excuse for not getting outdoors is lack of time, then you need to reclaim your weekends—and that bit of time between dinner and sundown—by wielding your pen and your day planner. Here's how.

Use weeknights more effectively. Why do so many of us spend our weekends shopping, cleaning, and cooking? Not only are the stores most crowded then, but we sacrifice our days off to chores that are easily and more efficiently done during the week. Assign weekend tasks to particular evenings of the week. For example, do your grocery shopping on Monday night, spend Tuesday night cooking dinners for the rest of the week, and designate Thursday night for vacuuming. Your goal: to wake up on Saturday with as few mandatory chores as possible.

Spread out the work. Do you know what the perfect gardening schedule is? Fifteen minutes of work, first thing every single morning. Do that, and we guarantee your garden will never be better tended—and your body will thank you for it, too. Saving up all the yard work for intense, hours-long sessions is not only tough on your muscles, patience, and schedule, it isn't great for the flowers, either! Instead, create a daily routine of planting, weeding, feeding, and watering one small area at a time. Over time, you and your garden will flourish. The same holds true for housecleaning, by the way—15 minutes a day may make your house less cluttered and cleaner than ever!

Schedule, schedule, schedule. Does the following conversation sound familiar?

"What do you want to do today?"

"Uh, I don't know. What do *you* want to do?"

"I don't know, either. I asked you first—what do you want to do?"

If your family regularly gets into this kind of cycle of indecision come weekend mornings, it's time to break out of it. The method: During the previous week, be specific in your planning for the upcoming weekend. Don't just suggest a nature walk on Sunday afternoon. Pick a time and place. Think through what

Help!

I simply don't like being outdoors. I'm bothered by bugs, find it unpleasant to wear sunscreen, and don't enjoy sweating. What can I do?

Ease into it by creating a comfortable "outdoor room" that is strictly for your relaxation. Your space should have a few comfortable lawn chairs, a chaise lounge, or a picnic table with padded benches or dining chairs.

To deal with the bugs, consider buying Buzz-Off clothing, which is made to repel biting insects. (It really works!) Also get citronella candles or a bug zapper to discourage flying critters.

Put on a wide-brimmed hat for protection from sun and glare. Make yourself some iced tea and put it in a sealed cup or travel mug. Then settle into your outdoor room with something fun to read and see what happens. We bet you'll discover the sounds of birds and wind to be relaxing and the breeze refreshing. In time, you'll come around to the pleasures of outdoor activity.

you'll need to have and whether preparations or reservations are in order. Having a set agenda and being prepared for it is the best way to avoid inactivity due to indecision.

Say No to Excuses

When the temperature's a pleasant 70 degrees, the humidity's a perfect 50 percent, the sun's shining, and it's a Saturday afternoon with absolutely nothing else on your agenda, you don't need too many extra enticements to get you out the door. In less than perfect conditions, though, it's sometimes tough to get going. Here's how to get motivated when time's short, the weather's challenging, or the great indoors is pulling you toward the couch.

If you've got just a few minutes: Pour your coffee into a travel mug with a lid and wander in the backyard or down the street. Grab garden shears and create a bouquet for the table or pinch off all those past-their-prime blooms in your border garden. Pull out a tennis racquet, golf club, or baseball bat and practice your stroke for a few moments. Crunch through autumn leaves or rake the front yard. If you have just a little time to spare at work, walk to a place 5 minutes from your office for lunch, then walk back. Or head over to a playground for 10 minutes of silliness with a friend. Keep a Frisbee and a ball in the trunk for quick fun.

If you're with the kids: Go out for miniature golf; stay home for badminton, backyard baseball or kickball; bounce on a trampoline; or teach 'em your favorite old summer street games—jump rope, kick the can, red light-green light, or Green Hornet. (An hour of tag burns more than 300 calories, too)! Dust off your bike and take a ride. Go hiking in a park with a simple set of trails and let the kids be in charge of the map— an experience that builds confidence. Play every sport in the book—soccer, flag football, baseball; the good news is, most kids will get more exercise and have more fun in vigorous backyard play than in an organized league, where less skilled athletes often meet with discouragement. Or try an old-time favorite: family yard work interspersed with fun, silly breaks.

If it's cold out: Dress in layers. For example, don a moisture-wicking T-shirt, a wool shirt, a fleece pullover, and a snow jacket; for your bottom half, start with thermal

1,001 Things to Do

If you put your mind to it, we're sure there's no shortage of things you'd enjoy doing outside. But few of us bother to put our minds to it. We say, just do it! Once you list ideas, pick a few of the best and schedule them. Here are some to get you started.

If you prefer activities with practical results, inspect your home's exterior and yard and list tasks that would make you feel better once they're completed. Examples: repaint the mailbox post, hang a window box, move the trashcans to a different storage location, paint the back steps.

If you love sports or solo activities, join a hiking club or scour the newspaper for a masters' level sports group. Or spend an evening at the sporting goods store buying a bat and ball, a tennis racquet, or skates—equipment for whatever you once enjoyed. It's time to revive the activities of your youth!

If you love wandering in nature, pick a park, mountain, beach, or lake that's close by. Find a map and check if there's an admission fee. Also consider cultivating an interest in birds. Bird-watching is one of America's hottest hobbies, thanks to the wonderful diversity of colors, shapes, songs, and personalities among American birds.

If you're social, schedule and plan fun outdoor events. If you have kids, consider water parks, sledding hills, playgrounds, pools, and zoos. If you don't have children, have barbecues, parties, and hikes or go to outdoor craft shows or music festivals. Or combine an outdoor activity with a treat: Fix up the yard, then have the neighbors over for a sunset barbecue. Invite your guests to play old-fashioned, grown-up lawn games. Bocce or croquet, anyone?

underwear or tights or panty hose, then wool pants, and finally waterproof rain or snow pants. The same goes for your feet—moisture-wicking socks, then wool socks, then water-proof boots. Cover your head and ears effectively, then completely forget about the temperature. Go sledding or skating. Rent cross-country skis and take a Saturday afternoon ski class at a local park or sporting goods store, then ski until sunset. Make snow angels or go snowshoeing instead of taking your regular walk. Shovel snow or chop ice off the front walk.

If it's raining: Wear waterproof outer clothes, grab the umbrella, and walk! Enjoy the sights and sounds of the city or country during a shower. It's surprisingly fun and sensual.

If it's windy: Fly a kite! Any type will do, but for a great upper-body workout, use a stunt kite. Don't have a kite? Then just walk into the wind. It's fun, silly, and strenuous, and you'll never feel more awake.

Get
Stronger

Once, building muscle was the nearly exclusive domain of big, sweaty guys working out in smelly gyms filled with the sounds of grunts and clanging iron. Their ultimate goal: cartoonish, overpumped, muscleman physiques.

The notable exception: Marilyn Monroe. This blond bombshell reportedly performed muscle-toning exercises several times a week and credited her curves to her strength-training routine. She had the right idea. Muscles are far too important to leave to the bodybuilders. Compelling research shows that a short, easy, fun strengthening and stretching routine won't leave you with Popeye-style arms. Instead, you'll look and feel more like Marilyn (or if you're a guy, a young Kirk Douglas)—lean, sexy, and strong.

In this chapter, you'll discover three 10-minute routines that harness the amazing weight-loss power locked inside your muscles.

This gentle strengthening and stretching will tone your body, boost your energy levels, and help you burn more calories 'round the clock.

What Marilyn Knew

Left to their own devices, your muscles begin to diminish in size and strength in your thirties or forties. At first, the change is so gradual that you may barely detect it. You may weigh the same but somehow look rounder, puffier—or your favorite jeans may no longer zip shut.

What's happening? As long, lean muscle mass shrinks, puffy, blobby fat moves in. Then weight gain accelerates. Muscle is metabolically active; that is, it uses up calories even when at rest. Each pound of muscle burns about 30 to 50 calories per day. Fat, in contrast, burns next to none. So when you replace muscle with fat, your metabolism slows down, and you begin gaining weight even if your diet and exercise habits haven't changed. A pound here, a pound there...it may seem like nothing. But after age 35 or so, you lose ⅓ to ½ pound of muscle each year—a loss that could eventually add up to an extra 300 to 450 calories a day that your metabolism *isn't* burning off! The result? Weight begins to climb. An unfair fact: This metabolic decline hits women harder than men, probably because men have more muscle mass to begin with.

Trying to lose those extra pounds just by cutting calories can backfire or prove amazingly difficult. Why? Because your metabolism is already running slowly, and eating less only further reduces muscle mass.

That's where the *ChangeOne* Fitness strengthening/stretching plan comes in.

You'll use resistance, in this case your own body weight and sometimes small dumbbells, to put a little healthy stress on the muscles in your upper and lower body and at your core—the key muscles of your abdomen and back. During resistance exercise, muscle fibers actually experience microscopic tears; as they heal, they grow denser and larger. You'll also stretch so your muscles and joints become more limber.

What you get: more muscle, less fat, and the ability to move with youthful ease and grace. Since muscle takes up less space than fat, you look trimmer even if you don't lose a pound. In fact, some people actually

Help!

Strength training is supposed to hurt, right? How else could it build my muscles? The trouble is, I don't want to do exercise that causes pain.

"No pain, no gain" is an outdated exercise myth perpetuated by competitive muscle builders and athletes. Strength training should never cause pain. In fact, research shows that a gentle routine can alleviate backaches, fibromyalgia and arthritis pain, and chronic neck discomfort.

As you get started with this routine, your muscles may feel a *bit* sore for a few days, and you may feel a little tired. That's normal. It's quite likely that your muscles haven't been used in these ways in a long time. Imagine they are being awakened after a long slumber. But if you're exhausted, your joints are sore, or your muscles feel as if they're cramped or pulled, you're overdoing it and need to go easier on yourself. Proceed slowly, with fewer repetitions of each exercise, and slowly build up.

gain a little weight when they begin strength training because they're building muscle—and muscle weighs more than fat. But they also notice that their clothes fit more loosely, or they even drop a dress size or two. Over time, weight loss speeds up as the extra muscle burns more calories all day long.

Five Big Benefits of Strengthening and Stretching

The bottom line? A little strength training is a girl's (and guy's) best friend. It's motivating. As one *ChangeOne* participant says, "Just feeling my muscles as I move the rest of the day reminds me that I am working on being healthy, and it makes me think twice before sabotaging it with a bad 'treat.' " Here's a rundown of what's in it for you.

A firmer, more shapely figure: Muscle is smooth, lean, hard, and small; fat is lumpy, flabby, soft, and big. Experts say that compared to a pound of fat, a pound of muscle takes up about 22 percent less space. In one Tufts University study of 40 postmenopausal women ages 50 to 70, those who performed easy strength-training exercises for about 80 minutes a week were significantly leaner and trimmer than those who didn't do the exercises.

A metabolic tune-up: In a University of Alabama study, women and men who strength-trained three times a week for six months gained 4½ pounds of lean muscle, lost 6 pounds of fat, and increased their metabolisms by 12 percent. Their bodies burned an extra 230 calories per day, even on days when they weren't working out.

More energy and a more active life: The Tufts researchers noticed something interesting about the women who strength-trained in their study: They increased their activity levels by 25 percent. In the year after the study ended, nonexercisers grew less active, but the muscle-strengthening group was on to new things: One woman went whitewater rafting with her family; another moved 4 tons of topsoil, one load at a time, in a wheelbarrow as she spruced up her yard; others took up in-line skating, mountain biking, and ballroom dancing. One even outscored the lead researcher at bowling. The study authors suspect that added strength—

the women were eventually as strong as or stronger than their own daughters—made all these activities easy to do.

Better posture; more everyday power: By doing a routine that targets all areas of your body, you will improve your posture, and handling heavy stuff—from grocery bags loaded with canned goods to toddlers to heavy furniture—will be a breeze.

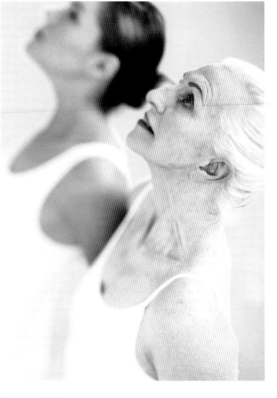

A more limber, graceful, ache-free body: Each of our *ChangeOne* strengthening routines ends with a couple of refreshing stretches. These are more than just feel-good moves (although stretching can help you relax, physically and mentally). While strength training contracts and flexes your muscles, stretching lengthens them, increasing your flexibility and range of motion and improving blood flow to your muscles. This means more oxygen and blood sugar for nourishment and more efficient whisking-away of waste products. "Each morning before I get dressed for the day, I do gentle stretching exercises," notes one *ChangeOne* participant. "What a difference for stiff joints! The flexibility lasts for quite a while."

Get Ready, Get Set, Go!

Some strength-training programs require serious equipment. Not *ChangeOne.* Our routines are just as effective and much more convenient. In total, we ask you to have two light dumbbells, a chair, a towel, a step, and a wall. These routines are designed for the home, although you can do them while traveling, either using a purse or briefcase in place of the dumbbell or just doing the movements without a weight but with your muscles tensed.

For even more convenience, we've broken the program into three 10-minute routines—an upper-body routine, a lower-body routine, and a core routine (the core being the back, abdomen, and hips). Do one routine each and every day. We recommend that you do it first thing in the morning, but for those who are night owls, evening or before bed is fine, too. The important thing is to do it—don't skip a day! If you don't like the idea of an "exercise period," just think of it as a quick household errand, like moving the laundry from the washer to the dryer. That's what one *ChangeOne* participant does to get herself going. "It's easier to say to myself, 'It's just ten minutes.' It doesn't seem so hard mentally to fit in that way when I really don't feel like exercising."

Check-In

We've asked you to fit four kinds of physical activity into your week: Walking, strengthening and stretching, outdoor fun, and extra everyday movements. Have you found time for all four—and does it feel relatively easy? Or has fitness become a source of stress? If so, go back to basics—with a twist. Start with fitting extra steps and movements into your everyday life. After a week or so, add 20 minutes of brisk walking a day. Once that's a regular part of your life, find time for 10 minutes of strengthening and stretching. You'll be feeling great—and ready to look for some outdoor fun.

Now let's be honest. At first, some of these exercises will feel a little awkward. Some will be more challenging than others. Constantly remind yourself that this is not a contest or a race or a program you'll be graded on. You are doing this for *you*, at your rate of speed, at your rate of progress. If you're struggling with a few of the moves, that's fine. Make the movement a little smaller or do it without the hand weight. If merely getting onto and off the floor is challenging, fine; start by just getting down on the floor and then back up again, skipping the exercise for now. We're sure that in time, you will not only be able to get through each routine comfortably but will also enjoy them immensely. Some final tips:

Don't fixate on time. At first, you may want a little longer rest period between movements, or you may choose to do fewer repetitions of each exercise. What's important is that you learn to do the routines correctly. Over time, you'll get more efficient.

Do the exercises slowly. Count 2 to 4 seconds as you perform the first half of each exercise and another 2 to 4 as you do the second half. That way your muscles work harder. Take time to perform each exercise slowly and correctly so that you get the best results.

Breathe right. Inhale before you begin each move so you can exhale during the first part (usually the more strenuous part of the exercise) and inhale during the second part.

Remember to rotate the routines! A key component of strength training is giving your muscles a day or two to rest, heal, and grow. By rotating through our three routines, you'll exercise each major muscle group at least twice a week, which is exactly the right amount. Never repeat the same routine two days in a row.

Try to do the exercises in the order listed. It's a sensible progression. Most important, though, always stretch after strengthening. Experts agree that it's best to stretch muscles when they're warm, not at the start of your routine when they're cold and tight.

As with the exercises, do the stretches slowly and deliberately. Hold each one for 10 to 30 seconds, as indicated. Move smoothly—never bounce or jerk your muscles. Inhale before you start, then exhale going into the stretch and inhale again as you release it. Breathe slowly to encourage relaxation. Never stretch to the point of pain. You may feel slight discomfort, but anything more means it's time to back off.

The Upper-Body ROUTINE

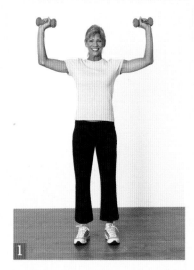

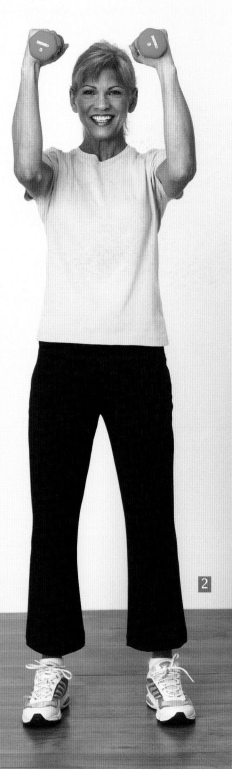

■ EXERCISE ONE

Cross-Over Chest Squeeze

1 Stand holding a light dumbbell in each hand. Bend your arms at 90-degree angles and hold them out to your sides so your upper arms are parallel to the floor with your palms facing forward.

2 Squeezing your chest muscles, move your elbows toward each other until they're about shoulder-width apart. Return to the starting position. Slowly do 8 to 12 repetitions.

■ EXERCISE TWO **Pec Pull**

1 Holding a dumbbell in your left hand, stand with
your right leg one huge step in front of your left,
with your back heel lifted off the floor. Rest your right
hand on your right thigh for support and lean forward
slightly. Hold your left arm across your chest so your
palm faces back.

2 Keeping your elbow bent, move it out to the side
until your upper arm is extended even with your
shoulder. Pause, then return to the starting position.
After doing 8 to 12 repetitions, repeat the exercise with
your other arm.

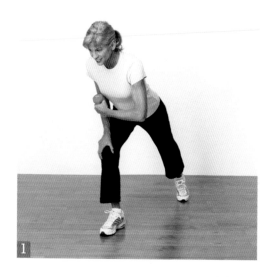

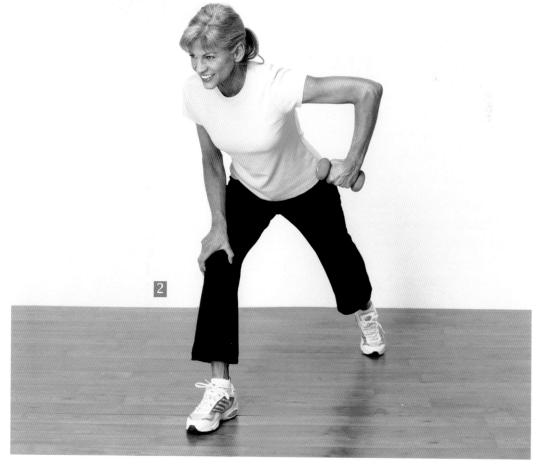

The Upper-Body ROUTINE

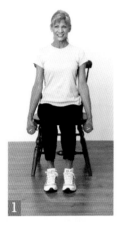

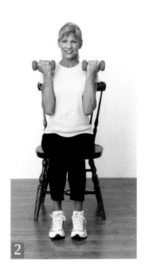

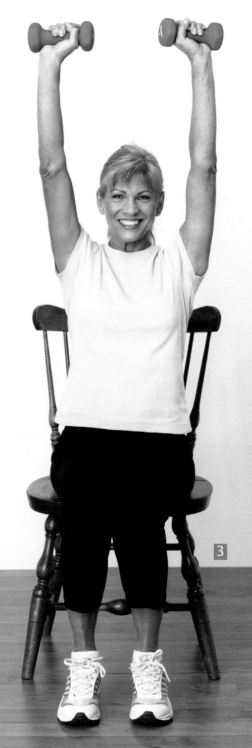

■ EXERCISE THREE
Curl and Press

1 Sit on a chair (preferably one without arms) with your feet flat on the floor. Hold a light dumbbell in each hand with your arms extended down at your sides.

2 Keeping your upper body stable, bend your elbows and curl the weights up toward your shoulders.

3 Immediately rotate your wrists so your palms are facing away from you and press the weights overhead. Pause, then reverse the move, lowering the weights to your shoulders, rotating your palms in toward your body, and lowering the weights back down to your sides. Do 8 to 12 repetitions.

■ EXERCISE FOUR

Triceps Kickback

1 Grasp a dumbbell in your left hand and place your right knee and hand on a chair seat so your back is parallel to the floor, as shown. Hold your left elbow at your side so your arm is bent at a 90-degree angle and your forearm is perpendicular to the floor.

2 Extend your elbow and move your hand backward until your forearm is parallel to the floor. Pause, then lower to the starting position. Complete 8 to 12 repetitions, then switch arms.

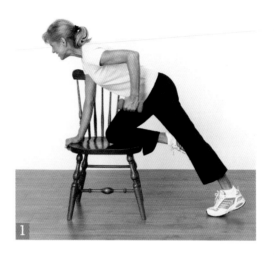

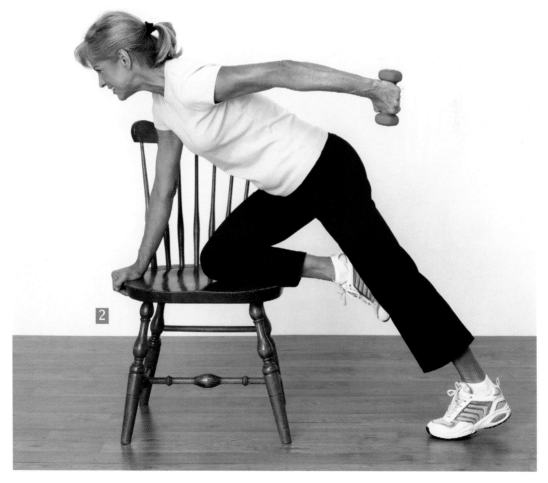

243

The Upper-Body ROUTINE

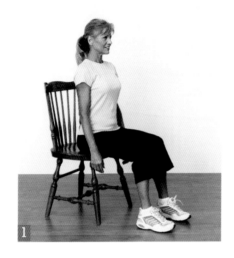

■ STRETCH ONE **Rag Doll**

1 Sit on the edge of a chair with your knees spread slightly and your feet directly below your knees.

2 Slump your body forward over your legs so your chest rests on or above your knees and your arms hang down. Wrap your arms under your knees and press your back up toward the ceiling. Hold this position for 20 to 30 seconds.

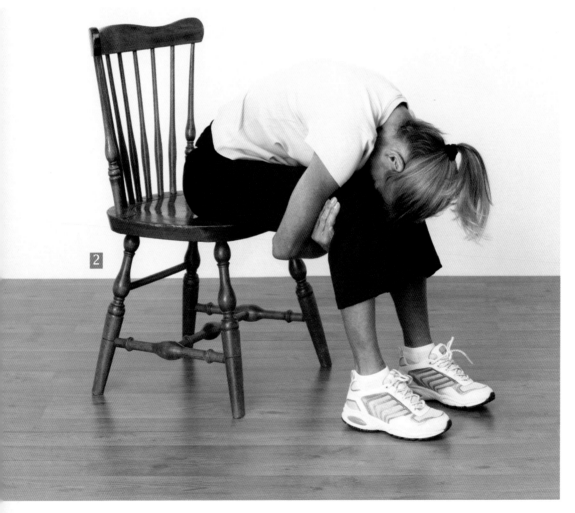

■ STRETCH TWO **De-Hunch**

1 Sit on the edge of a chair with your legs spread and your pelvis tilted slightly forward. Lift your chest and squeeze your shoulder blades together and down away from your ears.

2 Extend your arms at 45-degree angles from your body and reach slightly behind you with your palms facing forward. Hold 10 seconds, then relax for a few seconds. Repeat 3 times.

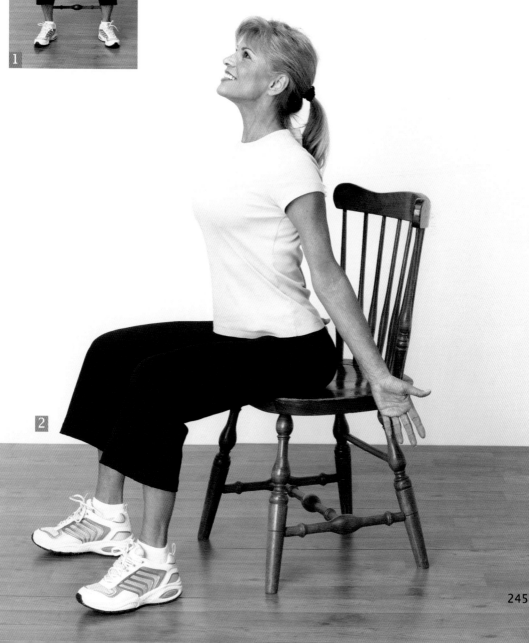

The Upper-Body ROUTINE

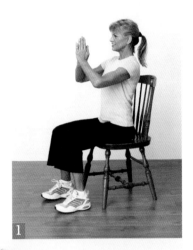

■ STRETCH THREE **Hand Press**

1 Sit on a chair with your feet flat on the floor. Press your palms together in front of your chest so your elbows are pointed out to the sides.

2 Keeping your hands pressed together, drop them down and slightly away from your body until you feel a stretch in your wrists and forearms. Hold for 20 seconds.

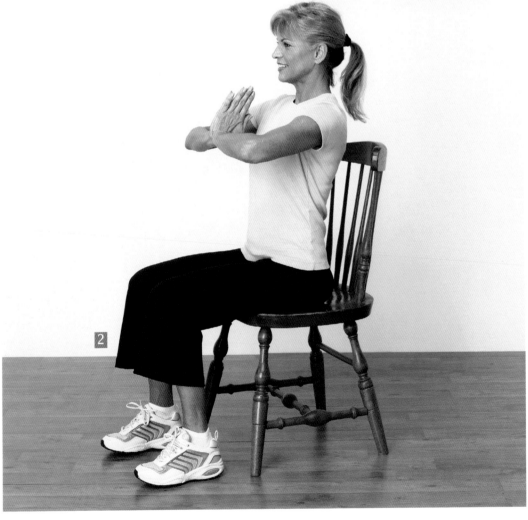

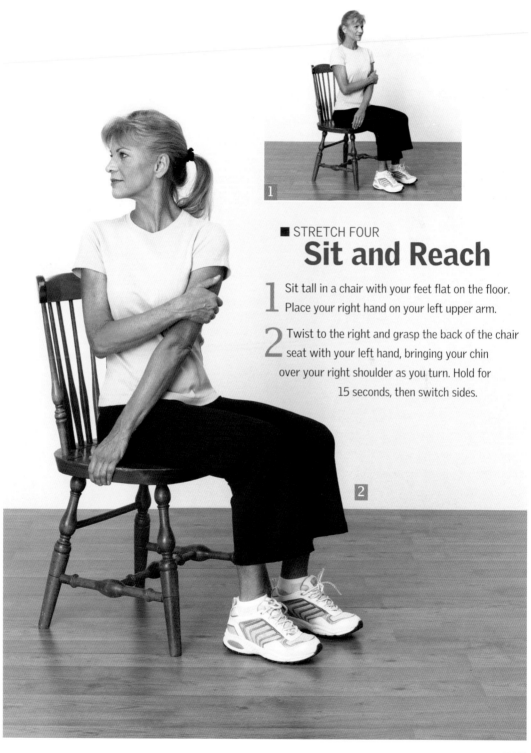

■ STRETCH FOUR
Sit and Reach

1 Sit tall in a chair with your feet flat on the floor.
Place your right hand on your left upper arm.

2 Twist to the right and grasp the back of the chair
seat with your left hand, bringing your chin
over your right shoulder as you turn. Hold for
15 seconds, then switch sides.

The Lower-Body ROUTINE

■ EXERCISE ONE Lawn-Mower Pull

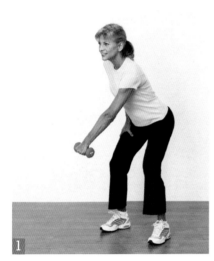

1 Stand with your feet hip-width apart, holding a light dumbbell in your left hand. Squat slightly until your legs are bent at about 45 degrees and place your right hand on your right thigh for support. Reach across your body with your left arm, holding the dumbbell in front of your right knee.

2 In one smooth motion, pull your arm back across your body (as though pulling a lawn mower cord) and stand up slightly, though not fully. Squat back down and repeat 5 times, slowly and carefully. Then switch sides.

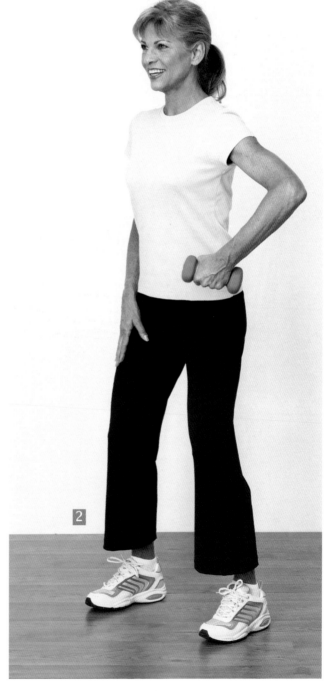

■ EXERCISE TWO **Chair Taps**

1 Stand tall, facing a chair, with your feet about hip-width apart and your hands on your hips. (You can place one hand on a wall for balance if you need to.)

2 Keeping your abdominal muscles tensed to support your back, lift your right foot and tap the seat of the chair with your toes. Return to the starting position. Repeat 10 times, then switch sides.

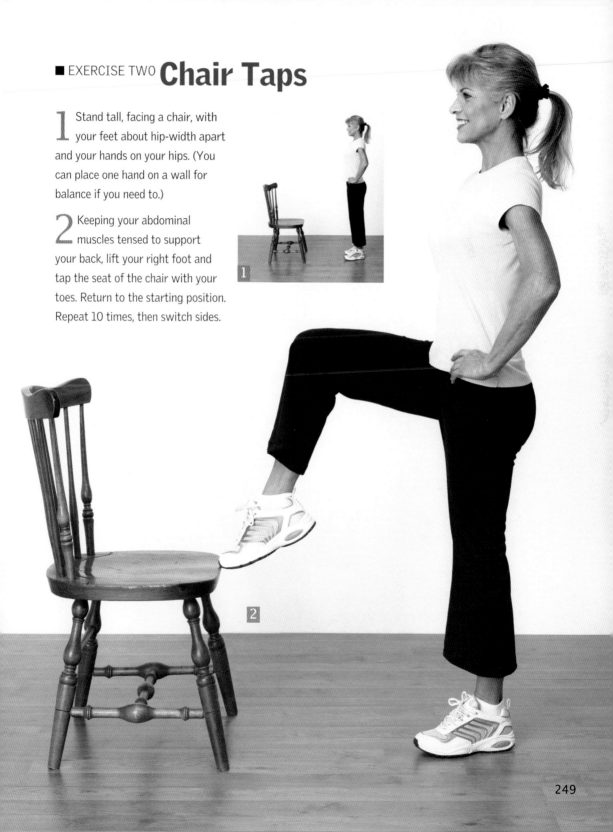

The Lower-Body ROUTINE

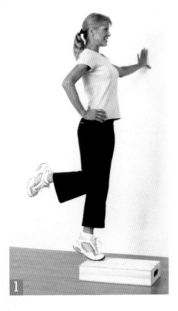

■ EXERCISE THREE

Heel Drop

1 Stand on the bottom step of a flight of stairs, or, if you have one, an exercise step. Lightly grasp the banister, or place your hand on a wall if using a step, for support. Bend your right leg and place the toes of your left foot on the edge of the step.

2 Let your left heel drop as far as comfortably possible. Press into the ball of your left foot and raise yourself onto your toes. Pause, then return to the starting position. Complete 8 to 12 repetitions, then switch legs.

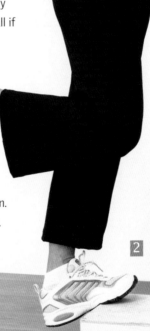

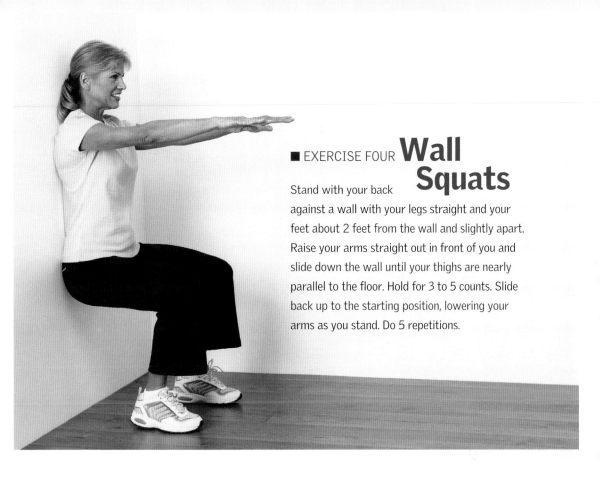

■ EXERCISE FOUR **Wall Squats**

Stand with your back against a wall with your legs straight and your feet about 2 feet from the wall and slightly apart. Raise your arms straight out in front of you and slide down the wall until your thighs are nearly parallel to the floor. Hold for 3 to 5 counts. Slide back up to the starting position, lowering your arms as you stand. Do 5 repetitions.

■ EXERCISE FIVE
Seated Leg Lift

Sit on the floor with your legs extended in front of you, your back straight, and your feet flexed. Place your hands on your lap or on the floor behind you for support. Keeping your foot flexed, tighten your left thigh and slowly raise your left heel off the floor. Pause, then slowly return to the starting position. Complete 8 to 12 repetitions, then switch legs.

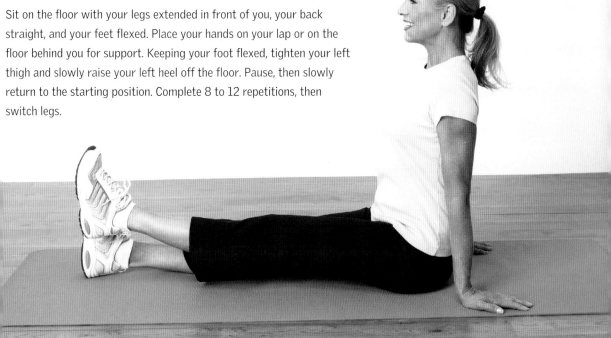

The Lower-Body ROUTINE

■ STRETCH ONE **Wall Stretch**

Stand at arm's length from a wall and place your palms flat against it. Extend your left leg behind you about 2 to 3 feet and press your left heel to the floor. (Your right knee will bend naturally as you extend the other leg.) Keeping both heels flat against the floor, press against the wall until you feel a nice stretch in your calf. Hold for 15 seconds, then repeat with the other leg.

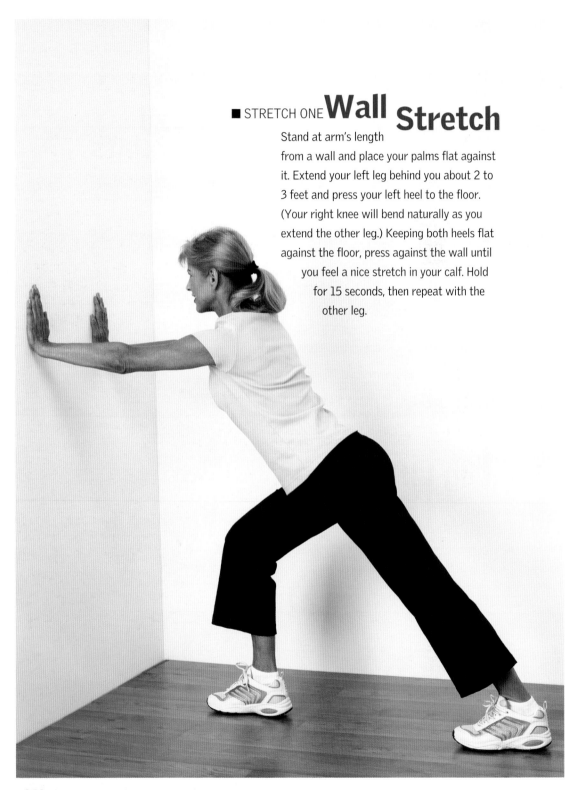

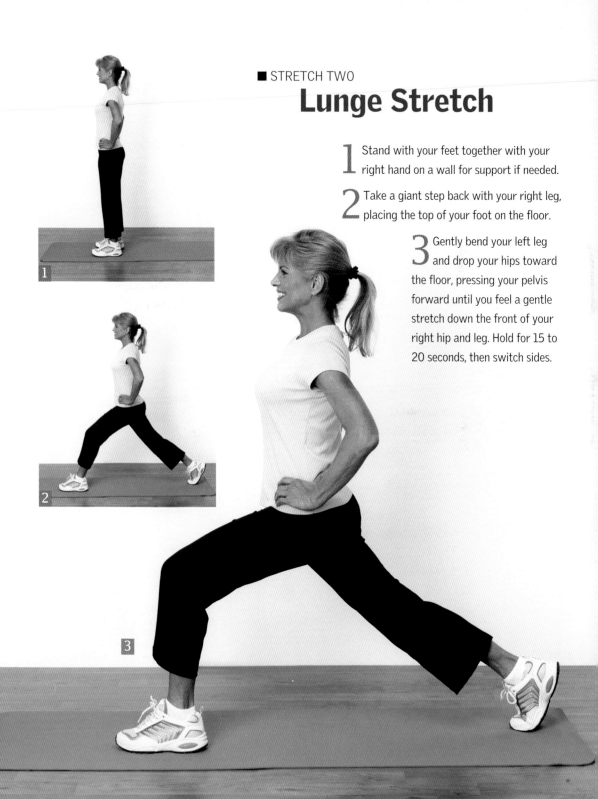

■ STRETCH TWO

Lunge Stretch

1 Stand with your feet together with your right hand on a wall for support if needed.

2 Take a giant step back with your right leg, placing the top of your foot on the floor.

3 Gently bend your left leg and drop your hips toward the floor, pressing your pelvis forward until you feel a gentle stretch down the front of your right hip and leg. Hold for 15 to 20 seconds, then switch sides.

The Lower-Body ROUTINE

■ STRETCH THREE
Butterfly

Sit on the floor with your back
straight, your knees bent, and the
soles of your feet touching so your
knees fall out to the sides. Grasp your
ankles with your hands. Keeping your
back straight (don't hunch over),
gently bend forward from the hips as
you press your knees down toward
the floor as far as comfortably
possible. Hold for 20 to 30 seconds.

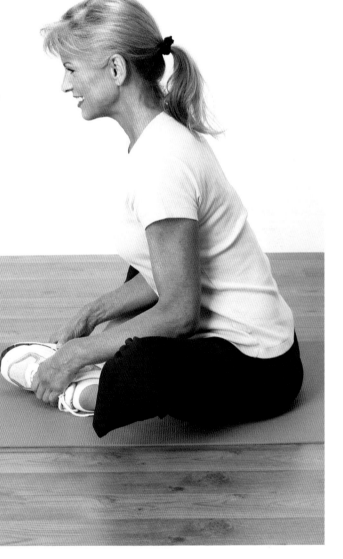

■ STRETCH FOUR **Standing Hamstring Stretch**

1 Standing upright, place your left heel about a foot in front of you and point your toes up. Place your hands on your right thigh for support.

2 Bend your right knee and gently bend forward from the hips, pressing your weight back until you feel a stretch in the back of your left leg. Hold 15 seconds, then switch legs.

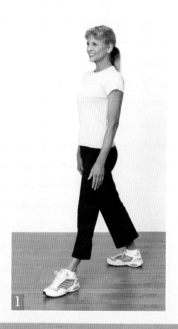

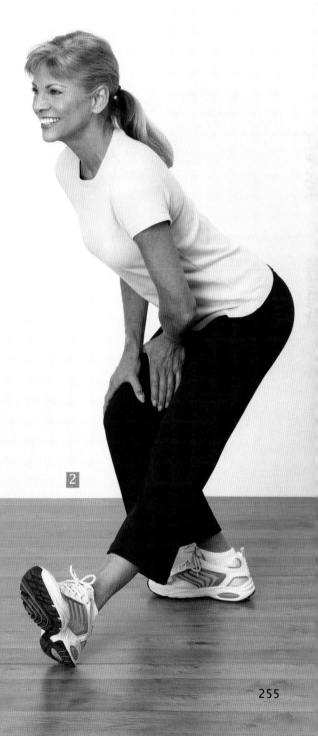

The Core-Body ROUTINE

■ EXERCISE ONE **Knee Drop**

1 Lie on your back with your knees bent, feet on the floor, arms straight out to the sides and hands resting on the floor, palms down.

2 Lift your legs so your knees are above your hips and your lower legs are parallel to the floor.

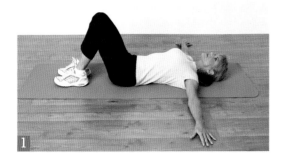

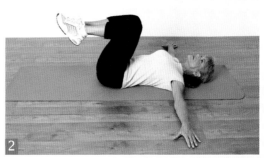

3 Contract your stomach muscles and drop both knees to the left as far as comfortably possible while keeping both shoulders on the floor. Pause, then return to the starting position. Repeat to the other side. That's 1 repetition. Alternate for a complete set of 10 reps.

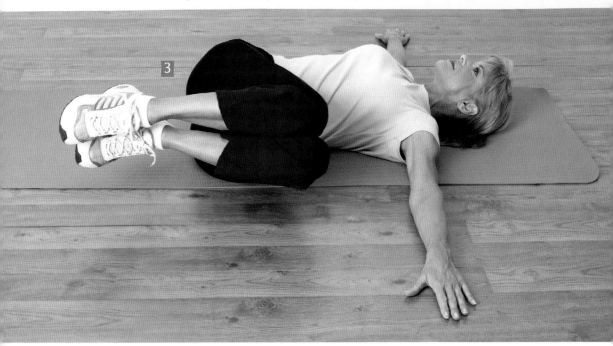

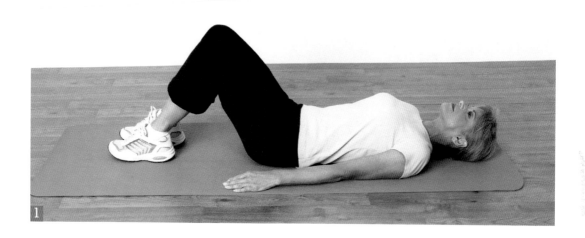

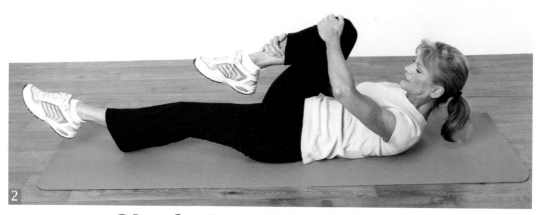

■ EXERCISE TWO **Single-Leg Stretch**

1 Despite the name, this is a strengthening exercise. Lie on your back with your knees bent. Tuck your chin to your chest and place your right hand on your right ankle and your left hand on your right knee.

2 Lift your left leg a few inches off the floor and pull your right knee toward your chest. Keeping your abdominals tight, switch sides, pulling your left knee toward your chest and lifting your right leg. Alternate 10 times for 1 set.

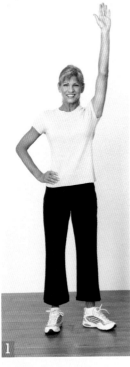

■ EXERCISE THREE
Standing
Side Crunch

1 Stand with your feet hip-width apart and your
left foot pointed slightly out to the side. Place
your right hand on your hip and extend your left
arm straight overhead.

2 Lift your left knee up and out to the side at
waist height as you move your left elbow
down to meet your knee. Repeat 10 times, then
switch sides.

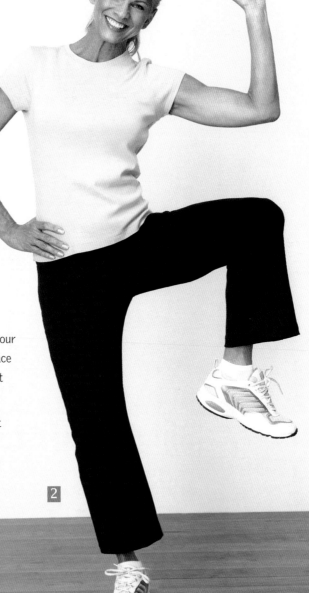

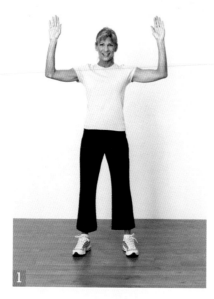

■ EXERCISE FOUR
Standing Crossover

1 Stand with your feet a few inches apart. Bend your arms at right angles and hold them out to your sides with your upper arms parallel to the floor and your palms facing forward.

2 Contract your stomach muscles and pull your left knee and right elbow toward each other. Pause, then return to the starting position. Do 8 to 12 repetitions, then switch sides.

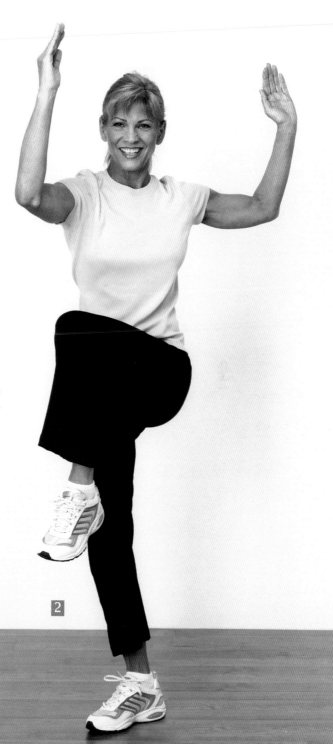

The Core-Body ROUTINE

■ STRETCH ONE Cat Stretch

1 Kneel on all fours with your hands directly below your shoulders and your knees directly below your hips. Pull your abdominal muscles in, drop your head, and press your back up, rounding it toward the ceiling.

2 Hold for 15 seconds, then raise your head and drop your belly toward the floor, arching your back in the opposite direction. Hold for 15 seconds.

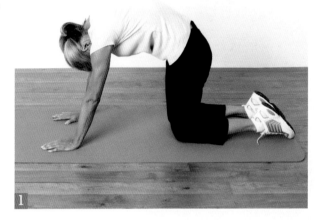

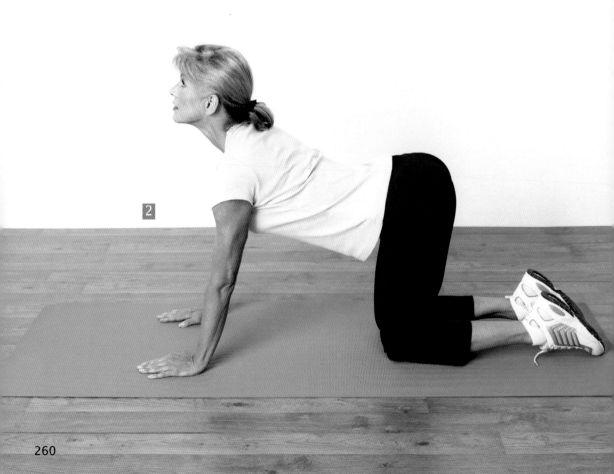

■ STRETCH TWO
Spinal
Twist

1 Kneel on all fours with your hands directly below your shoulders and your knees directly below your hips.

2 Extend your right arm under and across your body (your left arm will bend slightly) until your right shoulder is near or on the floor. Hold for 15 seconds, then switch sides.

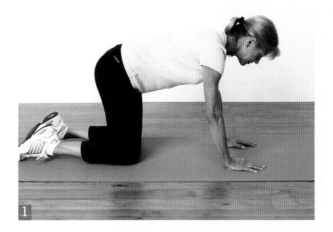

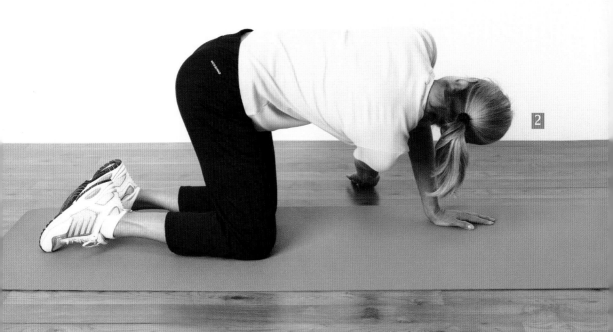

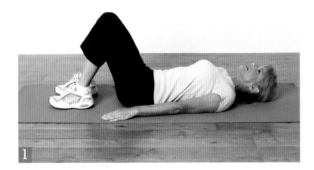

■ STRETCH THREE
Lower-Back Stretch

1 Lie on your back with your legs straight, then bend your knees toward your chest.

2 Clasp your right hand behind your right knee and your left hand behind your left knee and pull gently. Hold for 30 seconds.

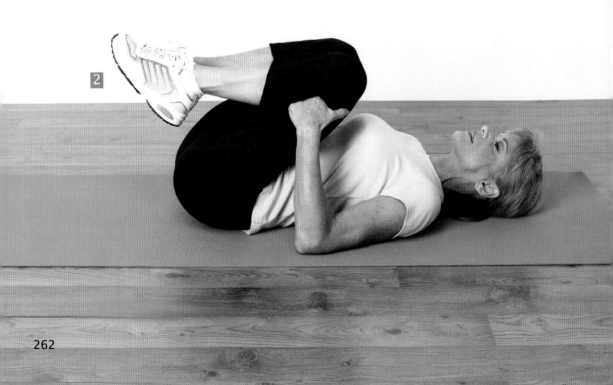

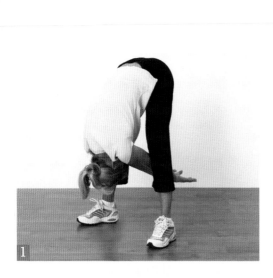

■ STRETCH FOUR Bend and Reach

1 Stand with your feet shoulder-width apart.
Contract your stomach muscles and bend
forward at the hips and knees, reaching your hands
between your knees, if possible.

2 Pause, then use your hips to straighten up,
extending your arms overhead and slightly
behind you. Hold for 10 seconds, then repeat. (If
you have back pain, skip the first part of this
stretch and simply stretch overhead.)

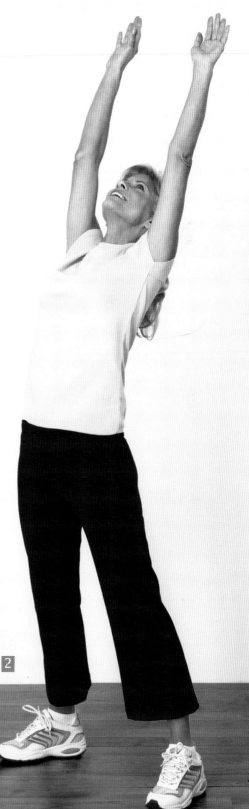

Get
Active

Move more, weigh less. That adage is so simple, so obvious, such a "Duh, I already knew that" statement that it barely seems worth repeating. That is, until you consider this: When Mayo Clinic scientists compared the minute-by-minute activity levels of overweight and skinny "couch potatoes," they discovered that the lean people were actually on their feet, moving around, for 152 more minutes every day than the others.

"Calories burned in everyday activities are far, far more important in obesity than we previously imagined," notes lead researcher James Levine, M.D., whose discovery inspired him to attach his computer to a low-speed treadmill and stash his telephone in a desk drawer so he would move more during the workday.

Now it's your turn. In the pages ahead, we'll help you find easy, fun, habit-forming ways to add more activity to your day.

You'll be surprised at how a little pacing, a little fidgeting, and a few extra steps can contribute to lasting weight loss.

Change One quiz

Does Daily Activity *Really* Matter?

For each question, choose True or False.

1. Sometimes the only difference between overweight and thin is the amount of "lifestyle activity"—standing, moving, or even twiddling your thumbs or flipping your hair out of the way a person gets.
☐ True ☐ False

2. Communicating with coworkers in person—by walking to their desk or office—rather than via e-mail or phone could, over time, save you two dress sizes.
☐ True ☐ False

3. Little "extra activities"—beating the cake batter by hand, walking from the farthest spot in the supermarket parking lot, scrubbing the floor by hand—can help you keep weight off better than a formal exercise routine can.
☐ True ☐ False

4. The reason people were thinner 50 years ago isn't just that they ate less. They moved more—so much more that few needed formal exercise programs to stay thin.
☐ True ☐ False

5. Walking upstairs can burn more calories faster than setting out on a fitness walk.
☐ True ☐ False

6. You could find a baby sitter for the kids while you work out, but you can burn just as many calories, and work your muscles just as hard, if you do some yard work with your family and then play a game of catch or kickball.
☐ True ☐ False

7. The following are great pieces of exercise equipment: a cast-iron skillet, a kitchen cleaver, a push lawn mower, a hose and a bucket of sudsy water to wash the car.
☐ True ☐ False

8. Even small amounts of activity can boost your energy quotient because movement sends more oxygen- and glucose-rich blood to your brain and muscles.
☐ True ☐ False

9. Who needs barbells? If you have a dog, you have a built-in arm-strengthening buddy living at your house. Just find a rope and start your workout!
☐ True ☐ False

Score

The answer to each question is emphatically "True." Lifestyle activity is a big part of the *ChangeOne* Fitness approach because it's both effective and versatile. It works all your muscle groups, it's easy to fit into your day, it requires no special clothes or equipment, and usually, it requires just slight adjustments to whatever you're doing now. Lifestyle activity also burns more calories than you might think—in one study, it kept weight off better than step aerobics!

Motionless in America

Ever wonder why folks in 1950s-era snapshots look so slim? Most of them (except perhaps Jack LaLanne) weren't pumping iron, training for a local 5K race, or dashing to the gym for Pilates class. The truth is, everyday life was packed with hundreds of activities that added up to a big calorie burn.

Among them, doing the laundry often meant using a hand-cranked wringer to squeeze excess water out of the wash (most machines didn't have automatic spin cycles), and drying it meant hauling baskets of heavy, wet clothes, sheets, and towels outside to hang on the line; car windows opened only if you rolled them down; and the only way to tune in Ed Sullivan on Sunday night was to get off the couch, cross the room, and turn the knob to switch channels. Corner grocery stores were commonplace, making it convenient to walk over for milk or an ice-cream cone—and most families had just one car, so daytime errands were often performed on foot.

Modern conveniences help us burn 700 fewer calories a day.

At work, communicating with coworkers required walking to their desks, and sending a message outside the company meant typing a letter on a manual typewriter, often with stiff keys that only responded to very muscular banging. The kids played outside, so moms and dads would wander out, too, to talk with the neighbors. Few families owned riding lawn mowers, so cutting the grass entailed lots of pushing.

Now, fast-forward to the 21st century—the era of the motionless American.

Thanks to modern technology, we've engineered so many old-fashioned "inconveniences" out of our lives that we burn an astonishing 700 *fewer* calories a day now. You can deposit your paycheck, buy a cheeseburger, pick up prescriptions, grab a cappuccino, and even (in some states) purchase a six-pack of beer at a drive-through. Remote controls operate our TVs and CD players; at the push of a button (a movement that burns a half calorie at best), you can wash the dishes, shop online, roll up your car window, heat dinner in the microwave (no preparation required either), or e-mail your neighbor. Vacuum cleaners and lawn mowers are self-propelled.

As the number of TV channels grows into the thousands, we're glued to the tube for hours each day—entering a trancelike state that Harvard University researchers say requires even fewer calories than reading a magazine, sewing, or playing a board game.

Trouble? You bet. Even if you add more dedicated exercise time to your day, you still won't compensate for all that inactivity. And this round-the-clock inaction only perpetuates itself. After all, inactivity leads to feeling lethargic. When you're feeling lethargic and low on energy, the last thing you want to do is get up and do something, so you feel more lethargic, and...well, you see how this leads to more couch time and even less activity.

The answer: Rediscover the joys of an active lifestyle—defined here as a daily routine in which you embrace as much movement as possible, whenever possible. It means standing and pacing while on the phone; opting for the stairs rather than the elevator; stretching your muscles while standing in line; and getting on your feet whenever possible.

ChangeOne Fitness will help you engineer activity back into your day in clever, enjoyable ways that add up to a significant, slimming calorie burn. It's your insurance policy against overweight—and a strategy that top weight-loss researchers say is proven to work. Combine a more active lifestyle with 10 minutes of daily strengthening/stretching moves and a daily walk, and you will be well on your way to a leaner, healthier, more energized you.

Getting active has multiple bonuses, too. Among them:

No need to leave home. If you're taking care of the kids or staying home with an elderly or ill loved one, it's not easy finding time to take a walk or head to the gym. But washing the car, scrubbing a floor, putting on a silly CD and dancing around the living room, or weeding an overgrown flower bed are possible.

Instant gratification-doubled. Finish one of our recommended "get active" activities, and you'll burn an extra 100 to 300 calories and have something to show for it: A clean, organized coat closet. A shiny kitchen floor. A beautiful flower bed. Or a bunch of smiling, happy kids (because they've been dancing or running around with you)!

5 Rules of Active Living

1. Never sit when you can stand.

2. Never stand when you can walk.

3. Always have some part of your body in motion.

4. Carry things more often and farther.

5. Use your feet for transportation whenever possible.

Help!

I'm too tired after work to move more! What can I do?

We'll assume that you are watching television come evening. Our recommendation: Do a little bit of exercise at every commercial break or every 10 minutes of viewing. (We won't let channel flipping be an excuse not to do this!) At first, limit yourself to stretching. Roll your ankles in circles, clockwise and then counterclockwise. Then draw big imaginary letters with your big toes; spell out your full name. Sit up straight, raise your arms over your head, clasp your hands, and reach higher to stretch your shoulders.

Feeling more ambitious? Up the exertion level during commercials: Walk around the house; do sit-ups; or assign each character in your favorite show an exercise, then do that move 10 times during the commercial break after the character first appears. Also do chores during commercials. Emptying wastebaskets, vacuuming a room, putting in a load of wash, or cleaning the casserole dish that's been soaking in the sink can all add up to plenty of calorie-burning chore time every hour. When you're finished, your home will shine—and you will have saved hundreds of calories by not snacking.

Watching TV with the kids? Announce a new rule: Everybody dances during commercials.

A guaranteed energy boost. Moving more helps cut stress and improves the flow of blood—and oxygen and blood sugar—to your muscles and brain.

It Really Works!

Researchers have long known that fitting more tidbits of activity into every hour of the day can help you lose weight as effectively as formal exercise—and seems to be even better for keeping it off.

When 40 overweight women either followed a low-calorie diet and added step aerobics classes three times a week or tried to squeeze more lifestyle activity into every day, both groups lost about 16 pounds after 16 weeks. After one year, the aerobics group had regained about 3½ pounds, but the lifestyle group had put on less than ¼ pound, reported University of Pennsylvania weight-loss researchers.

When scientists at the Cooper Institute for Aerobics Research in Dallas assigned 235 overweight women and men to either two years of formal exercise or a plan of stepped-up daily activity, both groups got fitter—and the lifestyle group lost more body fat.

At the Mayo Clinic, Dr. Levine's research team not only measured the daily activities of lean and overweight study volunteers (to record the measurements, the participants wore specially wired undergarments). They also put both groups on diets so the overweight people would slim down and the lean people would gain weight. The result? Even when at their new weights, naturally active people moved around more and naturally sedentary people remained...more motionless. The take-home lesson? If you tend to sit around, you'll have to resolve to get out of your seat more frequently.

That's where we come in. The rest of this chapter will give you dozens of ways to do just that.

At Home: Slimming Chores

How would you like to burn 250 calories in an hour, maybe more, and have a sparkling clean house afterward? You can if you see the hidden activity opportunity in housework. You'll also use most, if not all, of your major muscle groups—in your arms, legs, torso, and back. Here are some ways to maximize the burn.

Don't just wait; do something. Instead of pausing while the microwave heats something or waiting for the washer or dryer to finish a cycle, do squats or push-ups against a wall or just march in place. Walk around the first or second floor of your house or jog lightly in place.

Get a Chinese cleaver. These big knives, favored by chefs due to their heft and sharp blades, weigh more than almost any other kitchen knife, and therefore, you'll burn more calories every time you wield one instead of a puny vegetable knife. And you just might feel like an Iron Chef.

Cook as if it's 1904. Chop veggies by hand instead of in the food processor, whip eggs with a fork or whisk, mix cake batter with a big spoon instead of the mixer, dig out your manual can opener and get rid of the electric model, and, if you have time, wash and dry the dishes by hand. Use a cast-iron skillet—it's heavy! You'll get a bonus workout if you store it in a low cabinet and lift it up to the stove each time you plan to use it.

Make more trips. Stop fretting about making extra trips up and down the stairs and view them as your real-world Stairmaster routine. Skip the laundry chute and carry the clothes down to the basement in a basket. On weekends, consider resurrecting the lost art of drying

That's Amazing!

Just 10 minutes of doing an everyday activity may burn more calories than you'd expect.

Activity	Calories burned*
Walking downstairs	78-111
Walking upstairs	202-288
Making beds	46-65
Washing windows	48-69
Dusting	31-44
Washing floors	53-75
Gardening	42-59
Weeding	68-98
Using a push mower	52-74
Preparing a meal	46-65
Washing or dressing	37-53
Shoveling snow	89-130
Painting a house	40-55
Chopping firewood	84-121
Repairing a car	43-59
Caring for babies or toddlers	41-63
Playing the piano	32-47
Electrical work/plumbing	45-65

*Calorie range is for weights of 175-250 pounds.

clothes on a clothesline; your sheets will smell like sunshine and fresh air. Volunteer to take the trash out or empty the car after a vacation.

Scrub it. Washing floors by hand—the very old-fashioned way, on your knees—works your arm, back, and abdominal muscles. Just be sure to keep your tummy muscles tight so they help support your back.

Chew gum while you're working. The simple act of moving your jaws uses up about 11 calories per hour.

Bake bread once a week. Kneading dough is soothing and works muscles in your arms and shoulders. And the taste? Divine.

Outdoors: The Whittle-Your-Waist Work Party

Here are more ways to use the great outdoors as your personal gym.

Automatic Activity

When the phone rings...talk standing up and move around your house.

When sitting at a desk...tap your toes, bounce your knee, and do leg lifts.

When standing in line...stand on your heels and lift your toes as high as they can go.

When washing dishes...repeatedly rise onto your toes.

When bored...put the palms of your hands together in front of your chest and push them into each other as hard as you can.

When using a laptop computer...put it on a high counter and stand up to work.

While watching TV...walk in place.

While waiting at a red light...fully stretch your legs, arms, and neck.

Rake leaves. You'll burn 50 extra calories per half hour when you rake by hand rather than using a leaf blower.

Spiff up your ride. Wash your car by hand. You'll save money by not going to the car wash and burn up to 280 calories in an hour. Why not vacuum the upholstery and carpeting, wash the plastic trim on the insides of the doors, and do the insides of the windows, too?

Sweep the steps. Since you're not using the leaf blower, haul out the broom to clear your steps. Gee, wouldn't it be nice to give 'em a scrubbing, too? Got an extra 15 minutes? How about washing down the front door and the doorsill while you're at it.

Trim the old-time way. Leave the electric edger and trimmer in the garage and grab your old hand tools. Comfort hint: Use thick foam or an old carpet square to cushion your knees.

Change One success stories
Choosing to Be Healthy

It's hard to imagine how, as a mother of four, Cindy Bonsteel finds the time to exercise and make healthy meals. But, thanks to *ChangeOne* and her hard work and determination, she's already lost 110 pounds and is well on her way to her ultimate weight-loss goal.

"My husband and I have been married for 18½ years and have four beautiful children who are 17, 14, 3, and 2 years old," she says. "I had decided that I needed time for me first, and by doing that, I have gotten healthier and now have more energy for the children and my husband."

Even with the demands of caring for her large family, Cindy finds time to exercise. "I started to do step aerobics in the afternoons when my little ones were napping," she says. "As I got more healthy and lost more weight, I started to add miles to my walks, and now I am power walking. Three days a week, I go 1 hour early to pick up my 3-year-old at his preschool, and I do my walk there. We purchased a Bowflex machine, and I do strength training three or four days a week with that, and I also use it when my little ones are napping."

Her entire family has picked up on her new healthy habits. "The family likes *ChangeOne* meals, and they don't have any problem adjusting to that," she says. "We also have plenty of fresh fruits and pretzels on hand to snack on."

A mother of four, Cindy Bonsteel lost 110 pounds and now her whole family practices new healthy habits.

She recommends that people just starting *ChangeOne* stick with the program and try to remember they're making changes that will become new habits. "Before you know it, the weight will start coming off, and that really motivates you to keep sticking with it," she says.

"I don't like to call this a diet, as everyone in the world has a 'diet,'" she says. "You can have a junk-food diet or a healthy diet, and I choose to be healthy."

For more ChangeOne *success stories, go to www.changeone.com/successstories*

Rehab the push mower. Revive a lovely summer sound: the whisk-whisk-whisk of a muscle-powered push mower. Buy one and consider it an investment in a piece of exercise equipment, or rehabilitate the old one stashed way in the back of the garage. Sharpen the blades, oil the mechanism, and go. Ah! No exhaust fumes, no ugly power-motor noise.

Double-dig. Gardeners know that the best soil is double-dug. When you put in a new bed or turn over the soil in your vegetable patch in the spring, leave the power tiller in the shed and get out there with a sharp shovel. Dig each row twice—first to a single shovel's depth, then down one more shovel's worth. Refill the row by putting the first digging's soil in the bottom and the second's on top. You'll have more fertile soil on top and fluffy dirt down deep, so tender roots can grow strong, creating beautiful, healthy plants.

Plant bulbs. Garden catalogs start advertising sales of fall bulbs in midsummer. That's the time to think about daffodils, daylilies, tulips, and a host of other gorgeous spring and summer flowers for next year. Order a bunch and plant them over several fall weekends. Your efforts will be rewarded with a stunning display once winter's gone.

Stop buying weed killer. Be a friend to the earth and to your own muscles: Pull, dig out, and cut back weeds yourself. Your arms and back will get a workout.

On the Job: Don't Be Desk-Bound

It's easy to stay seated at work, jump up for lunch, and then plunk down again until quitting time rolls around. Here's how to burn more calories and add more energy to your day.

Get more "face time." Instead of sending e-mails or calling coworkers, stop by their desks to ask a question or figure out a solution to a work issue. Doing this instead of sending just one e-mail a day could save you 11 pounds over 10 years!

Take energy breaks. Every half hour, walk around your office or down the hall for 5 minutes. Jump up and down in your own office. Do push-ups with your hands resting against your desk. Do 10 leg lifts, then stand up and rise on your toes 10 times. Stretch your arms high 10 times, too.

Get a rolling chair. Try sitting on a large exercise ball instead of a desk chair. You'll use your abdominal and back muscles all day to help you balance.

Go the long way. Circle the building before heading to lunch. Use the bathroom or copy machine farthest from your desk. Volunteer to help coworkers move boxes or carry files or books.

Take the stairs, of course. *ChangeOne* recommends taking the steps at least twice a day. Just two flights daily could help you melt 6 pounds in a year! Climbing the stairs for just 2 minutes five days a week gives you the same calorie-burning, heart-rate-quickening results as a 36-minute walk!

Plan a walking meeting. Need to schedule a small meeting? Suggest a walking meeting instead of a confab in an airless conference room. Take a small notebook and a pen. Chances are, you'll have better ideas and forge a better relationship with your fellow walkers.

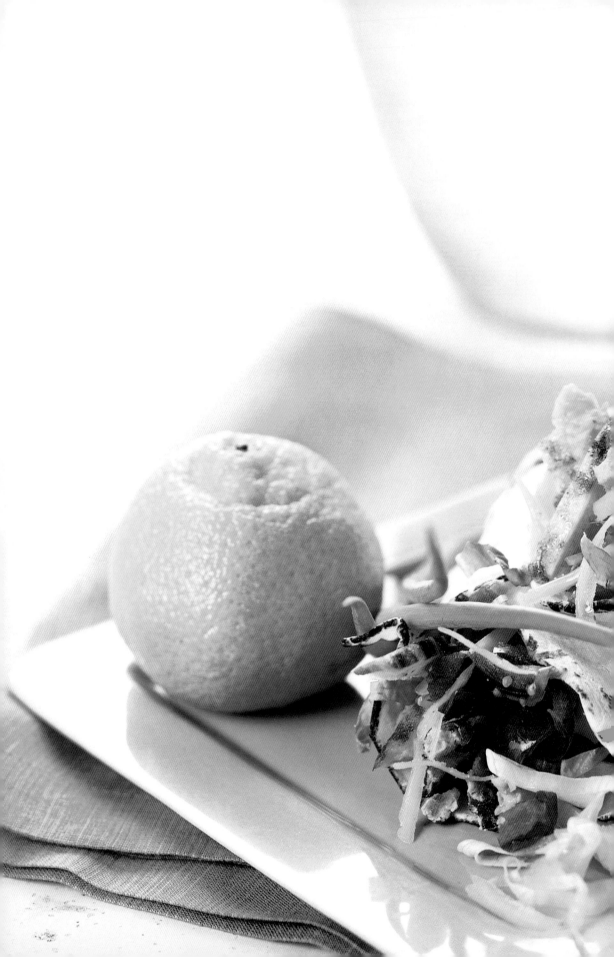

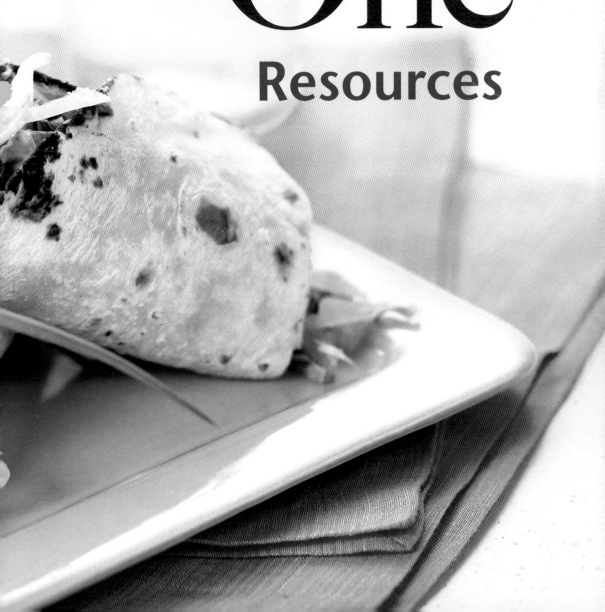

Part 3

Change
One

Resources

ChangeOne
Meals

Want to know the perfect dinner recipe? Here's the ingredient list:

- 1 smart shopping trip
- 1 well-stocked pantry
- 30 minutes free time
- 1 healthy dose of motivation
- 1 small pinch of cooking know-how

Have these ingredients? Then delicious, healthy *ChangeOne* meals are pretty much guaranteed!

In the pages ahead you'll find more than 60 fresh and easy recipes for *ChangeOne* dishes. But that's just a start. We also provide sample meal plans, shopping strategies, and more—enough kitchen know-how to make *ChangeOne* eating a snap!

You'll also find wonderful food photos, all showing proper *ChangeOne* portion sizes. Each recipe was developed to meet the *ChangeOne* calorie and nutrition guidelines as closely as possible. Want more recipes? There are cookbooks' worth at changeone.com.

Breakfast RECIPES

Silver Dollar Pancakes

SERVES 4

- ½ **cup self-rising flour**
- ½ **tablespoon sugar**
- ¼ **teaspoon baking soda**
- ¾ **cup buttermilk**
- 1 **tablespoon vegetable oil**
- 1 **large egg**
- ½ **teaspoon vanilla extract**

1. In a medium bowl, whisk the flour, sugar, and baking soda. In a small bowl, whisk the buttermilk, oil, egg, and vanilla until blended. Make a well in the flour mixture, pour in the buttermilk mixture, and whisk just until moistened. Let stand for 5 minutes.

2. Meanwhile, coat a large nonstick skillet with cooking spray and set over medium heat until hot but not smoking.

3. For each pancake, pour 1 tablespoon of batter into the skillet. Cook until bubbles appear all over the surface and begin to burst, about 3 minutes. Turn and cook until the undersides are golden, about 1 to 2 minutes.

Note: Make 4 pancakes for yourself. If not cooking for others, you can cover the extra batter and refrigerate for the next day or cook the entire recipe, wrap extra pancakes in foil, and refrigerate for a day or freeze for a week. To reheat, place wrapped pancakes in a 350°F oven for about 10 minutes.

The *ChangeOne* breakfast

4 silver dollar pancakes, 1 tablespoon light maple syrup, ½ cup sliced strawberries (2 golf balls), 8 ounces fat-free or low-fat milk

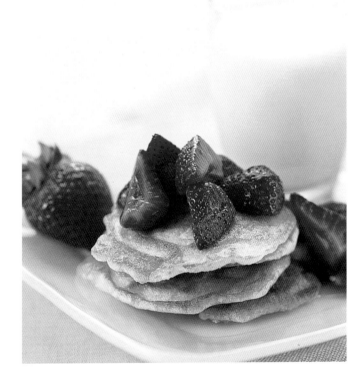

Breakfast RECIPES

Dried Cranberry Scones with Orange Glaze

MAKES 18

- 3 cups all-purpose flour
- 1½ teaspoons baking powder
- ½ teaspoon salt
- ¼ cup sugar
- 1¼ cups fat-free plain yogurt
- 3 tablespoons butter, melted
- 3 tablespoons margarine, melted
- 1 egg, lightly beaten
- 1 cup sweetened dried cranberries
- ½ cup sifted confectioners' sugar
- 1 teaspoon orange zest (grated rind)
- 1 tablespoon fresh orange juice

1. Preheat the oven to 400°F. Line 2 baking sheets with parchment paper.

2. In a large bowl, combine the flour, baking powder, salt, and sugar. In a small bowl, mix the yogurt, butter, margarine, and egg.

3. Make a well in the center of the flour mixture, pour in the yogurt mixture, and blend with a fork until moistened. Stir in the cranberries. Flour your hands and gently knead the dough in the bowl just until it comes together.

4. Turn the dough out onto a floured work surface and pat into a 9-inch square about 1 inch thick. With a small knife, cut into 9 squares, then cut each square into 2 triangles. Place the triangles 1 inch apart on the baking sheets and bake until golden, about 15 minutes.

5. In a small bowl, combine the confectioners' sugar, orange rind, and orange juice. When the scones are cool, transfer in batches to a wire rack set on a piece of wax paper, parchment, or foil and drizzle the glaze over them with a small spoon.

The *ChangeOne* breakfast

1 Blueberry Muffin with Lemon Glaze or 1 Dried Cranberry Scone with Orange Glaze, 1 wedge cantaloupe (about ⅛ whole cantaloupe), ¾ cup steaming latte (½ cup fat-free milk plus ¼ cup strong coffee)

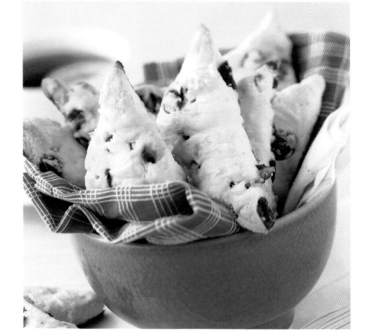

Blueberry Muffins with Lemon Glaze

MAKES 12

- 2 cups all-purpose flour
- 1 tablespoon baking powder
- ½ teaspoon salt
- ½ cup granulated sugar
- 2 eggs
- 4 tablespoons butter or margarine, melted
- ⅓ cup reduced-fat sour cream
- 2 teaspoons vanilla extract
- 1 cup plus 1 tablespoon fat-free or low-fat milk
- 1½ cups fresh or frozen blueberries
- ½ cup sifted confectioners' sugar
- 2 teaspoons lemon zest (grated rind)

1. Preheat the oven to 400°F. Put paper liners in a 12-cup muffin pan.

2. In a large bowl, mix the flour, baking powder, salt, and granulated sugar. In a medium bowl, combine the eggs, butter, sour cream, vanilla, and 1 cup of the milk.

3. Make a well in the center of the flour mixture. Pour in the egg mixture and stir with a fork until just blended; don't overmix. Fold in 1 cup of the blueberries.

4. Spoon the batter into the muffin cups and sprinkle evenly with the remaining blueberries. Bake until a toothpick inserted in the center of a muffin comes out clean, about 20 minutes. Cool on a wire rack for 10 minutes.

5. In a small bowl, combine the confectioners' sugar, lemon rind, and enough of the remaining milk to make the glaze liquid enough to drizzle over the cooled muffins.

Variation: Instead of blueberries, try sliced strawberries; 1 cup banana slices with ½ cup walnuts (no glaze); 1 cup chopped apple with ½ cup pecans (no glaze); or 1 cup pumpkin and 1 teaspoon pumpkin pie spice (no glaze).

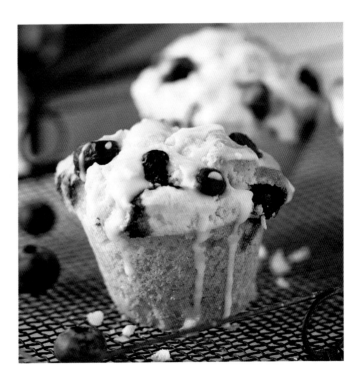

Breakfast RECIPES

Peach Quick Bread

SERVES 16

 2   medium peaches
1½   cups all-purpose flour
 ¾   cup whole wheat flour
 ¼   cup toasted wheat germ
 ¾   cup sugar
 1   teaspoon baking soda
 ½   teaspoon salt
 ½   cup fat-free plain yogurt
 1   egg
 2   egg whites
 2   tablespoons canola oil
 1   teaspoon almond
     extract

1. Preheat the oven to 350°F. Coat a 9- by 5-inch loaf pan with cooking spray.

2. In a medium saucepan, blanch the peaches in boiling water for 20 seconds. Peel, pit, and finely chop the peaches (you should have about 1 cup).

3. In a large bowl, combine the all-purpose flour, whole wheat flour, wheat germ, sugar, baking soda, and salt. In a small bowl, combine the yogurt, egg, egg whites, oil, and almond extract. Make a well in the flour mixture, pour in the yogurt mixture, and stir just until combined; do not overmix. Fold in the peaches.

4. Spoon the batter into the pan and smooth the top. Bake until a toothpick inserted in the center comes out clean, about 1 hour. Cool in the pan on a wire rack for 10 minutes, then turn out onto the rack to cool completely. Cut into 16 equal slices.

The *ChangeOne* breakfast

1 slice Peach Quick Bread (about ½ inch thick), ½ cup fresh raspberries (2 golf balls), 8 ounces fat-free milk, 1 cup coffee or tea

---

Vegetable-Cheddar Omelet

SERVES 1

 2   eggs
 1   teaspoon water
 2   teaspoons chopped
     fresh herbs (such as dill,
     basil, and parsley)
 ⅛   teaspoon salt
 ⅛   teaspoon fresh-ground
     black pepper
 ½   cup loosely packed
     thinly sliced fresh
     spinach
 1   plum tomato, chopped
 2   tablespoons shredded
     reduced-fat cheddar
     cheese

1. In a medium bowl, whisk the eggs, water, herbs, salt, and pepper. In a small bowl, toss together the spinach, tomato, and cheese; set aside.

2. Lightly coat a nonstick omelet pan or small skillet with cooking spray and set over medium heat for 1 minute. Pour in the egg mixture and cook until it begins to set on the bottom. Lift the edge with a spatula, pushing the cooked part toward the center of the pan and letting the uncooked portion run underneath. Cook until the top is almost set and the bottom is lightly browned.

3. Spread the spinach mixture over half of the omelet, leaving a ½-inch border around the edge and reserving 1 tablespoon of filling. Lift the omelet at the edge and fold in half. Cook for 2 minutes. Slide onto a plate and garnish with the reserved filling.

The *ChangeOne* breakfast

1 Vegetable-Cheddar Omelet, ¾ cup oven-baked potato wedges (lightly brush potatoes with oil, season, and bake at 375°F for 40 minutes), 1 wedge cantaloupe (about ⅛ of the canteloupe)

Zesty Cheddar-Asparagus Quiche

SERVES 6

1 tablespoon plain dried
bread crumbs

½ pound small all-purpose
potatoes, peeled and
very thinly sliced

2 teaspoons olive oil

1 pound asparagus,
trimmed

½ teaspoon salt

¾ cup shredded reduced-
fat sharp cheddar cheese

3 scallions, sliced

1 can (12 ounces) fat-free
evaporated milk

2 eggs

2 egg whites

2 teaspoons butter, melted

1 teaspoon dry mustard

¼ teaspoon fresh-ground
black pepper

1. Preheat the oven to 400°F. Coat a 9-inch pie pan with cooking spray and sprinkle with the bread crumbs. Beginning in the center, arrange the potato slices in slightly overlapping circles out to the sides. Lightly brush with the oil and press down gently. Bake for 10 minutes.

2. Set 8 to 12 asparagus spears aside. Cut the remaining spears into 1-inch pieces.

3. Sprinkle the crust with ¼ teaspoon of the salt and ¼ cup of the cheese. Cover with the asparagus pieces, then sprinkle with the scallions and another ¼ cup of the cheese. Arrange the whole asparagus spears on top.

4. In a medium bowl, beat the milk, eggs, egg whites, butter, mustard, pepper, and the remaining salt. Pour into the pan and sprinkle with the remaining cheese. Bake until a knife inserted in center comes out clean, about 35 minutes.

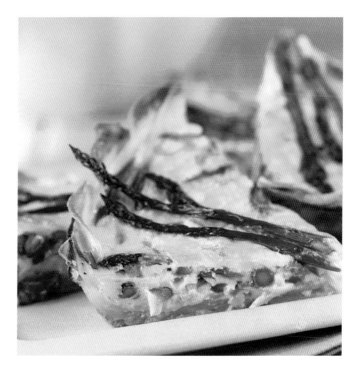

**The *ChangeOne*
breakfast**

1 slice Zesty Cheddar-
Asparagus Quiche, 1 slice
Peach Quick Bread (recipe
on page 280), 6 ounces
orange juice

Breakfast RECIPES

Vegetable Frittata

SERVES 4

- 4 ounces white mush-rooms, washed, trimmed, and thinly sliced
- ⅓ cup sliced red onion
- 5 eggs
- 4 egg whites
- 1 teaspoon chopped fresh herbs (thyme, oregano, or basil)
- ¼ teaspoon salt
- ¼ teaspoon fresh-ground black pepper
- 4 small plum tomatoes, thinly sliced
- 8 tablespoons shredded part-skim mozzarella cheese

1. Preheat the broiler. Coat a 10-inch nonstick, ovenproof skillet with cooking spray and set over medium-high heat. Add mushrooms and onion and sauté until tender, about 5 minutes. Transfer to a plate. Wipe out the skillet, coat with cooking spray, and return to the heat.

3. In a medium bowl, whisk the eggs, egg whites, herbs, salt, and pepper. Pour into the skillet and cook until the eggs begin to set, about 2 minutes. Don't stir, but lift the edge with a heatproof spatula and tilt the skillet to let the uncooked portion flow underneath.

4. Arrange the tomatoes and sautéed vegetables in concentric circles on top. Cook until the frittata is golden on the bottom and almost set on top, 2 to 3 minutes.

5. Sprinkle the cheese around the edges of the frittata. Transfer the skillet to the broiler and broil until the cheese melts and begins to brown, about 2 minutes. Cut into quarters.

The *ChangeOne* breakfast

1 wedge Vegetable Frittata (checkbook size), ½ cup fresh blueberries (2 golf balls), and 1 slice whole wheat toast

---

Chesapeake Crab Cakes

SERVES 4

- ½ cup fresh bread crumbs
- 1 celery stalk with leaves, finely chopped
- ⅓ cup finely chopped red bell pepper
- 2 tablespoons minced shallot
- 1 tablespoon finely chopped parsley
- 2 tablespoons coarse-grained mustard
- 2 tablespoons low-fat mayonnaise
- 1 egg
- 1 teaspoon Old Bay seasoning
- 1 pound lump crabmeat
- ⅓ cup all-purpose flour
- 2 teaspoons vegetable oil

1. In a large bowl, combine the bread crumbs, celery, pepper, shallot, parsley, mustard, mayonnaise, egg, and seasoning. Gently fold in the crabmeat.

2. Preheat oven to 350°F. Spread the flour on a piece of wax paper. Divide crab mixture into 8 equal portions, then form into patties with floured hands. Dredge in the flour.

3. Lightly coat a large nonstick, ovenproof skillet with cooking spray and set over medium-high heat until hot but not smoking. Cook 4 crab cakes until browned, about 2 minutes on each side. Drizzle 1 teaspoon of the oil around the crab cakes, turn the crab cakes, and gently shake the pan to spread the oil. Transfer to a plate lined with paper towels. Repeat with the remaining crab cakes and oil.

4. Lightly coat a baking sheet with cooking spray, transfer the crab cakes to the baking sheet, and bake until very hot in the center, 8 to 10 minutes.

The *ChangeOne* Sunday brunch (about 440 calories)

2 Chesapeake Crab Cakes, 1 green salad, 1 small crusty roll (2 golf balls), 1 cup seasonal berries (raspberries, strawberries, blueberries, or blackberries, as available) (baseball)

Breakfast CHOICES & TIPS

■ Bagel Delight

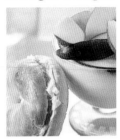

A bagel with cream cheese is perfectly fine for breakfast—if you eat the proper portion size and supplement it with fruit and dairy servings. Most deli bagels are two to four times the size you should eat. Choose a small (roughly 2-ounce) bagel and add just 2 teaspoons of cream cheese, about the size of half of your thumb. To round out the breakfast, have:

> 1 cup fat-free yogurt
> 1 teaspoon jam (either in the yogurt
>   or on the bagel)
> 1 peach (whole or sliced onto the bagel or into
>   the yogurt)

Tip: Cut bagels into correct portion sizes when you bring them home from the store, then freeze them in a resealable plastic bag.

■ About Eggs

Large eggs are the standard size for all *ChangeOne* recipes, but many cooks use extra-large eggs because they're more widely available. A large egg supplies 78 calories, an extra-large 90, and a jumbo 100. Most of the calories, fat, and cholesterol are in the egg yolk, which also contains beneficial compounds such as lutein, a pigment that aids eye health. According to research on eggs and blood cholesterol, most people can eat as many as seven whole eggs per week without increasing their cholesterol levels. To stretch your eggs, use additional egg whites. They are practically fat-free, and each one adds only 17 calories.

■ Choose Your Fruit

ChangeOne asks you to have a serving of fruit every morning. Since you can't always find wonderful fresh fruit in season, stock up on frozen unsweetened berries, peaches, and other types of fruit. No need to wash or defrost ahead of time. In general, one fruit can easily substitute

for another. A half-cup of blueberries, for example, contains 40 calories and 2 grams of fiber. By comparison, here's what the same amount of other fruits offer: apples (37 calories, 2 grams of fiber), oranges (42 calories, 2 grams of fiber), strawberries (25 calories, 2 grams of fiber), plums (91 calories, 1 gram of fiber), cantaloupe (30 calories, 1 gram of fiber).

■ An Alternative to Coffee

Try a vanilla steamer for a yummy alternative to your usual morning brew. Put ¾ cup of fat-free or low-fat milk in a microwave-safe mug and add ½ teaspoon of vanilla extract and artificial sweetener to taste. Heat in the microwave until warm, about 30 seconds. If you don't want to use vanilla, consider other extracts, such as almond or hazelnut.

■ Yogurt Cheese

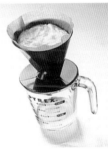

To make yogurt thicker so you can use it as a spread, line a drip-coffeemaker basket with a coffee filter and rest it on a bowl or measuring cup. Put 1 cup fat-free or low-fat plain yogurt (select a brand that does not contain gelatin) in the filter, cover, and refrigerate for at least 1 hour. The liquid in the yogurt will drip out through the filter.

■ About Muffins and Scones

Muffins are really just a quick bread (that is, a no-yeast bread) baked in a muffin tin. Scones, a kissing cousin to biscuits, are drier and flakier than muffins. *ChangeOne* muffins should fill a standard paper cupcake cup. Store-bought or diner muffins can be double that size, so share one of those with a friend or save half for another serving.

Tip: Buy or bake a batch of muffins and freeze in a resealable plastic bag. Pull one out in the morning for a quick breakfast.

Breakfast CHOICES & TIPS

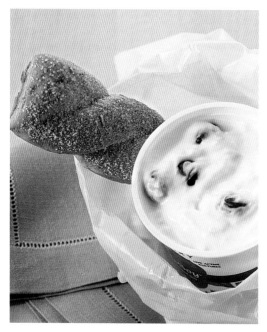

■ Breakfast on the Run

We love cereal bars for their convenience, healthfulness, crunch, and flavor. Soft-textured cereal bars are generally lower in calories and fat than crunchy granola bars, so check the nutritional information. We recommend bars in the 120- to 140-calorie range, but they may be a bit tougher to find than those in the 180- to 200-calorie range. With careful label reading, you'll find versions that are just right for you. Brands to try include Kellogg's Nutri-Grain Bars and Nutri-Grain Twists and Quaker Oats Fruit & Oatmeal Bars. Look for bars with at least 1 gram of fiber, but if you have a favorite that contains no fiber, go ahead and enjoy it—there's fiber in the fruit you eat with it.

For a perfect breakfast on the run, have 1 cereal bar (120 to 140 calories), ½ cup blueberries (2 golf balls), and 1 cup fat-free yogurt.

Tip: Pack a breakfast in a bag the night before so you can grab it and go in the morning.

■ A Smoothie Breakfast

Shakes, batidas, smoothies—no matter what you call them, these frosty combos of fruit and milk or yogurt refresh and nourish you. A smoothie and a piece of toast topped with peanut butter or a healthy margarine spread make a complete breakfast. For a delicious tropical smoothie, puree the following ingredients in a blender until completely smooth. This makes four servings (a serving should be 2 cups).

> 1 mango, cut into cubes
> 1 banana, cut into large chunks
> 1 cup pineapple chunks
> 1 kiwifruit, peeled and sliced
> 2 cups fat-free plain yogurt
> 1 cup ice cubes

Freeze leftovers in sealable plastic containers. To defrost, microwave for 30 to 60 seconds and stir.

Tip: At a restaurant, order the smallest smoothie available—12 ounces is ideal. And be sure to request that it's made with fat-free yogurt or fat-free or low-fat milk.

■ Cottage Cheese Melba

Cottage cheese is "fresh" cheese, meaning that its curds have not been aged or ripened. Its moist, loose texture and mild flavor make it ideal for all sorts of accompaniments, including fruits and jams, cereals, nuts, spices, and vegetables. It comes with different amounts of fat, ranging from none to 4 percent. *ChangeOne* recommends the medium range: low-fat. It tastes richer than fat-free and has fewer calories than regular 4 percent fat cottage cheese.

For a wonderful breakfast that's right at the *ChangeOne* calorie and nutrient targets, mix ½ cup of low-fat cottage cheese (2 golf balls) with an equal amount of sliced fruit and 1 teaspoon of fruit jam. We particularly like peach slices and raspberry jam together. Add a slice of raisin bread toast and a cup of coffee, and your day is off to a great start.

Tip: Ricotta cheese, a fresh cousin made from whey (the liquid drained off from the semisolid curds that make up cottage cheese), is smoother and creamier but higher in fat. Farmer and pot cheeses are drier than cottage cheese.

■ When Company Comes for Brunch

Looking for a way to provide a nice spread of food that's healthy and *ChangeOne* compatible? Try some or all of these ideas for your brunch menus.

Bread sampler:
- A basket of mini-muffins or crusty rolls

Salad variations:
- Spinach with reduced-fat dressing
- Sliced cucumbers tossed with rice wine vinegar, sesame oil, and a sprinkle of sugar
- Cubed tomatoes drizzled with balsamic vinegar and flavorful olive oil
- Baby lettuce and watercress

Cheese choices:
- Low-fat cottage cheese mixed with chopped cucumber, peppers, and radishes
- Part-skim ricotta flavored with vanilla extract, cinnamon, and sugar
- Assorted sliced reduced-fat cheeses

Fruit treats:
- Fresh fruit salad
- Tricolor melon ball salad (cantaloupe, watermelon, and honeydew)
- Sliced peaches drizzled with Amaretto

■ Lox and Bagels

We lighten the calorie load on this classic breakfast by using fat-free or reduced-fat cream cheese and only half a bagel. But you're not being short-changed: a deli or bagel-shop bagel weighs as much as five slices of bread. For a luscious Sunday brunch, have the following. It tallies roughly 600 calories, so it truly does cover both breakfast and lunch.

> ½ **deli bagel, any flavor, topped with:**
> **1 tablespoon reduced-fat cream cheese**
> **3 slices smoked salmon**
> **1 thick slice tomato**
> **1 slice red onion (optional)**
> **Capers (optional)**
> **1 cup fresh fruit salad (baseball)**
> **1 mimosa (equal parts orange juice and champagne or sparkling water)**
> **Coffee or tea**

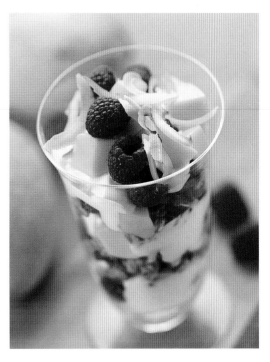

■ Yogurt Parfait

If you have children or grandchildren, you've probably seen the scene in the movie *Shrek* when Donkey rambles on about parfaits being the most perfect food in the world. He's not far from the truth. This parfait is an amazingly good breakfast and 100 percent in line with *ChangeOne* guidelines. Start with:

> ¾ **cup fat-free plain or artificially sweetened yogurt**
> ¼ **cup berries (1 golf ball)**
> ¼ **cup sliced mango (1 golf ball)**
> ¼ **cup low-fat granola (1 golf ball)**
> **1 tablespoon shredded coconut (thumb)**

In a tall parfait glass, layer one-third of the yogurt, half of the fruit, all of the granola, another one-third of the yogurt, the rest of the fruit, and the rest of the yogurt. Top with the coconut.

Tip: Don't like coconut? Chopped nuts are a perfect substitute. Likewise, peaches, cantaloupe, and even applesauce can substitute for the recommended fruit.

Lunch RECIPES

Hearty Split-Pea Soup

SERVES 6

- 1 teaspoon olive oil
- 1 tablespoon broth or stock
- 1 large onion, finely chopped
- 3 cloves garlic, minced
- 2 carrots, halved lengthwise and thinly sliced crosswise
- ¾ cup split peas
- 2 tablespoons tomato paste
- ½ pound smoked turkey breast, chopped
- ½ teaspoon salt
- ½ teaspoon fresh-ground black pepper
- ½ teaspoon rubbed or ground sage
- 4½ cups water
- ⅓ cup small pasta shapes
- ¼ cup grated Parmesan cheese

1. Heat the oil and broth in a nonstick Dutch oven over medium heat. Add the onion and garlic and cook, stirring frequently, until the onion is golden, about 7 minutes. Add the carrots and cook, stirring frequently, until crisp-tender, about 5 minutes.

2. Stir in the split peas, tomato paste, turkey, salt, pepper, sage, and water and bring to a boil. Reduce to a simmer, cover, and cook for 30 minutes.

3. Add the pasta and cook until the pasta and split peas are tender, about 15 minutes. Divide equally among 6 soup bowls. (Unused portions will keep for 3 or 4 days in the refrigerator and 2 to 3 months in the freezer.) Sprinkle with the Parmesan and serve.

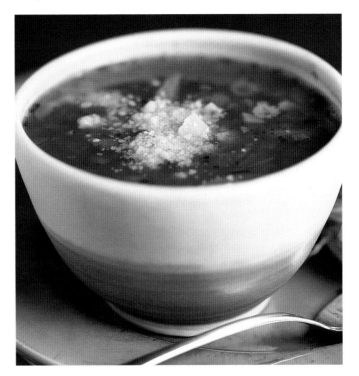

Cream of Asparagus Soup

SERVES 4

1¼	pounds asparagus, trimmed
1½	teaspoons olive oil
4	scallions, thinly sliced
½	pound all-purpose potatoes, peeled and thinly sliced
1¾	cups water
1	teaspoon tarragon
¾	teaspoon salt
¼	teaspoon fresh-ground black pepper
½	cup 1% milk

1. Cut 10 thin asparagus spears into 3 pieces each and set aside. Cut the remaining asparagus into ½-inch pieces.

2. Heat the oil in a medium nonstick saucepan over low heat. Add the scallions and cook, stirring frequently, until tender, about 2 minutes. Add the potatoes and ½-inch asparagus pieces and stir to combine.

3. Add the water, tarragon, salt, and pepper and bring to a boil. Reduce to a simmer, cover, and cook until the potatoes and asparagus are tender, about 10 minutes.

4. Transfer the soup to a food processor and puree. Return to the saucepan and stir in the milk and reserved asparagus. Cook over low heat until the soup is heated through and the asparagus is tender, about 3 minutes.

The *ChangeOne* lunch

1½ cups Hearty Split-Pea or Cream of Asparagus Soup, 1 slice hearty bread with ½ ounce sharp cheddar cheese, 1 orange, apple, or peach

---

Pete's Chopped Salad

SERVES 6

½	cup chopped red bell pepper
½	cup chopped green bell pepper
½	cup chopped cucumber
½	cup chopped red onion
1½	cups chopped tomatoes
1	cup fresh, canned, or frozen corn kernels
1	cup rinsed and drained canned black beans
2	tablespoons red wine vinegar
1	tablespoon olive oil
1	tablespoon lime juice
2	tablespoons minced cilantro
1	jalapeño pepper, minced (optional)

1. In a large bowl, combine the red pepper, green pepper, cucumber, onion, tomatoes, corn, beans, vinegar, oil, lime juice, cilantro, and jalapeño (if using).

Variation: Feel free to substitute ingredients to taste, particularly among the vegetables. Instead of black beans, consider using baby shrimp, diced ham, smoked turkey breast, or chickpeas.

The *ChangeOne* lunch

1 cup Pete's Chopped Salad (baseball), 1 medium whole wheat pita bread, ½ cup grapes (8 to 12)

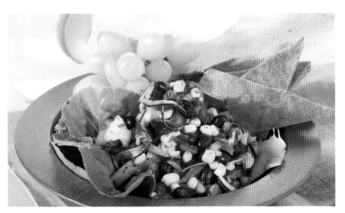

Lunch RECIPES

Meatless Chili Pots con Queso

SERVES 4

- 1 medium green bell pepper, finely chopped
- 1 medium onion, finely chopped
- 2 large cloves garlic, minced
- 2 cans (15 ounces each) red kidney beans, rinsed and drained
- 1 can (28 ounces) no-salt-added crushed tomatoes in puree
- ½ teaspoon chili powder
- ½ teaspoon fresh-ground black pepper
- ½ teaspoon ground cumin
- ¼ teaspoon ground cinnamon
- ½ cup shredded reduced-fat cheddar cheese
- ¼ cup plain low-fat yogurt
- ½ cup chopped avocado

1. Lightly coat a large nonstick skillet with cooking spray and set over medium-high heat. Add the green pepper, onion, and garlic and sauté until the onion is browned, about 5 minutes.

2. Stir in the beans, tomatoes and puree, chili powder, black pepper, cumin, and cinnamon. Simmer for 5 minutes.

3. Ladle into 4 bowls and sprinkle each portion with 2 tablespoons of the cheese. Garnish with the yogurt and avocado.

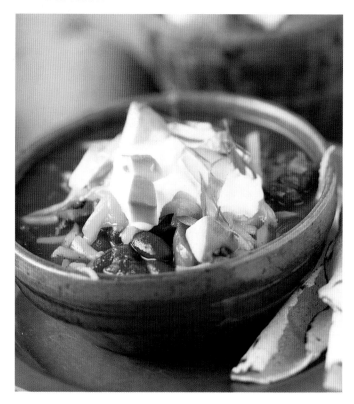

The *ChangeOne* lunch

2 cups Meatless Chili Pots con Queso (2 baseballs), 1 corn tortilla, 1 green salad with fat-free dressing

Roasted Vegetable Wraps with Chive Sauce

SERVES 4

1 tablespoon olive oil

1 tablespoon rice wine vinegar

1 teaspoon chopped fresh rosemary

1 clove garlic, minced

¼ teaspoon salt

2 medium zucchini (total 1 pound)

2 large red bell peppers

1 large red onion

4 7-inch flour tortillas

¾ cup Yogurt cheese (see page 283)

¼ teaspoon onion salt

1 tablespoon snipped fresh chives

1. Preheat the oven to 450ºF. Lightly coat a jelly-roll pan or shallow-sided baking pan with cooking spray.

2. In a small bowl, whisk the oil, vinegar, rosemary, garlic, and salt.

3. Cut each zucchini crosswise in half, then lengthwise into ¼-inch slices. Cut each red pepper into 8 strips. Cut the onion into 16 wedges.

4. Pour the oil mixture into the pan and add the vegetables. Bake, tossing frequently, until browned and tender, about 30 minutes. Sprinkle the tortillas with a little water, wrap in foil, and place in the oven during the last 5 minutes of cooking.

5. In a small bowl, combine the yogurt cheese, onion salt, and chives. Spread evenly on each tortilla and top with the vegetables. Fold in the sides of the tortillas and roll up.

The *ChangeOne* lunch

1 Roasted Vegetable Wrap with Chive Sauce, 1 green salad with non-fat dressing, ½ cup honeydew melon (2 golf balls) topped with mint leaf

---

Grilled Turkey Caesar Salad

SERVES 4

2 cloves garlic, peeled

3 tablespoons fresh lemon juice

2 tablespoons fat-free plain yogurt

1 tablespoon olive oil

¾ pound boneless, skinless turkey breast

¼ teaspoon salt

½ teaspoon fresh-ground black pepper

8 cups romaine lettuce, torn into bite-size pieces

½ cup garlic croutons

1 ounce piece Parmesan cheese

1. Preheat the grill. In a mini-processor or with the side of chef's knife, mash the garlic until paste-like. Place the garlic paste, lemon juice, yogurt, and oil into a jar with a tight-fitting lid and shake until blended.

2. Sprinkle the turkey with the salt and pepper and lightly coat with cooking spray. Grill until cooked through, 4 to 5 minutes per side. Cut across the grain into ½-inch-thick slices.

3. In a large bowl, toss together the lettuce, croutons, and turkey until well mixed. Shake the dressing, drizzle on the salad, and toss lightly.

4. Divide the salad equally among 4 plates. With a vegetable peeler, shave strips of cheese evenly over each portion.

The *ChangeOne* lunch

2 cups Grilled Turkey Caesar Salad (2 baseballs), 3 Ak-Mak flatbread crackers, ½ cup fresh fruit salad (2 golf balls)

Lunch CHOICES & TIPS

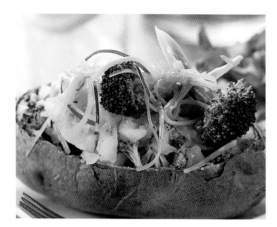

■ Ode to a Baked Potato

With the right toppings, potatoes can go from a side dish to a tasty, healthy entrée. Always start with a medium (6-ounce) baked potato, which is about the size of a tennis ball. Add to it unlimited vegetables, such as steamed broccoli, chopped tomatoes, chopped onions, steamed spinach, or grilled mushrooms. For protein and richer flavor, add ¼ cup (about a palmful) of grated cheddar cheese or ½ cup of canned beans, cottage cheese, or chili. Skip the butter and sour cream; if you want a finishing touch, add salsa. For lunch, have your stuffed potato with a green salad and ½ cup of berries (2 golf balls) in season.

■ Cooking with Beans

Beans, as we've said, are an outstanding food for health and weight. Buying them in cans makes the most sense if you're pressed for time when cooking, but canned beans have one drawback: their saltiness. Rather than buying low-sodium beans—which often lack flavor, can be mushy, and are more expensive—just remember to drain and rinse canned beans before adding them to your salad, soup, chili, or casserole.

Dried beans are great, too, with their firmer, more pleasing texture, but they take much longer to prepare. To soak dried beans, place them in a large pot with enough water to cover. Bring the water to a boil, then remove from the heat and let the beans soak for several hours or overnight. Discard the water. One cup of dried beans yields 3 cups cooked.

■ Soup in an Instant

Soup is so wonderful that it qualifies as a *ChangeOne* superfood. Not only is it nutritious and delectable, but it fills you up fast, making it the perfect starter for any lunch or dinner. It's also surprisingly easy to make. Keep a large supply of low-sodium chicken broth at home for anytime you want a quick bowl of soup. A few add-ins, and you have lunch ready to go. Some examples:

• Combine a can of chicken broth, one bunch of well-cleaned watercress, and a slice of fresh ginger. Heat for 5 minutes for a super quick and easy soup with a Chinese flair.

• Slice a carrot, a celery stalk, and any other green vegetable you have and add them to a can of broth. Add dried dill, salt, and pepper to taste and cook for 10 minutes. Throw in a fistful of egg noodles, cook for 5 minutes or until the noodles are soft, and voilà—instant homemade chicken noodle soup.

• Similarly, for a Japanese-style bowl of noodles, add a package of ramen noodles, vegetables, and a teaspoon of soy sauce to a can of chicken broth. Cook until the noodles are soft.

• Have leftover vegetables from last night? For a quick, colorful bowl of vegetable chowder, puree the veggies with a can of broth until smooth, then transfer to a saucepan and heat until simmering. Season to taste.

Tip: Canned soups are a mixed bag. Some are healthy and yummy, but many are way too high in salt, fat, and calories. Read the nutritional information carefully before buying. Also consider diluting canned soup with water to lower the calorie/sodium content per serving.

■ Making Soup Into a Meal

Want a soup that's substantial enough to be a meal in itself? Make sure it has a serving of protein, some kind of carbohydrate (such as rice, noodles, or potatoes), and plenty of vegetables. Legumes (split peas, beans, or lentils) are particularly good sources of protein and fiber. Or add strips of leftover chicken, beef, pork, or fish to broth-based vegetable soup to turn it into a complete nutritional package.

On the other hand, if you prefer your soup with more broth and fewer chunks of food, you'll want to pair it with a sandwich or salad. And what about "cream of" soups? Unless you're certain they're made with low-fat milk, assume that they are indeed made with cream and thus overly high in fat and calories.

Tip: To make a homemade soup creamy without the cream, try one of these methods.

- Add up to 1 cup of fat-free evaporated milk and cook just until heated through.
- Stir in ½ cup of plain low-fat yogurt or reduced-fat sour cream immediately before serving.
- Cut up 2 slices of American cheese and stir into the soup shortly before serving.

■ About Caesar Salad

Legend has it that the Caesar salad was invented by Caesar Cardini, a Tijuana, Mexico, restaurant owner, for a group of visiting movie stars. Others credit Caesar's brother Alex with the concoction. Whoever dreamed it up, the salad has become a classic. Today, variations abound, some healthy and some not. Too much cheese, too much oil in the dressing, oil-drenched croutons, and overly salty anchovies and Worcestershire sauce can make a Caesar salad a bad choice for weight loss. But if you're judicious with the heavier ingredients, this salad is a delight. Ask for half amounts of grated cheese and dressing, and you'll probably be right in line with *ChangeOne* targets.

To turn a Caesar salad into a full meal, just add a 3-ounce portion of meat, poultry, or seafood. A good idea: Wrap and refrigerate left-over grilled meat or fish for a Caesar salad the next day. Other choices include tofu cubes, tuna, salmon, or shrimp.

Tip: To make delicious, healthy croutons: Brush day-old bread lightly with olive oil (or coat with cooking spray), cut into ½-inch cubes, dust with dried basil or other favorite herbs and spices (we like chili powder on ours!). Place on a baking sheet and bake at 250°F until crisp, about 20 minutes. Store in an airtight container.

■ A Perfect Bowl of Chili

Classic chili contains beans and ground beef in seasoned tomato sauce. Texas chili is all meat and chili peppers, no beans or tomatoes. Cincinnati chili is served on a bed of spaghetti and covered with cheddar cheese. White chili has white beans, chicken or turkey breast, and no tomatoes. We say, forget all the formal categories and be creative. Make your chili with at least one-half vegetables by adding small chunks of peppers, onions, tomatoes, zucchini, green beans, and even carrots. Always include beans; they're filled with fiber and nutrition. If you use meat, cook it separately and drain the fat completely before adding it to the chili pot. For spices, we like oregano and a little bit of cumin in addition to the usual chili powder, salt, and pepper.

■ A Piece of Pita

We like pita breads for their diversity. You can open them up for fun and creative pocket sandwiches; fill them with bean sprouts, cucumbers, chopped carrots, lettuce, and tomatoes, then 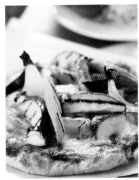 drizzle in some low-fat Italian dressing for a wonderfully healthy and filling sandwich. We also like putting things on pita bread. For a wonderful lunch in 10 minutes, make a pita pizza. Spread 2 tablespoons of tomato sauce, ¼ cup of grated part-skim mozzarella cheese, and unlimited grilled or raw vegetables on top of a small pita bread. Bake at 350°F until the cheese bubbles, about 5 minutes. Serve with a green salad and an apple for the perfect *ChangeOne* lunch.

Tip: Topping suggestions for a pita pizza include broccoli, mushrooms, onion, peppers, salad greens, spinach, tomato, or zucchini. If you want a little meat on top, cut the cheese portion in half.

Dinner RECIPES

Chicken and Broccoli Stir-Fry, Italian Style

SERVES 4

 1 tablespoon peanut oil

 3 scallions, thinly sliced

 ¾ pound boneless, skinless chicken breasts, cut across the grain into ½-inch-wide pieces

 1½ pounds broccoli florets

 1 cup chopped red bell pepper

 ½ cup chicken broth

 ½ teaspoon grated lemon zest

 ½ teaspoon salt

 ½ cup water

 1 teaspoon cornstarch dissolved in 1 table- spoon water

 1 tablespoon olive oil

 ½ cup slivered fresh basil or ½ teaspoon dried basil

 1⅓ cups orzo pasta

1. Heat 2 teaspoons of the peanut oil in a large nonstick wok or skillet over medium heat. Add the scallions and sauté until wilted, about 1 minute. Add the chicken and sauté until no longer pink, about 3 minutes. Add the remaining peanut oil and the broccoli and sauté for 2 minutes.

2. Add the pepper, broth, lemon zest, salt, and water. Bring to a boil, then reduce the heat and simmer until the chicken and broccoli are just cooked through, about 2 minutes.

3. Stir in the dissolved cornstarch, olive oil, and basil. Cook, stirring, until the sauce is slightly thickened, about 1 minute.

4. Cook the orzo according to package directions; drain. Divide equally among 4 plates. Divide the stir-fry into 4 equal portions (refrigerate any extra portions) and serve over the orzo.

Variation: For an equal number of calories, you can substitute one of the following: 9 ounces salmon fillet; 10 ounces pork tenderloin; 9 ounces firm tofu; 8 ounces beef tenderloin; 8 ounces boneless leg of lamb; ½ cup cashews.

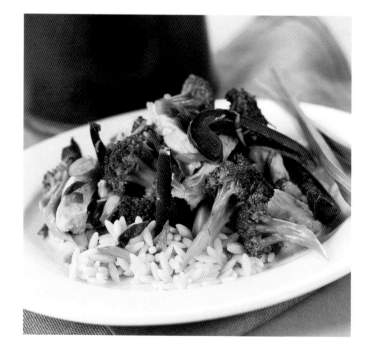

The *ChangeOne* dinner
2 cups) Chicken and Broccoli Stir-Fry (2 baseballs), 1 cup orzo (baseball)

Sautéed Chicken with Caramelized Onions

SERVES 4

1½ pounds medium onions

4 boneless, skinless chicken breast halves, 4 to 5 ounces each

½ teaspoon salt

½ teaspoon fresh-ground black pepper

4 teaspoons olive oil

2 tablespoons sugar

⅓ cup reduced-sodium chicken broth

1 teaspoon chopped fresh rosemary

1 teaspoon chopped fresh thyme

1 tablespoon red wine vinegar

1. Cut the onions into 6 wedges each. Sprinkle the chicken with ¼ teaspoon of the salt and ¼ teaspoon of pepper.

2. Coat a large nonstick skillet with cooking spray. Add 2 teaspoons of the oil and heat over medium-high heat for about 30 seconds. Add the chicken and sauté until browned, about 3 minutes on each side. Transfer to a plate.

3. Reduce the heat to medium and add the remaining oil. Sauté the onions, 1 tablespoon of the sugar, and the remaining salt and pepper until the onions turn golden and caramelize, about 8 minutes. Stir frequently, breaking the onions apart as they cook. Add the broth and boil until it evaporates, about 2 minutes.

4. Stir in the rosemary, thyme, and the remaining sugar. Return the chicken to the skillet and sprinkle with the vinegar. Cook until the chicken juices run clear, about 4 minutes. Place 1 chicken breast on each of 4 plates and top with about ½ cup onions.

The *ChangeOne* dinner

1 serving Sautéed Chicken with Caramelized Onions, ⅔ cup spinach fettuccine (tennis ball), 1 green Mediterranean salad (unlimited romaine and assorted other lettuces topped with tomato wedges, fresh-ground black pepper, ½ teaspoon olive oil, and unlimited balsamic vinegar)

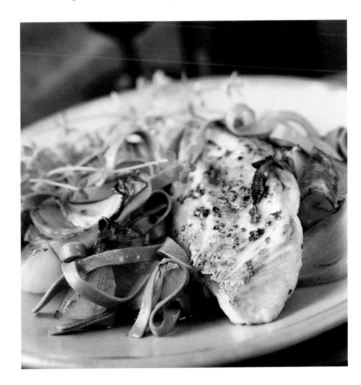

Dinner RECIPES

One-Crust Chicken Potpie

SERVES 4

- 1 **pound boneless, skinless chicken breasts**
- ¼ **teaspoon salt**
- 1 **package (15 ounces) refrigerated piecrust**
- 1 **egg white, lightly beaten with 1 teaspoon water**
- 2 **medium carrots, peeled and thinly sliced**
- 1 **cup frozen corn**
- 1 **cup frozen green peas**
- 1 **cup frozen small white onions**
- ½ **cup fat-free evaporated milk**
- 3 **tablespoons all-purpose flour**
- ½ **tablespoon butter**
- ¼ **teaspoon fresh-ground black pepper**

1. In a large saucepan, bring the chicken, ⅛ teaspoon of the salt, and enough water to cover to a simmer over medium-high heat. Reduce heat to low and gently poach the chicken until the juices run clear, about 15 minutes. Transfer to a cutting board, let cool, and cut into bite-size pieces. Reserve 1 cup of the poaching liquid.

2. Preheat the oven to 425°F. Lightly coat a baking sheet and four 1-cup baking dishes with cooking spray.

3. Dust a work surface lightly with flour. Unfold the piecrust, cut in half, and wrap the remaining half in foil or plastic wrap; refrigerate or freeze. Roll out the crust ⅛ inch thick, then cut out 4 squares to fit on top of the baking dishes. Brush the tops with the diluted egg white. Transfer the squares to the baking sheet and bake until crisp and golden, about 12 minutes. Transfer to a wire rack to cool.

4. Meanwhile, cook the carrots in boiling water until tender, about 5 minutes; drain. In a colander, rinse the corn, peas, and onions in hot water. In a small bowl, whisk the milk and flour until smooth.

5. Melt the butter in a medium saucepan over medium heat. Whisk in the milk mixture, then the reserved poaching liquid. Cook until the sauce thickens and boils, about 5 minutes. Stir in the chicken, carrots, corn, peas, onions, pepper, and the remaining salt. Cook until heated through, about 3 minutes. Divide among the 4 baking dishes and bake until the filling bubbles, about 15 minutes. Top each with a pastry square.

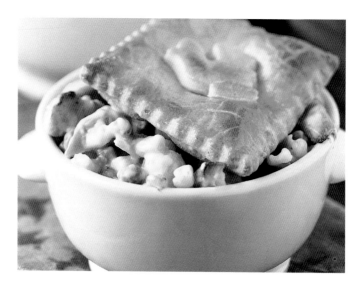

The *ChangeOne* dinner
1 serving One-Crust Chicken Potpie (baseball), 1 green salad with no-fat dressing

Grilled Beer-Can Chicken

SERVES 4

1   **roasting chicken**
    (2½ to 3 pounds)

3-4 **tablespoons dry spice
    rub (or make your own
    with equal parts
    paprika, onion powder,
    and garlic powder, plus
    salt and black pepper to
    taste)**

1   **can beer**

1. Prepare the grill. If using a charcoal grill, place the coals around the outside edge. If using a gas grill, leave one burner off.

2. Rub the chicken inside and out with the dry rub. Loosen the skin slightly and sprinkle a small amount of dry rub between the skin and the flesh.

3. Pour out half of the beer. Place the can in the center of the grill if using charcoal or over the unlit burner if using gas. Place the chicken on top of the can; the can should fit inside the chicken cavity so it and the chicken's legs form a "tripod" on the grill.

4. Close the grill lid and cook on medium heat until done, 45 minutes to 1 hour. Carefully remove the chicken and can from the grill.

5. Cut the chicken into 6 pieces—2 thighs, 2 drumsticks, and 2 breast halves. Remove the skin before eating.

The *ChangeOne* grilled dinner

Unlimited crudités (raw vegetables), 1 serving (1 breast or 1 drumstick and 1 thigh) Grilled Beer-Can Chicken, 1½ cups Grilled Summer Vegetables (recipe on page 304) (coffee mug), ½ cup German Potato Salad with Dijon Vinaigrette (recipe on page 309) (2 golf balls), 2 sesame breadsticks

Dinner RECIPES

Apple-Stuffed Turkey Breast with Orange Marmalade Glaze

1 whole bone-in turkey
breast (3 to 3½ pounds)

1½ teaspoons salt

1 teaspoon fresh-ground
black pepper

2 celery stalks, cut into
1-inch pieces

2 large apples, peeled and
thinly sliced

1 large onion,
thinly sliced

5 sprigs fresh thyme
plus 1 teaspoon
chopped thyme

2 teaspoons olive oil

2 cups apple juice

½ cup reduced-sugar
orange marmalade

½ cup dry white wine
or apple juice

1. Preheat the oven to 350ºF. Rinse the turkey, pat dry with paper towels, and rub the skin all over with the salt and pepper.

2. Combine the celery, half of the apples, half of the onion, and 3 of the thyme sprigs and form into a mound in the center of a roasting pan. In a medium bowl, toss the chopped thyme with the remaining apples and onion. Stuff half of the mixture under the turkey skin and place the remaining mixture in the neck cavity.

3. Place the turkey on top of the mound in the roasting pan. Lightly brush with the oil and top with the remaining thyme sprigs. Pour the apple juice into the pan and roast for 1 hour. Discard the thyme sprigs and baste with ¼ cup of the marmalade. Continue roasting until the turkey is browned and an instant-read thermometer inserted in the thickest part (not touching bone) registers 170ºF, basting twice with the remaining marmalade. Let stand for 10 minutes before transferring to a platter to slice. Remove the skin before serving.

4. Stir the wine into the apples and vegetables in the pan (do not strain). Bring to a boil over medium-high heat, scraping up browned bits from the bottom of the pan with a wooden spoon, until the liquid is reduced by half.

**The *ChangeOne*
holiday dinner**

3 ounces Apple-Stuffed Turkey Breast (deck of cards), ¼ cup gravy, 2 tablespoons cranberry sauce, ½ cup Orange-Glazed Carrots or Sweet Potatoes (recipe on page 310) (2 golf balls), 1 green salad with no-fat dressing, 1 small crusty roll

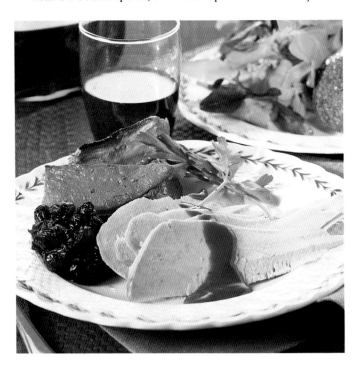

Beef Stew

SERVES 4

- 1 tablespoon olive oil
- ¾ pound lean stew beef, cubed
- 2 cups sliced carrots (1-inch pieces)
- 2 medium onions, cut into quarters
- 1 cup sliced parsnips (1-inch pieces)
- 1 cup sliced celery (1-inch pieces)
- 1 cup sliced potatoes (1-inch pieces)
- ½ teaspoon dried thyme
  Salt and pepper to taste
- 2 cups beef broth
- 4 cups egg noodles

1. Heat the oil over medium heat in a soup pot or baking dish large enough to hold all the ingredients. Brown the beef and drain off the excess fat.

2. Add the carrots, onions, parsnips, celery, potatoes, thyme, salt, pepper, and broth. Cover and simmer until the beef and vegetables are cooked through, about 45 minutes.

3. Cook the noodles according to package directions; drain. Divide into 4 equal portions (refrigerate any extra portions).

4. Before serving, divide the stew into 4 equal portions (refrigerate any extra portions). Serve over the noodles.

Note: If using a slow cooker, follow the manufacturer's directions.

The *ChangeOne* dinner
2 cups Beef Stew (2 baseballs), 1 cup egg noodles (baseball)

Barbecue Beef on a Bun

SERVES 4

- ⅓ cup ketchup
- 1 tablespoon red wine vinegar
- 2 teaspoons brown sugar
- ½ teaspoon ground ginger
- ½ teaspoon mustard
- 12 ounces sirloin steak
- 4 medium (2 ounces each) sandwich buns

1. Preheat the broiler. In a small bowl, combine the ketchup, vinegar, brown sugar, ginger, and mustard. Brush on one side of the steak.

2. Broil the steak 6 inches from the heat for 4 minutes. Turn, brush with the sauce, and broil for 3 to 4 minutes.

3. Slice the steak thinly and divide equally among the buns. Refrigerate any extra portions.

Variations: To make with chicken, use about 1 pound of boneless, skinless breast or thigh meat. Cut into strips and combine with the sauce. Heat in a 350°F oven or simmer on the stove until the sauce bubbles and the chicken is cooked through, about 15 minutes.

To make with pork, use about 1 pound of a lean cut, such as tenderloin. Prepare as with beef.

The *ChangeOne* dinner
1 serving Barbecue Beef on a Bun, 1 cup Colorful Coleslaw (recipe on page 305) (baseball), served separately or on the sandwich

Dinner RECIPES

All-American Pot Roast with Braised Vegetables

SERVES 12

1 boneless beef chuck
   roast (about 3 pounds),
   trimmed of all visible fat

1½ teaspoons salt

1½ teaspoons fresh-ground
   black pepper

8 large carrots, peeled
   and cut into 2-inch
   chunks

2 medium onions,
   coarsely chopped

4 cloves garlic, crushed

1 can (28 ounces) whole
   tomatoes in puree

1 cup chopped fresh basil

2 cups dry red wine or
   reduced-sodium beef
   broth

2 pounds small red or
   Yukon Gold potatoes,
   scrubbed

2 teaspoons cornstarch
   dissolved in 2 table-
   spoons water

1. Preheat the oven to 325ºF. Tie the roast and rub with 1 teaspoon of the salt and 1 teaspoon of the pepper. In a Dutch oven, sear the meat over medium-high heat until browned on all sides, about 8 minutes. Transfer to a plate.

2. Add the carrots, onions, and garlic to the pot and sauté in the meat drippings until the onions are browned, about 8 minutes. Stir in the tomatoes and puree, ½ cup of the basil, and the remaining salt and pepper. Cook for 5 minutes, breaking up the tomatoes with a spoon.

3. Return the meat to the pot. Add the wine and enough water to come 2 inches up the side of the pot. Bring to a boil. Cover with foil and then with a lid to create a tight seal. Roast for 1 hour, turning once.

4. Add the potatoes and the remaining basil to the pot, adding more water if needed to come 2 inches up the side. Roast until the meat and vegetables are tender, about 1 hour.

5. Cut meat into small chunks and arrange on a platter with the vegetables. Strain the braising liquid into a saucepan and bring to a simmer. Whisk in the dissolved cornstarch, bring to a boil, and cook until the gravy thickens, about 1 minute. Ladle over the meat and vegetables.

Note: Cover and refrigerate leftovers for 1 to 2 days, or divide into individual portions and freeze for up to 1 month.

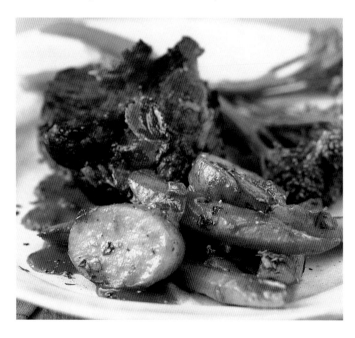

The *ChangeOne* dinner

3 ounces All-American Pot Roast (deck of cards), ¾ cup Braised Vegetables (tennis ball), 1 small slice crusty sourdough bread

Barbecued Halibut Steaks

SERVES 4

- 3 small scallions
- ¼ cup reduced-sodium soy sauce
- ⅓ cup reduced-sugar apricot jam
- 3 tablespoons ketchup
- 1 tablespoon red wine vinegar
- 4 halibut steaks (5 ounces each)

1. Preheat broiler or prepare grill. Thinly slice the scallions diagonally, transfer to a small bowl, and set aside.

2. In a small bowl, combine the soy sauce, jam, ketchup, and vinegar. Measure out ⅓ cup and set aside to be used as a sauce.

3. Place the fish on a broiler pan or grill rack and brush with the remaining soy sauce mixture. Broil 4 inches from the heat until browned and cooked through, about 5 minutes, or grill on 1 side just until cooked through, about 10 minutes. Spoon the reserved sauce over the fish. Pass the bowl of sliced scallions at the table to sprinkle over the fish.

The *ChangeOne* dinner

1 Barbecued Halibut Steak (checkbook), 1 serving Grilled Onion and Scallions (1 onion and 2 scallions, lightly oiled and broiled about 4 inches from the heat until browned), 1½ cups Ziti and Zucchini (recipe on page 309) (2 tennis balls)

Sweet-and-Sour Glazed Pork with Pineapple

SERVES 4

- 1 can (16 ounces) juice-packed pineapple chunks
- ⅓ cup red currant jelly
- 2 tablespoons plus 2 teaspoons Dijon mustard
- ¾ teaspoon salt
- 1 pound pork tenderloin, trimmed of all visible fat
- 1 tablespoon lemon juice

1. Preheat the oven to 400°F. Drain the pineapple, reserving the juice.

2. In a small saucepan, combine the pineapple juice, jelly, 2 tablespoons of the mustard, and ¼ teaspoon of the salt. Cook over medium heat, stirring frequently, until the jelly has melted and the mixture is slightly syrupy and reduced to ⅔ cup, about 5 minutes. Remove from the heat and let cool to room temperature. Measure out ½ cup and set aside to be used as a sauce. Reserve the remaining mixture for basting.

3. Place pork in a 7-by-11-inch baking dish. Sprinkle with the lemon juice and remaining salt and brush with the basting mixture. Roast, basting every 10 minutes with pan juices, until cooked through, about 30 minutes.

4. Meanwhile, in a small bowl, combine the pineapple chunks with the remaining mustard. Let the pork stand for 10 minutes before slicing into 4 equal portions. Serve with the reserved sauce and pineapple-mustard mixture on the side.

The *ChangeOne* dinner

3 ounces Sweet-and-Sour Glazed Pork with Pineapple (deck of cards), ⅔ cup basmati rice (tennis ball), unlimited steamed pattypan squash or other green vegetable

Dinner RECIPES

Heartland Meat Loaf

SERVES 8

- 2 large onions, chopped
- 2 large celery stalks, chopped
- 1 large green bell pepper, chopped
- 3 cloves garlic, minced
- 2 pounds 90% lean ground beef
- 1 cup fresh whole wheat bread crumbs (about 2 slices)
- 1 egg
- ½ teaspoon fresh-ground black pepper
- 2 cups chopped canned tomatoes in puree
- ¼ cup ketchup
- 1 bag (12 ounces) egg noodles
- ¼ cup parsley, chopped

1. Preheat the oven to 350ºF. Lightly coat a 13-by-9-inch baking dish and a large nonstick skillet with cooking spray.

2. Add the onions, celery, bell pepper, and garlic to the skillet and sauté over medium-high heat until soft, about 5 minutes. Transfer to a large bowl. Add the beef, bread crumbs, egg, and black pepper and mix with clean hands.

3. In a small bowl, combine the tomatoes and ketchup. Add half to the meat mixture and mix.

4. Transfer the meat mixture to the baking dish and shape into a loaf about 10 by 7 inches, mounding it slightly in the center. Make a lengthwise groove down the center and pour the remaining tomato mixture into it. Bake until an instant-read thermometer inserted in the center registers 165ºF, about 1 hour 15 minutes. Let stand for 10 minutes before slicing into 8 equal portions. Cover and refrigerate any extra for tomorrow's dinner, or wrap in foil and freeze for up to 1 month.

5. Cook the noodles according to package directions. Drain, reserving ⅓ cup of the cooking water. Place the noodles in a bowl, add the water and parsley, and toss to mix. Divide equally among 4 plates and top with the meat loaf.

The *ChangeOne* dinner

1 slice Heartland Meat Loaf (about 1 inch thick), ⅔ cup egg noodles (tennis ball), steamed baby zucchini or other vegetables drizzled with 1 teaspoon olive oil (thumb tip)

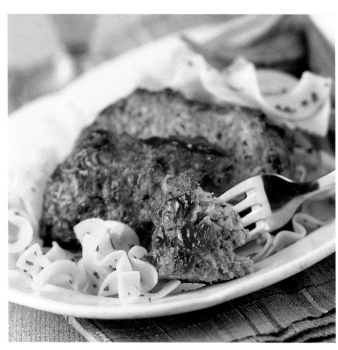

Homestyle Tuna Noodle Casserole

SERVES 4

- 2 cans (6 ounces each) water-packed tuna
- 1 can (14 ounces) fat-free cream of mushroom soup
- ½ cup fat-free evaporated milk
- ½ cup sliced black olives
- 1 can (4 ounces) chopped green chiles
- 2 cups cooked noodles

The *ChangeOne* dinner

1½ cups Homestyle Tuna Noodle Casserole (2 tennis balls), unlimited arugula salad with 1 teaspoon olive oil and balsamic vinegar to taste

1. Preheat the oven to 375ºF. Coat a medium baking dish with cooking spray.

2. Combine the tuna, soup, milk, olives, chiles, and noodles in the baking dish. Bake until bubbly, about 30 minutes.

Variation: You can substitute ingredients freely. Instead of tuna, try tofu or canned or leftover turkey or chicken. Instead of mushroom soup, try fat-free cream of broccoli soup or fat-free cream of tomato soup. Also consider adding vegetables such as broccoli, onions, zucchini, carrots, or celery.

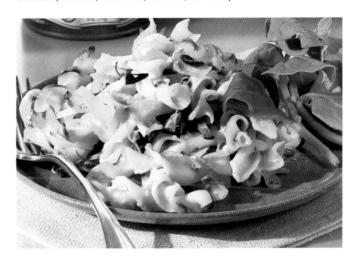

Red Snapper and Snaps in a Packet

SERVES 4

- 3 cups sugar snap peas or snow peas
- 2 tablespoons lemon juice
- 2 teaspoons olive oil
  Salt and fresh-ground black pepper to taste
- 4 red snapper filets (6 ounces each)

1. Preheat the oven to 400ºF or prepare the grill.

2. In a medium bowl, toss together the peas, lemon juice, oil, salt, and pepper.

3. Coat four 15-inch-long pieces of parchment or foil with cooking spray. Place a fillet on the bottom half of each piece and top with about ¾ cup of the pea mixture. Fold the parchment over the fish and peas and seal by folding over the edges.

4. Place the packets on a baking sheet in the oven or directly onto the grill and cook for 10 to 12 minutes.

The *ChangeOne* dinner

1 packet Snapper and Snaps, 1 cup Spanish Rice (recipe on page 310) (baseball)

Dinner RECIPES

Shrimp Kebabs

SERVES 4

- 1 pound shrimp, marinated for at least 1 hour in the refrigerator (see page 313 about marinades)
- 1 green bell pepper, seeded and cut into 1-inch squares
- 1 red bell pepper, seeded and cut into 1-inch squares
- 1 pound assorted vegetables, such as pearl onions, red or Vidalia onions cut into wedges, zucchini cut ino ¼-inch slices, cherry tomatoes, white or Portobello mushrooms, carrots cut into 1-inch pieces, or garlic cloves
- 12 skewers
- 2 teaspoons olive oil

1. Prepare the grill or preheat the broiler. Microwave the peppers and, if using, carrots and onions until softened, about 1 minute.

2. Thread the shrimp, peppers, and other vegetables onto the skewers and brush with the oil. Grill or broil until the shrimp are pink and cooked through, 5 to 7 minutes.

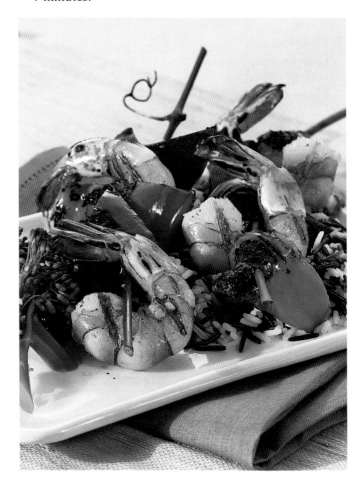

The *ChangeOne* dinner
2 or 3 Shrimp Kebabs, 1 cup White and Wild Rice, (recipe on page 311) (baseball), ½ cup Sesame Broccoli (recipe on page 307) (2 golf balls)

Pasta Primavera

SERVES 4

1⅓ cups small cauliflower florets

1⅓ cups small broccoli florets

7 ounces plain or spinach fettuccine

2 teaspoons olive oil

1 small red onion, diced

2 cloves garlic, minced

½ pound mushrooms, thinly sliced

½ teaspoon salt

½ teaspoon dried rosemary, crumbled

1 medium tomato, cut into ½-inch cubes

2 teaspoons all-purpose flour

1 cup fat-free or low-fat milk

¼ cup grated Parmesan cheese

¼ cup parsley

1. In a large pot of boiling water, blanch the cauliflower and broccoli for 2 minutes. Transfer to a plate with a slotted spoon.

2. Add the fettuccine to the boiling water and cook according to package directions. Drain and transfer to a large serving bowl.

3. Meanwhile, heat 1 teaspoon of the oil in a large nonstick skillet over medium heat. Add the onion and garlic and sauté until tender, about 5 minutes. Add the mushrooms and sauté until softened, about 3 minutes.

4. Add the remaining oil to the skillet. Add the cauliflower and broccoli, sprinkle with the salt and rosemary, and sauté until heated through, about 1 minute. Add the tomato and cook until softened, about 3 minutes.

5. Sprinkle the flour over the vegetables and stir to coat. Add the milk and bring to a boil, then reduce the heat and simmer, stirring, until slightly thickened, about 3 minutes. Stir in the cheese and parsley. Add to the pasta and toss to combine. Divide into 4 equal portions (refrigerate any extra portions).

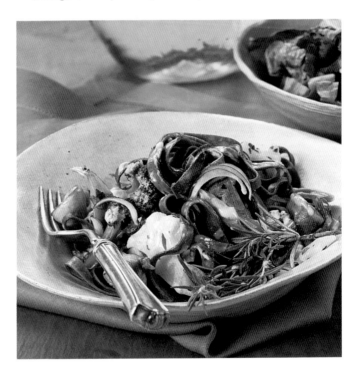

The *ChangeOne* dinner
2 cups Pasta Primavera
(2 baseballs), 3 cups Italian
Salad (recipe on page 308)
(3 baseballs)

Dinner RECIPES

Grilled Summer Vegetables

SERVES 4

- 2 small bulbs fennel (about 8 ounces each), cleaned
- 1 small eggplant (about 1 pound), cut lengthwise into ½-inch-thick slices
- 4 plum tomatoes, halved
- 3 large bell peppers (preferably 1 each green, red, and yellow), cut into ½-inch-wide strips
- 1 medium red onion, cut into 8 wedges
- ½ teaspoon salt
- ½ teaspoon fresh-ground black pepper
- 1 tablespoon orange juice
- 8 basil leaves, very thinly sliced
- 1 small clove garlic, minced
- 1 teaspoon grated orange zest

1. Preheat a gas grill to high or light a charcoal grill. Cut the fronds from the fennel and set aside. Peel the bulbs and cut vertically into ½-inch slices. Coat the fennel, eggplant, tomatoes, bell peppers, and onion with cooking spray or a very light coating of olive oil, then sprinkle with the salt and pepper.

2. Grill the vegetables, turning once, until tender and evenly browned, about 4 minutes on each side. Transfer to a serving platter and sprinkle with the orange juice.

3. Finely chop 1 tablespoon of the reserved fennel fronds. In a small bowl, combine with the basil, garlic, and orange zest. Sprinkle over the vegetables.

4. Divide into 4 equal portions (refrigerate any extra portions). One serving is 1½ cups (coffee mug).

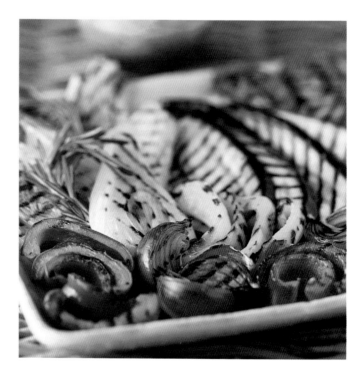

Side Dish RECIPES

Thai Noodle Salad

SERVES 4

- 8 ounces Asian rice noodles
- 1 teaspoon peanut oil
- 2 cloves garlic, minced
- 1 medium onion, thinly sliced
- ¼ cup vegetable broth
- ¼ cup sliced scallions
- 1½ cups bean sprouts, rinsed and drained
- ⅓ cup natural peanut butter
- ¼ cup light coconut milk
- 8 cups mixed greens
- ¼ cup fresh cilantro, chopped
  Juice of 2 limes
- 2 tablespoons peanuts

1. Cook the noodles according to package directions.

2. Meanwhile, heat the oil in a large nonstick skillet. Add the garlic and sauté for about 30 seconds. Add the onion and broth and cook until tender, about 5 minutes.

3. Drain the noodles and add to the skillet. Add the scallions and bean sprouts and toss gently until well mixed.

4. In a small bowl, combine the peanut butter and coconut milk. Add to the skillet and toss to coat.

5. Divide the noodles into 4 equal portions (refrigerate any extra portions). Place 2 cups of greens on each of 4 plates, top with the noodles, and garnish with the cilantro, lime juice, and chopped peanuts.

Colorful Coleslaw

SERVES 4

- 1 cup shredded green cabbage
- 1 cup shredded red cabbage
- ½ cup shredded Napa cabbage or other cabbage as available
- ½ cup shredded carrots
- ¼ cup low-fat mayonnaise
- ½ tablespoon deli or Dijon mustard
- 1 tablespoon red wine vinegar
- ½ tablespoon sugar
  Salt and fresh-ground black pepper to taste

1. In a large bowl, combine the green, red, and Napa cabbage with the carrots, mayonnaise, mustard, vinegar, sugar, salt, and pepper. Mix well. Refrigerate for at least 1 hour. (The cabbage will wilt and shrink when marinated.)

2. Divide into 4 equal portions (refrigerate any extra portions). One serving is 1 cup (baseball).

Side Dish RECIPES

Summer Ratatouille

SERVES 4

- 1 medium eggplant (about 1½ pounds)
- ¾ teaspoon salt
- 1 small bulb fennel
- 2 teaspoons olive oil
- 2 small yellow squash (6 ounces each), chopped
- 1 small onion, cut into thin wedges
- 2 tablespoons low-sodium chicken broth
- 2 large cloves garlic, minced
- 1 can (16 ounces) no-salt-added whole tomatoes
- 1 tablespoon chopped fresh oregano
- 1 teaspoon chopped fresh rosemary plus sprigs for garnish
- 1 green bell pepper, chopped

1. Slice the eggplant crosswise and sprinkle both sides with ½ teaspoon of the salt. Place on a double layer of paper towels and let stand for 15 minutes. Rinse, pat dry, and cut into cubes. Trim and chop the fennel.

2. Heat 1 teaspoon of the oil in a large nonstick skillet over medium-high heat. Add the squash and onion and sauté until the onion is softened, about 5 minutes. Transfer to a large bowl.

3. Add the broth and ½ teaspoon of the oil to the skillet. Stir in the eggplant and reduce the heat to medium. Cover and cook, stirring occasionally, until tender, about 12 minutes. Transfer to the bowl.

4. Add the garlic and the remaining oil to the skillet and cook for 30 seconds. Stir in the tomatoes, fennel, oregano, and chopped rosemary, breaking up the tomatoes with a spoon. Cover and simmer for 5 minutes, then stir in the pepper. Cover and simmer for 7 minutes.

5. Return the vegetables to the skillet. Sprinkle with the remaining salt, bring to a boil, and cook, stirring occasionally, for 3 minutes.

6. Divide into 4 equal portions (refrigerate any extra portions). One serving is approximately 1 cup (baseball). Serve warm or at room temperature, garnished with the rosemary sprigs.

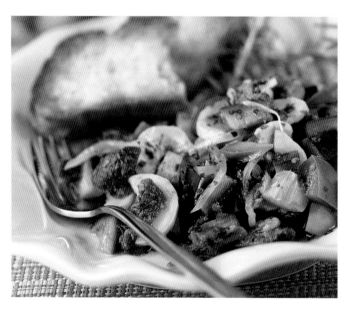

Asparagus with Confetti Vinaigrette

SERVES 4

1½ pounds asparagus

1¼ teaspoons salt

2 large red bell peppers

2 large yellow bell peppers

4 scallions, thinly sliced

2 teaspoons fresh thyme or ½ teaspoon dried thyme

⅓ cup low-sodium chicken broth

3 tablespoons white wine vinegar

½ teaspoon fresh-ground black pepper

1. Bring ½ inch of water to a simmer in large skillet over medium-high heat. Add the asparagus and 1 teaspoon of the salt. Simmer until tender, 3 to 4 minutes. Transfer to a platter and keep warm.

2. Very finely chop the red and yellow bell peppers.

3. Wipe the skillet dry with paper towels, coat with cooking spray, and set over medium-high heat. Add the bell peppers and sauté until tender, about 4 minutes. Stir in the scallions and thyme and cook for 1 minute.

4. Stir in the broth and vinegar and bring to a simmer. Sprinkle with the black pepper and the remaining salt and pour over the asparagus.

5. Divide into 4 equal portions (refrigerate any extra portions). One serving is approximately 5 asparagus spears.

Snow Peas and Apples with Ginger

SERVES 4

2 teaspoons olive oil

2 tablespoons finely slivered peeled fresh ginger

3 cloves garlic, minced

1 pound snow peas, strings removed

2 crisp red apples, cut into thin wedges

½ teaspoon salt

1. Heat the oil in a large nonstick skillet over low heat. Add the ginger and garlic and cook until tender, about 2 minutes.

2. Add the peas, apples, and salt and cook, stirring frequently, until the peas are crisp-tender, about 7 minutes.

3. Divide into 4 equal portions (refrigerate any extra portions). One serving is approximately ⅔ cup (tennis ball).

Sesame Broccoli

SERVES 4

2 cups broccoli florets

4 tablespoons chicken stock or broth

2 teaspoons sesame oil

1½ tablespoons sesame seeds

1. Set a medium nonstick saucepan on medium heat until warm. Add the broccoli and broth and sauté until softened, 7 to 10 minutes. Remove from the heat, drizzle with the oil, and sprinkle with the seeds.

2. Divide into 4 equal portions (refrigerate any extra portions). One serving is ½ cup (2 golf balls).

Side Dish RECIPES

Barley Pilaf with Herbs

SERVES 4

1½	teaspoons olive oil
2	slices turkey bacon, coarsely chopped
1	medium onion, finely chopped
2	cloves garlic, minced
2	carrots, thinly sliced
½	cup pearled barley
½	teaspoon salt
½	teaspoon rubbed sage
½	teaspoon thyme
2¼	cups water
½	teaspoon grated lemon zest
½	teaspoon fresh-ground black pepper
¼	cup grated Parmesan cheese

1. Heat the oil in a medium saucepan over medium heat. Add the bacon and cook for 2 minutes. Add the onion and garlic and cook until the onion is tender and golden, about 5 minutes. Add the carrots and cook until tender, about 5 minutes.

2. Add the barley and stir to combine. Add the salt, sage, thyme, and water and bring to a boil. Reduce the heat and simmer, stirring frequently, until the barley is tender, about 45 minutes. Add the lemon zest, pepper, and cheese and stir until combined.

3. Divide into 4 equal portions (refrigerate any extra portions). One serving is approximately ⅔ cup (tennis ball).

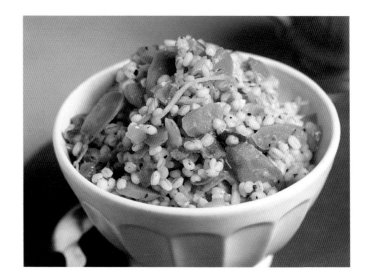

Italian Salad

SERVES 4

1	head romaine lettuce, torn into bite-size pieces
½	cup chopped olives
⅔	cup finely chopped red bell peppers
⅔	cup finely chopped green bell peppers
¼	cup pine nuts
½	cup canned or cooked chickpeas

1. In a large salad bowl, toss together the lettuce, olives, peppers, pine nuts, and chickpeas. Dress with 2 tablespoons fat-free or low-fat Italian dressing (low-fat dressing adds about 30 calories per serving).

2. Divide into 4 equal portions (refrigerate any extra portions). One serving is 3 cups (3 baseballs).

German Potato Salad with Dijon Vinaigrette

SERVES 4

1 pound small red potatoes, scrubbed and quartered

½ teaspoon salt

3 slices turkey bacon

1 small onion, chopped

3 tablespoons cider vinegar

1½ tablespoons sugar

1 tablespoon country-style Dijon mustard

½ teaspoon olive oil

½ teaspoon fresh-ground black pepper

¼ cup finely chopped sweet pickles

¼ cup finely chopped red bell pepper

¼ cup minced parsley

1. Place the potatoes, enough water to cover, and ¼ teaspoon of the salt in a large saucepan and bring to a boil over high heat. Reduce the heat to medium and cook until tender, about 10 minutes. Drain and keep warm.

2. Cut the bacon in half crosswise. Cook in a large, deep nonstick skillet until crisp, transfer to paper towels to drain, and crumble. Add the onion to the skillet and sauté in the pan drippings until golden, about 7 minutes.

3. Place the vinegar, sugar, mustard, oil, black pepper, and the remaining salt in a jar and shake. Whisk into the skillet, bring to a simmer, and cook until fragrant, about 2 minutes. Add the potatoes, pickles, bell pepper, and half of the bacon. Cook, stirring, until the potatoes are coated and heated through, about 2 minutes. Sprinkle with the parsley and remaining bacon.

4. Divide into 4 equal portions (refrigerate any extra portions). One serving is ½ cup (2 golf balls).

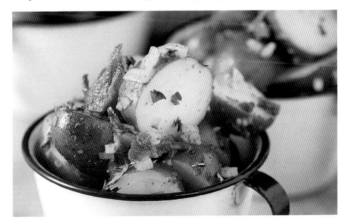

Ziti and Zucchini

SERVES 4

6 ounces ziti

2 medium zucchini

2 teaspoons olive oil

2 tablespoons slivered basil

2 tablespoons grated Parmesan cheese

1. Cook the ziti according to package directions; drain.

2. Meanwhile, slice each zucchini in half crosswise, then slice each half into eighths lengthwise. Place in a medium bowl and microwave just until softened, about 3 minutes.

3. Add the ziti, oil, basil, and cheese and toss to combine.

4. Divide into 4 equal portions (refrigerate any extra portions). One serving is 1½ cups (2 tennis balls).

Side Dish RECIPES

Orange-Glazed Carrots or Sweet Potatoes

SERVES 4

- 2 pounds carrots or sweet potatoes, peeled
- 1 can (6 ounces) frozen orange juice concentrate, thawed
- 2½ teaspoons ground coriander
- 1 teaspoon salt
- ¾ cup water
- 1 tablespoon olive oil
- ⅓ cup chopped fresh mint

1. If using carrots, halve lengthwise and cut into 2-inch strips. If using sweet potatoes, cut into eighths lengthwise and cut into 2-inch strips.

2. In a large skillet, combine the vegetables, orange juice concentrate, coriander, and salt. Add the water and bring to a boil over medium heat. Reduce the heat, cover, and simmer until crisp-tender, about 15 minutes. Uncover, increase the heat to high, and cook until tender, about 7 minutes.

3. Add the oil and cook, swirling the skillet until the vegetables are glossy and the sauce is creamy, about 1 minute. Stir in the mint.

4. Divide into 4 equal portions (refrigerate any extra portions). One serving is ½ cup (2 golf balls).

Spanish Rice

SERVES 4

- 1 medium onion, finely chopped
- 1 medium green bell pepper, finely chopped
- 1 celery stalk, finely chopped
- 2 cloves garlic, minced
- 4 ounces mushrooms, sliced
- ⅔ cup long-grain white rice
- 1 cup low-sodium tomato juice
- 1 cup low-sodium chicken broth
- ½ teaspoon salt
- ¼ teaspoon fresh-ground black pepper
- 1 bay leaf
- 4 plum tomatoes, halved, seeded, and finely chopped

1. Lightly coat a deep nonstick skillet with cooking spray. Add the onion, bell pepper, celery, and garlic and sauté until the onion is almost soft, about 3 minutes. Stir in the mushrooms and rice and sauté until the rice is golden, about 2 minutes.

2. Stir in the tomato juice, broth, salt, black pepper, and bay leaf and bring to a boil over medium-high heat. Reduce the heat, cover, and simmer, stirring occasionally, for 15 minutes. Stir in the tomatoes.

3. Cover and cook until the rice is tender and the liquid is absorbed, about 10 minutes. Fluff with a fork to keep the rice from sticking. Remove from the heat and discard the bay leaf.

4. Divide into 4 equal portions (refrigerate any extra portions). One serving is 1 cup (baseball).

Quick Black Beans and Rice

SERVES 4

- 2 teaspoons olive oil
- 1 red bell pepper, finely chopped
- ½ medium onion, finely chopped
- 1 celery stalk, chopped
- 1 clove garlic, minced
- 1 can (16 ounces) black beans, rinsed and drained
- 1 tablespoon chopped chipotle peppers in adobo, 1 teaspoon chopped jalapeño pepper, 1 tablespoon chopped green chiles, or 1 teaspoon hot sauce (optional)
- 2 cups cooked brown rice

1. Heat the oil in a large nonstick skillet. Add the pepper, onion, celery, and garlic and sauté until softened, about 5 minutes. Add the beans and seasoning of choice (if using) and heat until warmed. Combine with the rice.

2. Divide into 4 equal portions (refrigerate any extra portions). One serving is one cup (baseball).

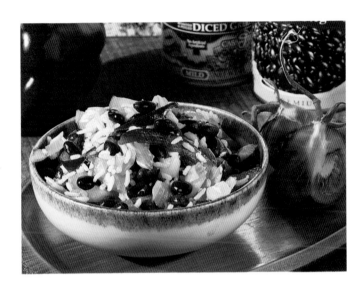

Wild and White Rice

SERVES 4

- 2⅔ cups water
- Pinch of salt
- ⅔ cup wild rice
- ⅔ cup long-grain white rice

1. Place the water, salt and wild rice in a medium saucepan and bring to a boil. Cover, reduce the heat, and simmer for about 20 minutes.

2. Add the white rice and stir to combine. Cover and simmer for 20 minutes, until the rice is cooked.

3. Divide into 4 equal portions (refrigerate any extra portions). One serving is 1 cup (baseball).

Dinner CHOICES & TIPS

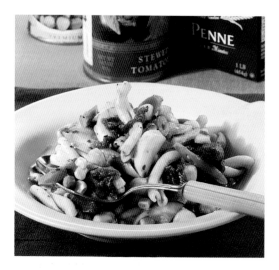

■ Kitchen Sink Stew

Yes, you can still eat well when you're low on fresh foods. Here's a Kitchen Sink Stew that's surprisingly good. To a medium soup pot, add:

- 1 can (28 ounces) stewed tomatoes
- 1 can (28 ounces) chickpeas or other beans
- 2 cups frozen mixed vegetables
- 1 cup pasta (preferably elbow macaroni or small shells)
- 1 teaspoon dried herbs of your choice (we like half oregano and half basil)
- 2 cups water

Bring to a boil over medium-high heat. Reduce the heat to low and simmer until the pasta is cooked, about 20 to 30 minutes, depending on pasta size. Dinner is 2 cups (2 baseballs) of stew and a slice of garlic bread.

■ Making a Perfect Pot Roast

Lower-fat, muscular cuts of meat such as chuck and round require moist roasting to make them tender. The best cuts to buy for pot roast are round rump roast, bottom round roast, eye round roast, and round tip roast. For freshness, choose roasts that feel firm to the touch, not soft. To make your roast tender:

- Keep liquid in the cooking pot at all times.
- Cover the pot and lid with foil to create a tighter seal.

- Roast in the oven at a low temperature (325°F) or on the stove on low heat.

- Allow enough cooking time; don't turn up the heat to speed cooking.

- Cook until "fork tender." Insert a double-pronged grill fork into the thickest part of the roast. If it goes in easily and pulls out easily, the meat is done.

Tip: Use pot roast cooking juices for gravy. Just be sure to remove the liquid fat, using either a turkey baster or a gravy separator. Want thicker gravy? Whisk 1 to 2 tablespoons of cornstarch or flour with a few tablespoons of gravy, pour the mixture into the remaining gravy, and gently simmer.

■ Pork Ideas

Hogs have been put on a diet, meaning that today's cuts are leaner than ever. Pork loin, chops, and tenderloin are the leanest. What's good news for lowering calories, though, can be bad news for taste. Lean cuts are easy to overcook because they have very little fat to keep them moist. It's best to buy thicker cuts that are less apt to dry out during cooking. We particularly like coating a whole tenderloin with olive oil, garlic, and rosemary and roasting at 300˚F until the meat is cooked through (the time will vary based on the size of the tenderloin). Slice thinly and serve with the juices for a wonderful entrée. We also like using thin strips of pork in stir-fries with loads of vegetables and Asian seasonings. Boneless country-style ribs are more fatty, but used sparingly, they are particularly delicious when sliced and cooked in a wok.

Tip: Believe it or not, a slice of well-cooked bacon has fewer calories than one link of pork sausage. Neither is healthy, though; if you must have a breakfast meat, opt for Canadian bacon, or better yet, switch to turkey sausage or bacon.

■ The Pleasures of Poultry

While beef remains America's most popular entrée (Americans eat an average of 62 pounds of it each year, thanks to all those hamburgers), chicken is a close second (57.5 pounds), followed by pork (48.5 pounds) and seafood (16.3 pounds). While we admit we love a good steak on occasion, chicken is definitely the *ChangeOne* favorite because of its flexibility, leanness, and great taste. Even better is turkey, which is lowest in fat among poultry. Here's a calorie and fat comparison, based on a 3-ounce cooked portion without skin.

Item	Calories	Fat (g)
Turkey breast	114	0.6
Duck breast	119	2.1
Chicken breast	140	3.0
Duck leg meat	151	5.1
Turkey leg meat	159	6.1
Chicken leg meat	174	8.2
Goose	202	10.8

For great everyday eating, stock your freezer with boneless, skinless chicken breast halves—the most convenient cut of chicken you can buy. Slice while frozen for stir-frying, thaw and use whole, or pound into cutlets. Pair with sauce to keep the meat moist. Here's a tried-and-true cooking method for four servings:

1. Place four breast halves, about 6 ounces (checkbook) each, on a broiler pan. Sprinkle with lemon juice, fresh-ground black pepper, and olive oil so the chicken is well coated.

2. Broil about 4 inches from the heat, turning after about 3 minutes. Cook until done, 6 to 10 minutes, depending on the thickness. Alternatively, you can grill the chicken for about the same time.

Tip: When roasting a chicken, leave the skin on while cooking but remove it before serving. Chicken skin is a vice worth skipping: It adds a teaspoon of fat to every 3-ounce serving.

■ About Marinades

A marinade is a seasoned liquid used to flavor, tenderize, and moisten food (typically meat, fish, or poultry). Marinades often contain ingredients such as oil, vinegar, lemon or fruit juice, soy sauce, yogurt, herbs, and spices. Marinating imparts great flavor without many calories. It

also may fend off the cancer-promoting compounds that form when meat and other animal proteins are grilled at high temperatures.

Most supermarkets stock a wide selection of marinades, but as always, check the label to make sure the calorie and fat counts aren't exorbitant. Or make your own, incorporating your favorite flavors. Marinades are perfect for improvisation, so don't get hung up on following recipes to the letter.

To marinate, place the food in a bowl or resealable plastic bag. Pour in about ¼ cup of your favorite marinade—such as teriyaki, lemon-pepper, or lime-ginger—and mix well. Refrigerate for at least 1 hour.

Tip: To ensure food safety, discard remaining marinade after removing the food from the container.

■ *ChangeOne* Essentials: Stock and Broth

Stock and broth are must-have ingredients for healthy cooking. Use them for quick soups, as substitutes for oil when sautéing, or to add flavor and moisture to roasts and vegetable dishes. On rainy weekends, make large batches at home and freeze in quart containers.

• Stock, made by simmering bones (chicken, beef, veal, or fish stock), shells (seafood stock), or vegetables in just enough water to cover, has a rich flavor and texture. Concentrated stock can be purchased at many supermarkets and specialty food stores, and most general cookbooks have standard stock recipes.

• The best vegetables for stock include carrots, onions, leeks, celery, and garlic. Avoid cabbage, broccoli, and other members of the cabbage family; they will make the stock bitter.

• Broth is often made by adding water and seasonings—salt, herbs, and black pepper—to stock. Because it's more watery than stock, the flavor is less intense.

• When buying canned broth, look for reduced-sodium varieties; regular canned broths are often quite salty.

Dinner CHOICES & TIPS

■ Tips for Stir-Frying

Most of us associate stir-frying with Chinese cooking, but this low-fat cooking method can be used to create healthful meals with flavors from around the world. On page 292, we give you a recipe for an Italian-themed stir-fry. Use it as a basis for other international delights by substituting as follows:

Cuisine	Instead of Broccoli and Red Bell Pepper	Instead of Olive Oil and Basil
Mexican	Assorted peppers and corn	Squeeze of lime juice and ¼ cup cilantro
Chinese	Green beans and mushrooms	1 tablespoon soysauce, ½ teaspoon sesame oil
Thai	Unchanged	2 tablespoons lime juice and peanut butter
Greek	Eggplant and assorted peppers	2 tablespoons lemon juice and olives

■ About Woks

If you don't have a wok, is it worth getting one? Absolutely. A wok is perfectly designed for low-calorie cooking because it uses little oil and cooks vegetables and meats so quickly that they keep their flavor and nutrition. A wok is not just for Asian cooking; you can use it anytime you need to sauté something quickly. When shopping for a wok, you'll have several choices.

Nonstick, flat bottom: This is our favorite because it fits on any stove and cleanup is a breeze. Downside: It doesn't conduct heat as well as traditional steel woks do.

Traditional steel: This version conducts heat extremely well, and the concave design makes it simple to keep the food cooking evenly. Downside: It requires regular seasoning with oil and careful drying after each use to avoid rust.

Grill-top: Made from coated steel, this wok has small holes all over it so that smoky flavor penetrates the food. Downside: Foods can over-cook or burn easily.

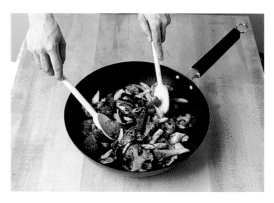

Tip: Be sure you can handle the weight of the wok with one hand. The more you use it, the more you'll discover that you'll be picking it up frequently while cooking and to pour finished dishes onto serving plates.

■ The Joys of Asian Seasonings

Countries that share a continent don't necessarily share a cooking style, as we see in Asia. Each country uses its own unique combination of sauces and seasonings. Our Asian noodle recipe on page 305 features the classic flavors of Thailand: coconut, peanut, cilantro, and lime. To travel through the other cuisines of Asia, consider the flavors of:

China: Soy sauce, five-spice powder, hoisin sauce, oyster sauce, garlic

Japan: Soy sauce, rice wine, sugar, fish stock, ginger

Korea: Soy sauce, sesame oil, garlic, chile peppers, fermented soy paste

Vietnam: Fish sauce, lemongrass, cilantro, garlic, shrimp paste

Indonesia: Tamarind, ginger, thick soy sauce, coconut, lemongrass

The Philippines: Coconut milk, garlic, ginger, vinegar, fermented shrimp paste

■ Tips for Cooking Fish

With the exception of grilled tuna, which is often served rare, most fish should be cooked all the way through, until the flesh is flaky but still moist. The 10-minute rule is helpful: Cook for a total of 10 minutes per inch of thickness. Steaks and large fillets may take longer, while thin fillets cook in a matter of minutes. Be sure to match fish to a cooking method appropriate to its texture. Here are a few guidelines.

Steaks: Grilling is good for fish steaks such as halibut, salmon, shark, swordfish, and tuna, which hold together well when you turn them.

Fillets: Higher-fat fillets such as salmon, sea bass, and trout won't fall apart on the grill, especially if you invest in a special grill basket for fish. Baking or pan-sautéing is best for thin fillets such as sole, flounder, red snapper, mahi mahi, tilapia, and other varieties. They're more apt to fall apart on the grill.

Whole fish and large fillets: These can be grilled, steamed in a wok or fish steamer, baked, or poached.

■ About Barbecuing

Let's be clear about language: When you quickly cook foods over hot charcoal or flames, it's actually *grilling*. Barbecuing means cooking meats at a low temperature, using indirect heat and smoke, for a very long time. Thanks to its use of intricate spice rubs, marinades, and sauces, barbecuing has emerged as one of the great American art forms (and trust us, a perfectly barbecued pork tenderloin is a work of art!). That said, both grilled and barbecued foods taste great and fit well into the *ChangeOne* eating approach, since both methods allow fat—with all its calories—to drip off the meat. Just choose lean meats and watch your portion sizes; it's easy to overindulge in grilled or barbecued meat. One solution: Have lots of grilled vegetables on the side.

One issue with grilling is food safety. It's all too common for meats and poultry to be burned on the outside and barely done on the inside. Undercooked meat can harbor harmful bacteria, and the charred parts of the skin contain cancer-causing compounds. The culprit is the intense direct heat—the hot coals or gas flames of outdoor grills. The solution? Cook with indirect heat. On a gas grill, turn on only one or two burners, leaving part of the grill top unheated. On a charcoal grill, arrange the coals along the wall of the grill. Place meat or poultry on the unlit side of a gas grill or in the center of a charcoal grill. You may want to place a drip pan under the meat. If desired, follow the manufacturer's directions for adding wood chips to your grill.

Close the grill and cook the meat until done (but open the lid to baste frequently). To ensure that the meat is properly cooked, use a meat thermometer. You want readings of 150°F for beef, 150°F to 160°F for pork, 160°F for chicken breast, and 170°F for chicken thighs.

Tip: Despite their sugar content, barbecue sauces add way more taste than calories. Lowest in calories are the vinegar-based sauces popular in North Carolina. We also love "dry" barbecuing, in which the meat is smothered in a "rub" of tangy spices and cooked without sauce; if you want sauce, you add it at the table. This is a style used for both Kansas City and Memphis barbecue.

■ Pasta Pleasures

Most of us love a big bowl of rich spaghetti. That's both a blessing and a curse, since, in moderation, pasta can be the perfect foundation for a meal, but in excess, is very high in calories without supplying much nutrition. As with every *ChangeOne* meal, make sure your pasta dinners feature more vegetables than noodles. We recommend whole grain noodles; they are much richer in fiber and more filling but are just mildly different in flavor than regular bleached pasta.

Toss with sauce immediately.

Tip: Always keep jars of marinara sauce in the cupboard. For a fast pasta dinner, put the noodles on to cook and then sauté garlic, onions, green peppers, mushrooms, and other vegetables with a little olive oil in a wok or large skillet. When the vegetables are softened, mix in a jar of marinara sauce; some extra herbs, such as oregano or basil; and a splash of cooking wine. Drain the noodles, and when the sauce is heated through, you're ready to serve!

Dinner CHOICES & TIPS

■ Try a Potpie

Potpies are perfect for *ChangeOne* because they're already portioned into individual servings. They're also easy to adapt. You can alternate among chicken, turkey, tuna, and even tofu without changing the wonderful flavor of the dish. Our recipe, found on page 294, calls for frozen vegetables—available year-round—so potpies always are in season. If you're serving a crowd, double the recipe and bake in a baking dish. Try these variations on our basic recipe.

Chicken breast: Boneless, skinless chicken thighs (¾ pound), Turkey breast chunks (1 pound), Drained water-packed tuna (3 cans), Firm tofu (¾ pound)

Piecrust: Refrigerated biscuit dough (½ biscuit per pie)

Frozen peas: Frozen edamame (soybeans), shelled, Frozen mixed vegetables

Frozen corn: Fresh corn, Fresh or frozen lima beans

Fat-free evaporated milk: Fat-free half-and-half

Tip: Skip the potpie when dining out or purchasing ready-made dishes. Traditional potpies are made with cream in the filling and crust, pushing them well beyond 500 calories per serving.

■ Planning for the Holidays

Holidays and food go hand in hand, and most of us look forward to enjoying the same family favorites year after year. It's okay if you choose to leave *ChangeOne* behind for a holiday meal. But if you want to stay with the program through the holidays, here's our plan for preparing food for a crowd.

• Select at least two appetizers: one vegetable (such as stuffed mushrooms or a platter of crudités) and one holiday favorite (such as a low-fat cheese log).

• Serve a green salad as a low-calorie filler.

• Offer a healthy, simple, broth-based soup, such as chicken broth with bay scallops and spinach, as a surprisingly refreshing third course.

• Include one or two entrées, a starch side dish (pasta, rice, or potatoes), rolls or bread, and at least two cooked vegetables.

• Think berries and fruit when it comes to dessert. A slice of angel food cake smothered with strawberries, blueberries, or peach slices would make almost anyone happy. Fruit sorbets are a nice alternative to ice cream.

• Prepare each recipe for about half the number of people at your dinner. For example, if you have 16 guests, prepare each dish to serve 8.

■ Exploring Root Vegetables

Carrots, parsnips ("blond" carrots), turnips, onions, and potatoes are particularly well suited for slow cooking because their fibrous flesh stays firm during the stewing process. They are abundant in the winter months, when fresh, locally grown vegetables may be in short supply. All supply fiber, along with an assortment of vitamins and minerals. Try these ways to prepare root vegetables.

Roast: Cut into 1-inch chunks, toss with a bit of olive oil, and roast in a shallow pan at 450°F until softened, 30 to 45 minutes.

Puree: Cut into 1-inch chunks and boil or microwave until softened, 3 to 5 minutes. Mash or puree with a little milk or broth, a pinch of salt, fresh-ground black pepper, and a teaspoon of butter until smooth.

Braise: Cut into 1-inch chunks, place in a pot with enough stock or broth to cover, and simmer, covered, until the liquid is absorbed and the vegetables are soft, about 15 minutes.

■ Exploring Leafy Greens

Cooking greens—popular varieties include kale, turnip greens, collard greens, mustard greens, dandelion greens, and Swiss chard—are among the healthiest foods in the supermarket. They are equally easy to cook and wonderfully good to eat. Yet there they sit forlornly in the vegetable section, too often passed up by shoppers who don't quite know what to do with a bundle of oversize edible leaves. So here's the answer: Buy 2 pounds of any variety of fresh, crisp greens. Clean them thoroughly, trim off the tough stalks and thick veins, and chop into large pieces. Fill a large pot with 6 to 7 quarts of water and boil for an hour or two (you can't overcook them). Near the end of cooking, add seasonings: salt, pepper, a little vinegar if you like a touch of sourness, a little hot sauce for kick. We sometimes sauté garlic, onions, and chopped turkey bacon and add them to the mix. Finally, taste and adjust the seasonings. It's that simple.

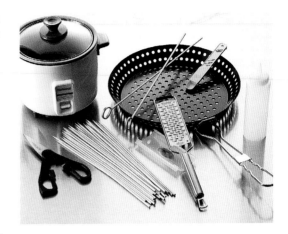

Clockwise from top left: rice steamer, grill pan, adjustable measuring spoon, squeeze bottle, microplane grater, skewers, and kitchen scissors.

■ Essential Tools

Well-chosen kitchen tools are a dieter's friend. Here are some top choices:

Quality knives: Any professional chef will tell you that good knives are crucial. If yours won't cut butter, it's time to sharpen them up or invest in a new set.

Kitchen scissors: Removing chicken skin, trimming string-bean tips—you'll be surprised how often these come in handy.

Measuring cups: Essential tools to prevent portion creep.

Timers: Accurate timers with loud alarms will keep watch over what's cooking and remind you when you're needed.

Adjustable measuring spoon: This simple tool will replace the clutter of spoons on your counter when you are baking or making a dish with lots of ingredients.

Kitchen scale: Another great way to keep portions in check. If you do a lot of cooking at home, a scale will also be handy for recipes that list ingredients in ounces or grams.

Nonstick frying pan or skillet: Here, too, the nonstick surface cuts down on the amount of oil needed for sautéing.

Grill pan: When you cook moist foods like fish filets or vegetables on the grill, they tend

to stick or break apart—but not when you use a grill pan. Consider a grill wok as well.

Skewers: Skewers are wonderful tools for grilling, of course, but they're useful other ways, from testing the doneness of cakes and muffins to tenderizing meat.

Salad spinner: A must for salad lovers. A spinner makes it easy to rinse and dry salad leaves without bruising them.

Vegetable steamer: Try a collapsible metal steamer rack that will fit into a saucepan, or buy a dedicated steamer. Make sure you have one big enough to handle a variety of vegetables.

Blender: With a decent blender you can whip up yogurt smoothies, fruit ices, savory sauces, and homemade soups.

Microplane grater: Super sharp, these graters make easy work out of grating high-flavor ingredients like hard cheese or chocolate. They're also perfect for zesting citrus.

Crock pot: Put together a simple meal early and let it cook all day. Perfect for chilis, stews, and other slow-cook items.

Dessert & Snack RECIPES

Chocolate Snacking Cake

MAKES 36 SQUARES

1⅓   cups all-purpose flour

1   cup plus 2 teaspoons unsweetened cocoa powder

1½   teaspoons baking powder

½   teaspoon salt

¼   cup fat-free buttermilk

1   tablespoon instant espresso powder

1   cup granulated sugar

½   cup packed light brown sugar

½   cup unsweetened applesauce

2   teaspoons vanilla extract

2   egg whites

½   cup semisweet mini chocolate chips

1   tablespoon confectioners' sugar

1. Preheat the oven to 325°F. Line an 8-inch square baking pan with foil, leaving a 1-inch overhang.

2. Sift the flour and 1 cup of the cocoa together into a small bowl, then add the baking powder and salt. In a small saucepan, heat the buttermilk and espresso over low heat until the espresso is dissolved.

3. In a medium bowl, mix the granulated sugar, brown sugar, applesauce, buttermilk mixture, and vanilla. Stir in the flour mixture just until blended.

4. In a large bowl, using an electric mixer on high speed, beat the egg whites just until soft peaks form. Fold into the batter and stir in the chocolate chips.

5. Pour the batter into the baking pan and bake just until set, about 35 minutes; do not overbake. Transfer the pan to a wire rack to cool for 15 minutes, then remove the cake from the pan and place on the rack to cool completely.

6. Sift the confectioners' sugar and the remaining cocoa over the cake. Cut into 36 pieces a little more than 1 inch square. One serving is 1 square. You can wrap leftovers in heavy-duty foil and freeze for up to 1 month. Well sealed, the cake can last at room temperature for about five days.

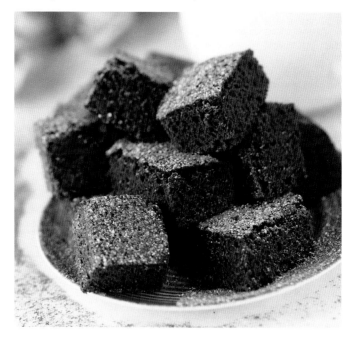

Brownie Bites

⅔ cup all-purpose flour

⅓ cup unsweetened cocoa powder

2 tablespoons cornstarch

1 teaspoon baking powder

¼ teaspoon baking soda

¼ teaspoon salt

1 cup packed light brown sugar

¼ cup prune butter

2 tablespoons fat-free plain yogurt

2 tablespoons vegetable oil

1 egg

3 tablespoons semisweet mini chocolate chips

½ cup coarsely chopped walnuts

1. Preheat the oven to 350°F. Coat an 8-inch square baking pan with cooking spray.

2. In a medium bowl, stir together the flour, cocoa, cornstarch, baking powder, baking soda, and salt. Set aside.

3. In a large bowl, using an electric mixer, beat together the brown sugar, prune butter, yogurt, oil, and egg. Stir in the flour mixture just until combined.

4. Pour the batter into the baking pan and scatter the chocolate chips and walnuts on top. Bake until a toothpick inserted in the center comes out with some crumbs and the sides of the brownie begin to pull away from the pan, 18 to 20 minutes. Transfer the pan to a wire rack to cool. Cut into 16 pieces about 2 inches square. One serving is 1 brownie. You can wrap leftovers in heavy foil and freeze for up to 1 month. Well sealed, these can last at room temperature for about five days.

Chocolate-Dipped Strawberries

SERVES 8-12
DEPENDING ON BERRY SIZE

⅔ cup semisweet chocolate chips

1 pint strawberries, rinsed and dried

1. Line a baking sheet with parchment.

2. In a small bowl, microwave the chocolate chips on medium until melted into a thick liquid, about 30 seconds. Stir well.

3. Using a fork or strawberry stem, dip each strawberry into the chocolate, allowing excess chocolate to drip off. Gently place on the baking sheet.

4. When all the strawberries have been dipped, refrigerate on the baking sheet until the chocolate hardens, about 30 minutes. One serving is 1 strawberry. You can store leftovers in the refrigerator for up to 1 day.

Dessert & Snack RECIPES

Cantaloupe Salad with Raspberry Vinaigrette

SERVES 4

1 tablespoon hulled pumpkin seeds

¼ cup seedless raspberry all-fruit spread

1 tablespoon balsamic vinegar

2 teaspoons fresh lemon juice

¼ teaspoon ground cinnamon

1 large cantaloupe, cut into 8 wedges

1 cup blueberries

1. Toast the pumpkin seeds in a small, heavy skillet over medium heat until they begin to pop, about 5 minutes. Set aside.

2. In a large bowl, whisk the raspberry spread, vinegar, lemon juice, and cinnamon.

3. Add the cantaloupe and blueberries and toss to combine. Sprinkle with the pumpkin seeds. One serving equals 2 cantaloupe wedges, ¼ cup blueberries (golf ball), and 1 teaspoon pumpkin seeds (thumb tip).

Blueberry Bonanza

SERVES 4

½ cup 1% milk

2 tablespoons nonfat dry milk

1 package (12 ounces) frozen blueberries, thawed

⅛ teaspoon salt

¼ cup plus 1 teaspoon sugar

½ cup fat-free plain yogurt

½ packet unflavored gelatin

2 tablespoons cold water

½ cup fresh blueberries

1. In a small bowl, combine the milk and dry milk and whisk until well blended. Place in the freezer for up to 30 minutes.

2. In a medium saucepan over low heat, combine the frozen blueberries, salt, and ¼ cup of the sugar. Bring to a simmer and cook until the sugar has dissolved, the berries have broken up, and the mixture has been reduced to 1 cup, about 10 minutes. Let cool to room temperature, then stir in ⅓ cup of the yogurt.

3. Sprinkle the gelatin over cold water in a heatproof measuring cup. Let stand for 5 minutes to soften. Set the measuring cup in a saucepan of simmering water until the gelatin has melted, about 2 minutes. Let cool.

4. With a hand mixer, beat the chilled milk until thick, soft peaks form. Beat in the remaining sugar, then the gelatin mixture. With a rubber spatula, fold the milk mixture into the blueberry mixture.

5. Spoon into 4 dessert bowls or glasses and refrigerate until set, about 2 hours. To serve, top each portion with a dollop of the remaining yogurt and the fresh blueberries. One serving is 1 bowl or glass.

Fruit Boats with Orange-Balsamic Glaze

SERVES 4

¼ cup balsamic vinegar

¼ teaspoon grated orange zest

2 tablespoons fresh orange juice

2 teaspoons brown sugar

1 large cantaloupe

1 pint strawberries, rinsed, hulled and quartered

½ pint blueberries, rinsed

½ pint raspberries, rinsed

2 kiwifruits, peeled, halved, and cut into thin wedges

1. In a small bowl, combine the vinegar, orange zest, juice, and brown sugar. Microwave on high until syrupy, 2 to 3 minutes, or cook in a small saucepan over medium-high heat for 4 to 5 minutes. Set aside.

2. Cut the cantaloupe into quarters and scoop out balls, leaving a thin layer of flesh on the rinds.

3. In a large bowl, combine the cantaloupe balls, strawberries, blueberries, raspberries, and kiwis. Drizzle with the glaze and toss to coat. Spoon into the 4 cantaloupe boats and serve immediately. One serving is 1 boat.

Chocolate Chip Oatmeal Cookies

MAKES 36

1 cup all-purpose flour

½ teaspoon baking soda

½ teaspoon salt

1 cup old-fashioned oats

4 tablespoons butter

⅔ cup packed light brown sugar

½ cup granulated sugar

1 egg

1½ teaspoons vanilla extract

⅓ cup reduced-fat sour cream

¾ cup semisweet chocolate chips

1. Preheat the oven to 375°F. Line 2 large baking sheets with parchment paper.

2. In a medium bowl, whisk the flour, baking soda, and salt. Stir in the oats.

3. In a large bowl, using an electric mixer on high speed, cream the butter, brown sugar, and granulated sugar until well blended. Add the egg and vanilla and beat until light and creamy, about 3 minutes. With a wooden spoon, blend in the sour cream, then add the flour mixture all at once and stir until combined (don't overmix, or the cookies may be tough). Stir in the chocolate chips.

4. Drop heaping teaspoonfuls of dough 2 inches apart on the baking sheets. Bake until golden, about 10 minutes. Cool on the baking sheets for 2 minutes, then transfer to wire racks to cool completely. One serving is 1 cookie. You can store the cookies in an airtight container for up to 2 weeks or freeze for up to 3 months.

Dessert & Snack RECIPES

Pecan Icebox Cookies

MAKES 72

- 1¾ cups all-purpose flour
- ½ teaspoon ground cinnamon
- ¼ teaspoon salt
- ¼ teaspoon baking soda
- ¼ cup (½ stick) butter, softened
- ⅔ cup granulated sugar
- ⅓ cup packed light brown sugar
- 1 egg
- 1 tablespoon vanilla extract
- ⅓ cup reduced-fat sour cream
- ⅓ cup chopped pecans, toasted

1. In a medium bowl, whisk the flour, cinnamon, salt, and baking soda.

2. In a large bowl, using at electric mixer on high speed, cream the butter, granulated sugar, and brown sugar until light and fluffy, about 4 minutes. Add the egg and vanilla and beat until well blended. Using a wooden spoon, stir in the flour mixture, then the sour cream and pecans.

3. Tear off a 20-inch sheet of plastic wrap and sprinkle lightly with flour. Transfer the dough to the plastic and shape into a 15-inch log. Roll tightly in the plastic and refrigerate until firm, about 2 hours.

4. Preheat the oven to 375°F. Unwrap the dough and cut into rounds ¼ inch thick, making about 72 cookies. Working in batches, place the rounds ½ inch apart on ungreased baking sheets. Bake just until crisp and golden around the edges, about 8 minutes. Transfer to wire racks to cool. One serving is 2 cookies. You can store the cookies in an airtight container for up to 2 weeks or freeze for up to 3 months.

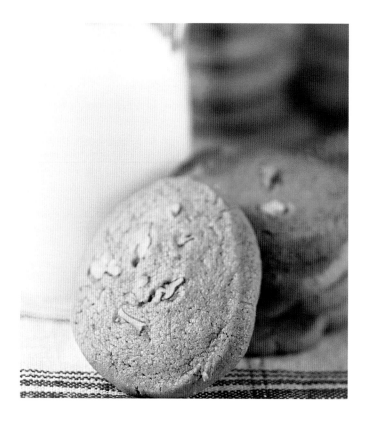

Meringue Nut Cookies

MAKES 36

⅓ cup walnuts

4 teaspoons unsweetened cocoa powder

¼ teaspoon ground cinnamon

½ cup plus 2 tablespoons confectioners' sugar

2 egg whites

⅛ teaspoon salt

1. Preheat the oven to 300°F. Line 2 baking sheets with parchment paper.

2. Toast the walnuts in a small skillet, stirring frequently, until crisp and fragrant, about 7 minutes. When cool enough to handle, chop coarsely.

3. Sift together the cocoa powder, cinnamon, and ½ cup of the confectioners' sugar onto a sheet of waxed paper.

4. In a large bowl, using an electric mixer, beat the egg whites and salt until stiff peaks form. With a rubber spatula, gently fold the cocoa mixture into the egg whites, then fold in the nuts.

5. Drop generous teaspoonfuls of batter 1 inch apart on the baking sheets. Bake until set, about 20 minutes. Transfer to a wire rack to cool. Dust with the remaining confectioners' sugar just before serving. One serving is 4 or 5 cookies. You can store the cookies in an airtight container.

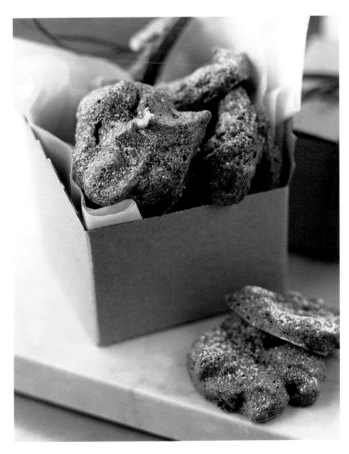

Dessert & Snack RECIPES

Ruby-Studded Trail Mix

MAKES 3 CUPS

1½   cups corn cereal squares

¾   cup thin pretzel sticks

2   tablespoons hulled
sunflower seeds

¼   teaspoon salt

¼   cup grated Parmesan
cheese

¾   cup dried cranberries,
coarsely chopped

1. Preheat the oven to 350ºF. In a large bowl, combine the cereal, pretzels, sunflower seeds, and salt. Coat lightly with cooking spray. Add the cheese and toss to combine.

2. Transfer to a jelly-roll pan and bake, stirring occasionally, until crisp and slightly crusty, about 15 minutes.

3. Let cool to room temperature, then transfer to a large bowl. Add the cranberries and toss to combine. One serving is ½ cup (2 golf balls). You can store leftovers in the refrigerator in an airtight container.

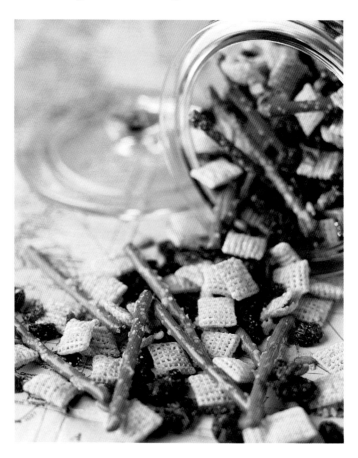

Roasted-Pepper Pinwheels

MAKES 8 PIECES

- 1 red bell pepper, seeded and cut lengthwise into flat slices (about 4, depending on shape of pepper)
- ½ cup canned chickpeas, rinsed and drained
- 1 tablespoon fat-free plain yogurt
- ½ teaspoon dark sesame oil
- ½ teaspoon grated lemon zest
- 2 teaspoons fresh lemon juice
- 2 teaspoons water
- Pinch of salt
- 1 8-inch spinach-flavored flour tortilla
- 1 cup mixed salad greens

1. Preheat the broiler. Broil the peppers, skin side up, 4 inches from the heat until charred, about 10 minutes. Transfer to a plate. When cool enough to handle, peel and cut into ½-inch-wide strips.

2. In a food processor, combine the chickpeas, yogurt, oil, lemon zest, lemon juice, water, and salt and puree until smooth.

3. Spread the mixture evenly over one side of the tortilla, leaving a ½-inch border all around. Top with the salad greens and peppers and roll up. Wrap tightly in foil or plastic wrap and refrigerate for at least 1 hour but no more than 4 hours. The roll will get softer and easier to slice while refrigerated.

4. To serve, unwrap and slice crosswise into eight 1-inch-wide pieces. One serving is 2 pieces. Send leftovers home with friends to eat that day—these pinwheels don't keep well.

Dessert & Snack RECIPES

MultiGrain Soft Pretzels

MAKES 12

- ¾ cup old-fashioned oats
- 1¾ cups all-purpose flour
- 1 cup whole wheat flour
- ½ cup toasted wheat germ
- 1 packet (¼ ounce) rapid-rise yeast
- 5 teaspoons sugar
- 1½ teaspoons table salt
- 1½ cups very warm water (120°F to 130°F)
- 3 tablespoons baking soda
- 1 tablespoon coarse or kosher salt

1. Toast the oats in a small skillet over low heat, stirring frequently, until golden, about 5 minutes. Transfer to a large bowl.

2. Add the all-purpose flour, whole wheat flour, wheat germ, yeast, 3 teaspoons of the sugar, and the table salt. Stir in the water. Transfer to a floured work surface and knead until smooth, about 5 minutes. Transfer to an ungreased bowl, cover, and let rise in a warm place until doubled in bulk, about 45 minutes.

3. Line 2 large baking sheets with parchment paper. Punch down the dough and cut into 12 equal portions. With clean hands, roll each portion into a 16- to 18-inch rope, then twist each rope into a pretzel shape. Place on the baking sheets, cover, and let rise until almost doubled in bulk, about 20 minutes.

4. Preheat the oven to 425°F. Bring a large skillet of water to a simmer and add the baking soda and the remaining sugar. Slide the pretzels into the water 3 at a time. Cook for 15 seconds, turn, and cook for 15 seconds longer. Blot dry on paper towels.

5. Transfer the pretzels to the baking sheets. Sprinkle with the coarse salt and bake until crisp and golden, 18 to 20 minutes. Transfer to a wire rack to cool. Serve warm or at room temperature. One serving is 1 pretzel. Allow leftovers to cool completely before storing in an airtight container.

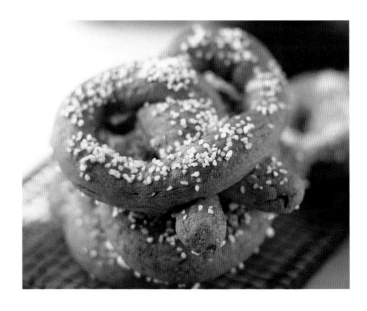

Sweet and Spicy Snack Mix

MAKES 8 CUPS

½ cup walnut halves

5 cups air-popped popcorn

1½ cups unsalted mini pretzel twists (about 2 ounces)

½ cup sugar

1 tablespoon lemon juice

3 tablespoons hulled pumpkin seeds

½ tablespoon ground cumin

½ teaspoon salt

¼ teaspoon cayenne pepper

1. Preheat the oven to 350ºF. Spread the walnuts on a baking sheet and bake until lightly crisp and fragrant, about 7 minutes. When cool enough to handle, chop coarsely.

2. Coat a large heatproof bowl with cooking spray. Add the popcorn and pretzels and toss well to combine.

3. In a large, heavy skillet, stir together the sugar and lemon juice. Cook, stirring, over medium heat, until the sugar has dissolved, about 5 minutes. Add the walnuts, pumpkin seeds, cumin, salt, and cayenne. Cook and stir until the nuts are well coated.

4. Transfer to the bowl with the popcorn and pretzels and stir quickly to combine. Let cool to room temperature. One serving is ½ cup (2 golf balls). You can store leftovers in an airtight container in the refrigerator.

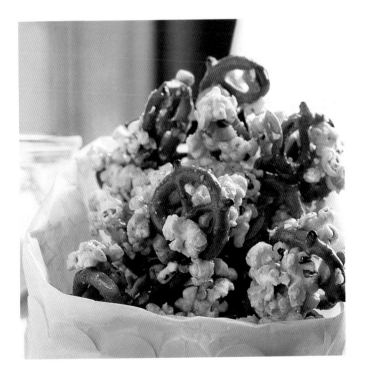

Dessert & Snack CHOICES & TIPS

■ Lightening Up Baked Desserts

The secret to decadent cakes and cookies can be revealed in just one word: fat. Want elaboration? Butter, margarine, oil, eggs, sour cream, whipping cream, nuts, and cream cheese. For healthier desserts, find ways to use less of these ingredients. Here are some tips.

• Don't try to eliminate fat entirely; it's needed for flavor and texture. Generally, you can successfully reduce the fat in a traditional dessert recipe by approximately 50 to 75 percent by using substitutions.

• Good substitutes for butter and cream are low-fat plain yogurt, low-fat or fat-free sour cream; buttermilk; low-fat evaporated milk; pureed raw fruits such as bananas or pineapple; and pureed cooked fruits such as dried dates, prunes, apricots, apples, and figs.

• In an egg, the fat is entirely in the yolk. If a recipe calls for one egg, go ahead and use it, since the yolk is important for flavor and texture. But for every two eggs in a recipe, we suggest using one whole egg and two egg whites.

• Egg substitutes can be used in breads, muffins, cakes, cookies, and puddings. Try different brands of liquid egg substitute; they don't all taste the same.

• Instead of buttery piecrusts, use cookie-crumb crusts held together with mostly water and just a smidgeon of canola oil.

• To make delicious crunchy toppings, use quick-cooking oats or a crunchy cereal like Grape-Nuts to replace the nuts traditionally used. Use a few nuts occasionally for taste, and always toast them to bring out their full flavor.

• Using low-fat evaporated milk or low-fat condensed milk instead of heavy cream gives desserts a creamy, rich consistency.

• Feel free to use light cream cheese instead of regular, but skip fat-free cream cheese, which doesn't cook well. You can also substitute yogurt cheese for cream cheese; see how to make it on page 283.

■ Beloved Berries

Berries have wonderful textures and exquisite flavors, and they pack a seriously healthful punch. For all these reasons, we consider berries to be a top *ChangeOne* food for snacks and desserts. From a health perspective, blueberries supply the most antioxidants, naturally occurring plant compounds that help protect the body's cells from damage by guarding against cancer and keeping blood vessels sound. Strawberries are lowest in calories and richest in vitamin C; raspberries and blackberries supply the most fiber.

Use berries to make cobblers, smoothies, and sorbets; serve fresh with a cookie or brownie or on top of sorbet or Italian ice for a simple dessert; add berries to sliced peaches and pour on a little orange juice for an instant fruit salad; or, easiest of all, eat them unadorned. Be sure to rinse thoroughly them before eating.

Tip: While berries are best fresh, most freeze well, particularly if you intend to use them for baking, in sauces, or in smoothies. You can buy frozen berries any time of year, but they're cheapest in summer, when customers are buying fresh instead. Better yet, find a pick-your-own berry farm near you, spend a fun day filling a bucket, and freeze your own. You'll have a year's supply for surprisingly little money.

■ About Melons

Melons—cantaloupe, honeydew, Crenshaw, watermelon, and a growing number of gourmet varieties—are among the lowest-calorie fruits. They have high water content and less sugar than other fruits, despite their sweet, fresh taste. We recommend having a melon or two in your refrigerator at all times. In particular, summer is watermelon season; a large slice makes a perfect dessert. From a health standpoint, cantaloupe is a standout for its vitamin C and vitamin A, two important nutrients that you get mainly from fruits and vegetables. A cup of melon contains 45 to 60 calories.

Meal Plans

It's a vicious circle: If you don't know what you're going to be cooking this coming week, you can't shop for food effectively. And if you're not shopping effectively, it's awfully hard to cook and eat well. As we've said a few times, eating the *ChangeOne* way takes a little planning.

We're here to help. The *ChangeOne* meal plans on the following pages are the perfect tool for organizing your daily meals and snacks.

Truth is, while we would be proud if you followed the plans closely, that's not what we expect. Following a rigid eating plan is both unappealing and unsustainable. But look these over carefully anyhow. You'll learn how much food you should eat in a day—an extremely important lesson—and perhaps will discover a few days worth of eating plans that you might actually enjoy.

Note that each day's meal plan falls right around our 1,300 calorie target. For those in the 1,600 Club, remember that you should double your grain portion at breakfast, and either double a grain or protein portion at lunch or dinner.

Week 1	MONDAY	TUESDAY	WEDNESDAY	
Breakfast	**Yogurt Parfait** (page 285) • Yogurt layered with granola, fruit, and coconut	**Bagel Delight** (page 283) • Mini-bagel topped with jam and reduced-fat cream cheese • Yogurt with sliced ripe peach	**Breakfast on the Run** (page 284) • Cereal bar • Yogurt topped with blueberries	
Lunch	**Caesar Salad Lunch** • Caesar Sald (page 291) • Medium whole grain roll • Cantaloupe cubes	**Soup and Sandwich** • Hearty Split-Pea Soup (page 286) • Tuna Salad Sandwich (page 44) • Seasonal fruit	**DINING OUT** **Friendly Fast-Food** (page 47) • Regular hamburger with lettuce, tomato, and condiments • Green salad	
Snack	Baked tortilla chips and salsa	Hot cocoa made with skim milk	Baked Apple (page 67)	
Dinner	**Barbecued Halibut Steak Dinner** (page 299) • Barbecued Halibut Steak • Grilled Onions and Scallions • Ziti and Zucchini (page 309)	**Beef Stew** (page 297) • Beef Stew • Egg noodles	**Kitchen Sink Stew** (page 312) • Kitchen Sink Stew • Garlic bread	
Snack/ Dessert	Blueberry Bonanza (page 320)	Fudgsicle	Yogurt smoothie	

THURSDAY	FRIDAY	SATURDAY	SUNDAY
A Perfect Bowl of Cereal (page 28) • Bran flakes topped with raisins and chopped nuts • Skim or low-fat milk	**Cottage Cheese Melba** (page 284) • Cottage cheese with peach slices • Raisin bread toast • Vanilla Steamer (page 283)	**Pancakes to Start** (page 277) • Silver Dollar Pancakes topped with light syrup and sliced strawberries • Skim or low-fat milk	• Dried Cranberry Scones with Orange Glaze (page 278) • Skim or low-fat milk ## Brunch (page 285) • Hummus and pita • Crudité platter • Vegetable-Cheddar Omelet (page 280) • Whole wheat toast with butter and jam • Cantaloupe wedge
The Perfect Deli Lunch (page 45) • Turkey and Swiss Cheese Sandwich on wheat bread • Italian pickled vegetable salad • Melon salad	**The Perfect Soup-and-Salad Lunch** (page 49) • Vegetable soup with breadsticks • Green salad topped with grilled chicken • Green or red grapes	**Pita Pizza and Salad** • Pita Pizza (page 291) • Green salad • Apple	
Frozen yogurt	Corn tortilla with melted cheese	Cup of yogurt topped with fruit	
DINING OUT **Italian Restaurant** (page 94) • Minestrone soup • Chicken breast cacciatore with pasta • Sautéed spinach and garlic • Fresh berries	**Sweet-and-Sour Pork Dinner** (page 299) • Sweet-and-Sour Glazed Pork with Pineapple • Basmati rice • Steamed patty-pan squash	**DINING OUT** **Chinese Restaurant** (page 96) • Wonton soup • Egg roll • Chicken chow mein • Steamed Chinese vegetables • Pineapple chunks	**Heartland Meat Loaf Dinner** (page 300) • Heartland Meat Loaf • Egg noodles • Steamed baby zucchini
Brownie Bites (page 319)	Skim or low-fat latte	Air-popped popcorn	

Week 2	MONDAY	TUESDAY	WEDNESDAY	
Breakfast	**A Smoothie Breakfast** • Tropical Smoothie (page 284) • Toasted English muffin half with peanut butter	**A Perfect Bowl of Cereal** (page 28) • Bran flakes topped with raisins and chopped nuts • Skim or low-fat milk	**Egg on a Roll Breakfast** (page 25) • Scrambled egg on a whole wheat roll • Fresh fruit salad • Skim or low-fat milk	
Lunch	**Tuna Salad Sandwich Lunch** • Tuna Salad Sandwich (page 44) • Carrot and celery sticks • Banana	**Turkey Caesar Lunch** (page 289) • Grilled Turkey Caesar Salad • Ak-Mak flatbread crackers • Fresh fruit salad	**Baked Potato and Salad Lunch** (page 290) • Baked potato stuffed with broccoli and cheese • Green salad • Seasonal berries	
Snack		Chocolate Chip Oatmeal Cookie (page 321) with skim or low-fat milk	Frozen yogurt	
Dinner	**Sautéed Chicken Dinner** (page 293) • Sautéed Chicken with Caramelized Onions • Spinach fettuccine • Green salad	**Sunday Roast Dinner** (page 298) • All-American Pot Roast • Braised Vegetables • Crusty sourdough bread	**Pasta Primavera** (page 303) • Pasta Primavera • Italian Salad (page 308)	
Snack/ Dessert	Fruit Boats with Orange-Balsamic Glaze (page 321)	Apple	Pineapple chunks	

THURSDAY	FRIDAY	SATURDAY	SUNDAY
Café-Style Breakfast (page 278) • Blueberry Muffin with Lemon Glaze (page 279) • Cantaloupe wedge • Steaming latte	**Breakfast on the Run** (page 284) • Cereal bar • Yogurt topped with blueberries	**Yogurt Parfait** (page 285) • Yogurt layered with granola, fruit, and coconut	**Pancakes to Start** (page 277) • Silver Dollar Pancakes topped with light syrup and sliced strawberries • Skim or low-fat milk
Chopped Salad Lunch (page 287) • Pete's Chopped Salad • Whole wheat pita • Grapes	**The Perfect Deli Lunch** (page 45) • Turkey and Swiss Cheese Sanwich on wheat bread • Italian pickled vegetable salad • Melon salad	**Burrito to Go** (page 104) • Chicken fajita with condiments • Orange	**Wrap Sandwich** (page 289) • Roasted Vegetable Wraps with Chive Sauce • Green salad • Honeydew melon
Peanut butter on a rice cake	Strawberry smoothie	Graham crackers with skim or low-fat milk	Pretzel sticks and reduced-fat string cheese
DINING OUT **Mexican Restaurant** (page 104) • Ceviche • Steak soft tacos with condiments	**Potpie Dinner** (page 294) • One-Crust Chicken Potpie • Green salad	**Dinner on the Grill** • Crudité platter • Grilled Beer-Can Chicken (page 295) • Grilled Summer Vegetables (page 304) • German Potato Salad with Dijon Vinaigrette (page 309) • Sesame breadsticks	**Barbecue Beef Picnic Dinner** (page 297) • Barbecue Beef on a Bun • Colorful Cole Slaw (page 305)
Almond-flavored milk	Brownie Bites (page 319)	Chocolate Snacking Cake (page 318)	Blueberry Bonanza (page 320)

Week 3	MONDAY	TUESDAY	WEDNESDAY	
Breakfast	**Quick Bread Delight** (page 280) • 1 slice Peach Quick Bread • Fresh raspberries • Skim or low-fat milk	**Café-Style Breakfast** (page 278) • Blueberry Muffin with Lemon Glaze (page 279) • Cantaloupe wedge • Steaming latte	**Yogurt Parfait** (page 285) • Yogurt layered with granola, fruit, and coconut	
Lunch	**Soup and Sandwich** • Hearty Split-Pea Soup (page 286) • Tuna Salad Sandwich (page 44) • Seasonal fruit	**Meatless Chili** (page 288) • Meatless Chili Pots con Queso • Corn tortilla • Green salad • Banana	**DINING OUT** **Friendly Fast-Food** (page 47) • Regular hamburger with lettuce, tomato, and condiments • Green salad • Orange	
Snack	Crackers with peanut butter	Graham crackers and hot cocoa with skim milk	Edamame (steamed soybeans)	
Dinner	**Red Snapper and Spanish Rice** (page 301) • Snapper and Snaps in a Packet • Spanish Rice (page 310)	**DINING OUT** **Diner** (page 102) • Chicken noodle soup • Green salad • Half a hot roast beef sandwich • Mashed potatoes • Cooked carrots • 2 butter cookies	**Italian-Style Stir-Fry** (page 292) • Chicken and Broccoli Stir-Fry, Italian Style • Orzo	
Snack/ Dessert	Brownie Bites (page 319)		Frozen yogurt	

THURSDAY	FRIDAY	SATURDAY	SUNDAY
Breakfast on the Run (page 284) • Cereal bar • Yogurt topped with blueberries	**Bagel Delight** (page 283) • Mini-bagel topped with jam and reduced-fat cream cheese • Yogurt with sliced ripe peach	**Hearty Frittata** (page 282) • Vegetable Frittata wedge • 1 slice wheat toast • Fresh blueberries	**Pancakes to Start** (page 277) • Silver Dollar Pancakes topped with light syrup and sliced strawberries • Skim or low-fat milk
Pita Pizza and Salad • Pita Pizza (page 291) • Green salad • Apple	**The Perfect Deli Lunch** (page 45) • Turkey and Swiss Cheese Sandwich on wheat bread • Italian pickled vegetable salad • Melon salad	**The Perfect Soup-and-Salad Lunch** (page 49) • Vegetable soup with breadsticks • Green salad topped with grilled chicken • Green or red grapes	# Brunch • Chesapeake Crab Cakes (page 282) • Green salad • Crusty roll • Seasonal berries • Pecan Icebox Cookies (page 322)
Mixed dried fruit	Ruby-Studded Trail Mix (page 324)	Container of nonfat yogurt	Mixed nuts
Quick Black Beans and Rice with Chicken • Marinated Grilled Chicken Breast Filet (page 313) • Quick Black Beans and Rice (page 311) • Green salad	**Noodles and Greens** (page 305) • Thai Noodle Salad with greens	**Casserole Dinner** (page 301) • Homestyle Tuna Noodle Casserole • Arugula salad	**DINING OUT** **Italian Restaurant** (page 94) • Green salad • Spaghetti with red clam sauce • Sautéed broccoli
Sorbet (page 69)	Fresh fruit	Air-popped popcorn	Fresh fruit salad

Shopping Smartly

Putting *ChangeOne* into action at the grocery store is a snap with our guide to sensible shopping lists that will ensure you're never without the essentials.

Chances are you already have many of the ingredients for the meals in the three weekly sample plans on the previous pages. They're drawn from the basic provisions—the pantry supplies and refrigerator items—that we detailed back in Week 7. As you think about shopping strategies, take some time to look back at that list of Kitchen Essentials on page 129, and keep it handy. You'll be referring to it often as you get comfortable with stocking a *ChangeOne* kitchen.

Our meals call for lots of perishable foods, especially fruits, vegetables, meats, and dairy products, so it's important to have a checklist to track these items and avoid waste. We've included two sample *ChangeOne* shopping lists on the next page that will help you track perishables.

Grocery stores stock produce separately from dairy, meats, and seafood, so start your list with that in mind. It's also helpful to divide the perishables into two groups: long-life items and short-life items.

Long-life items are those that can be stored in a cool pantry or in the refrigerator and will keep for a few weeks. Plan to check these items and restock as needed about twice a month. Short-life items will keep only a few days in the refrigerator and are best bought and used for a specific recipe. Check these once a week and restock as needed.

Okay, now it's time to tackle the whole store. Use the following shopping guidelines to stay on top of the master list on page 129, and to stay timely with perishable items.

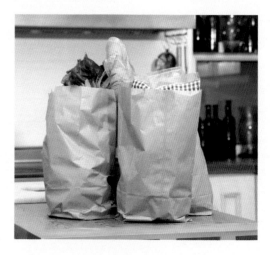

Monthly: Around the same time every month, check and restock your kitchen staples.

Twice monthly: Check and replenish long-life produce, dairy, meats, and seafood as needed.

Weekly: Pick up short-life items for that week's meals.

A few more general guidelines can simplify your shopping strategy even further:

- Plan a week's recipes, then check your pantry and refrigerator for items you will need that week and make sure they're on your list.

- You're the best judge of how much you'll need of each item, based on the number of people you're cooking for and the substitutions you make.

- You can substitute just about any fruit or vegetable for another, so buy the ones you like or those that are in season.

- If you find you're not going to use fresh meat, poultry, or fish within a day after you buy it, freeze it.

Twice-Monthly List

QTY	PRODUCE
	Apples
	Pears
	Oranges
	Lemons and limes
	Melons, uncut
	Kiwifruit
	Cabbage
	Carrots
	Celery
	Garlic
	Ginger
	Onions
	Potatoes
	Scallions
	Squash in season

QTY	DAIRY, MEAT, SEAFOOD
	Butter
	Cheeses, hard and dry (parmesan)
	Yogurt
	Beef (freezer)
	Chicken breasts (freezer)
	Roasting chicken (freezer)
	Salami, hard Italian
	Salmon (freezer)
	Cod fillets (freezer)

Weekly List

QTY	PRODUCE
	Berries
	Grapes
	Bananas
	Peaches
	Pears
	Mangoes
	Cantalope
	Cucumbers
	Edamame (soybeans)
	Lettuce and salad greens
	Red and green peppers
	Tomatoes
	Zucchini
	Broccoli
	String beans
	Sprouts

QTY	DAIRY, MEAT, SEAFOOD
	Cheeses, medium (cheddar, jack)
	Cheeses, soft (ricotta, cottage)
	Milk
	Deli meats
	Meats, uncooked
	Seafood, uncooked

Personal tools

Throughout *ChangeOne* we've asked you to write things down. How's the weight loss progressing? What are your current goals? What did you eat today? Were you active?

But truth is, few of us are in the habit of writing down such things. So we've tried to make it easier for you.

On the following pages are all the guides you need to progress through *ChangeOne*.

Each of these forms was conceived to be as simple to use as possible. They'll ask the tough questions, but they'll also lead to clear, concise answers. So give them a try; each one will take just a few minutes. Make as many copies of each form as you need to track your progress.

Here's what you'll find:

- The *ChangeOne* Contract
- Daily Food Diary
- Progress Log
- Hunger Profile
- Daily Activity Log
- Your Healthy Weight Calculator

And remember, for these and other interactive weight-loss tools, subscribe to our Web site, changeone.com/special.

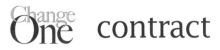 contract

ChangeOne begin date: _____

I VOW TO MYSELF that over the next three months I will learn and practice the eating and fitness habits necessary to lose weight and improve my health. I put forth the following goals:

Intermediate weight target: _____

Ultimate weight target: _____

HOW I EXPECT MY LIFE TO IMPROVE: _____

_____

_____

_____

HOW I EXPECT MY HEALTH TO IMPROVE: _____

_____

_____

_____

IN ADDITION to weekly weigh-ins on a scale, I will track my progress by the two methods I will list below (for example, clothing size, appearance, energy, notches in a belt, or self-confidence):

1. _____

2. _____

I HEREBY AFFIRM that the goals I have set meet the TRIM test. Each one is Time-bound, Realistic, Inspiring, and Measurable.

I agree to review my progress and reevaluate my strategies for reaching my goals every two weeks during the program.

I agree to keep this contract as a reminder of my commitment.

Signed: _____

Witnessed by (optional): _____

Date:

Hunger Profile

Instructions: Make a copy of this form and carry it with you during the day. Every time you get hungry, record the time, how you felt (tired, bored, ravenous, stressed-out, just plain hungry), what you ate, or what you did instead of eating (took a walk, distracted myself with work). This will help you determine your eating habits—both good and bad—and make it easier to adjust your meal and snack times for healthy weight loss.

	TIME	HOW I FELT	WHAT I ATE	WHAT I DID
MORNING				
AFTERNOON				
EVENING				

Date:

Daily Food Diary

Instructions: First, write down what you eat. Next, estimate portions as carefully as you can based on what you've learned throughout *ChangeOne*. For example, if one egg is the recommended portion at breakfast and you eat two, write in "two portions." Keep a copy of the form with you and fill it in as soon as you can after a snack or meal.

Finally, for each item you eat that either exceeded the proper portion size or is in excess of your ChangeOne daily eating targets—for example, a large third snack or an extra piece of chcken—check the column to the right. This will help you see where you are having the most trouble complying with the healthy eating guidelines you are learning to follow.

	WHAT I ATE	ESTIMATED PORTIONS	IN EXCESS?
BREAKFAST			
LUNCH			
DINNER			
SNACKS			

Date:

Daily Activity Log

Instructions: Use this form to track daily exercise. Include all activities of 5 minutes or more in duration and estimate their intensity. As general guidelines, light activities could be dusting, ironing, or playing croquet; moderate activities could be playing golf, raking the lawn, walking, or washing the car; and strenuous activities could be aerobic dance, jogging, bicycling, swimming, hiking, or playing tennis. When you're done, add up the number of minutes you spent doing light, moderate, and strenuous activities.

TIME	WHAT I DID	TIME SPENT IN MINUTES PER INTENSITY		
AM		Light	Moderate	Strenuous
6:00				
7:00				
8:00				
9:00				
10:00				
11:00				
PM				
12:00				
1:00				
2:00				
3:00				
4:00				
5:00				
6:00				
7:00				
8:00				
9:00				
10:00				
11:00				
AM				
12:00				
1:00				
2:00				
3:00				
4:00				
5:00				
TOTAL MINUTES				

Progress Log

Instructions: Once a week record your weight and estimate how much time you spend being active. Jot down notes on any problems or issues you're facing. Try to schedule the same time each week to weigh yourself and fill in the form.

Week of: _____ **Weight:** _____

NOTES

AVERAGE DAILY ACTIVITY
- ❏ 45 minutes or more
- ❏ 30 minutes
- ❏ Less than 30 minutes

HOW I'M FEELING
- ❏ Great
- ❏ Okay
- ❏ Stressed out
- ❏ Discouraged
- ❏ _____

_____
_____
_____
_____
_____
_____

Week of: _____ **Weight:** _____

NOTES

AVERAGE DAILY ACTIVITY
- ❏ 45 minutes or more
- ❏ 30 minutes
- ❏ Less than 30 minutes

HOW I'M FEELING
- ❏ Great
- ❏ Okay
- ❏ Stressed out
- ❏ Discouraged
- ❏ _____

_____
_____
_____
_____
_____
_____

Week of: _____ **Weight:** _____

NOTES

AVERAGE DAILY ACTIVITY
- ❏ 45 minutes or more
- ❏ 30 minutes
- ❏ Less than 30 minutes

HOW I'M FEELING
- ❏ Great
- ❏ Okay
- ❏ Stressed out
- ❏ Discouraged
- ❏ _____

_____
_____
_____
_____
_____
_____

Week of: _____ **Weight:** _____

NOTES

AVERAGE DAILY ACTIVITY
- ❏ 45 minutes or more
- ❏ 30 minutes
- ❏ Less than 30 minutes

HOW I'M FEELING
- ❏ Great
- ❏ Okay
- ❏ Stressed out
- ❏ Discouraged
- ❏ _____

_____
_____
_____
_____
_____
_____

At the end of each week use the graph at right to chart weight changes. Track it for four weeks.

_____ STARTING WEIGHT

	WEEK 1	WEEK 2	WEEK 3	WEEK 4
+8 lbs				
+6 lbs				
+4 lbs				
+2 lbs				
-2 lbs				
-4 lbs				
-6 lbs				
-8 lbs				

Your Healthy Weight Calculator

What's your ideal weight? The answer depends on your body type. Researchers use a scale called Body Mass Index, or BMI, which assigns a number based on a combination of height and weight. Essentially, the number indicates whether you are carrying a healthy or unhealthy level of body fat.

To find your BMI on the chart below, locate your height in inches in the column on the left. Then scan the horizontal row of numbers to find your weight. Finally, move up to locate the number directly above the column where your weight appears, in the row marked "BMI" at the top of the chart. (If you don't see your weight or height on the chart below, visit changeone.com/bmi to calculate your place on the BMI.)

You'll notice that the BMI chart gives a wide range of weights that fall within the normal category. The normal BMI weight range for someone who is 5 foot 7 inches (67 inches) is between 121 and 153 pounds, for instance. The reason for the 32-pound range: people have different body types, some slender, some stocky, some small-boned, some large.

The BMI index isn't foolproof. It tends to overestimate body fat in athletes and people with very muscular builds. And it tends to underestimate body fat in older people, who have usually lost muscle mass.

	NORMAL						OVERWEIGHT								OBESE					
BMI	19	20	21	22	23	24	25	26	27	28	29	30	31	32	33	34	35	36	37	38
HEIGHT (INCHES)	BODY WEIGHT IN POUNDS																			
58	91	96	100	105	110	115	119	124	129	134	138	143	148	153	158	162	167	172	177	181
59	94	99	104	109	114	119	124	128	133	138	143	148	153	158	163	168	173	178	183	188
60	97	102	107	112	118	123	128	133	138	143	148	153	158	163	168	174	179	184	189	194
61	100	106	111	116	122	127	132	137	143	148	153	158	164	169	174	180	185	190	195	201
62	104	109	115	120	126	131	136	142	147	153	158	164	169	175	180	186	191	196	202	207
63	107	113	118	124	130	135	141	146	152	158	163	169	175	180	186	191	197	203	208	214
64	110	116	122	128	134	140	145	151	157	163	169	174	180	186	192	197	204	209	215	221
65	114	120	126	132	138	144	150	156	162	168	174	180	186	192	198	204	210	216	222	228
66	118	124	130	136	142	148	155	161	167	173	179	186	192	198	204	210	216	223	229	235
67	121	127	134	140	146	153	159	166	172	178	185	191	198	204	211	217	223	230	236	242
68	125	131	138	144	151	158	164	171	177	184	190	197	203	210	216	223	230	236	243	249
69	128	135	142	149	155	162	169	176	182	189	196	203	209	216	223	230	236	243	250	257
70	132	139	146	153	160	167	174	181	188	195	202	209	216	222	229	236	243	250	257	264
71	136	143	150	157	165	172	179	186	193	200	208	215	222	229	236	243	250	257	265	272
72	140	147	154	162	169	177	184	191	199	206	213	221	228	235	242	250	258	265	272	279
73	144	151	159	166	174	182	189	197	204	212	219	227	235	242	250	257	265	272	280	288
74	148	155	163	171	179	186	194	202	210	218	225	233	241	249	256	264	272	280	287	295
75	152	160	168	176	184	192	200	208	216	224	232	240	248	256	264	272	279	287	295	303
76	156	164	172	180	189	197	205	213	221	230	238	246	254	263	271	279	287	295	304	312

Remember that losing even a few pounds when you're overweight will make you healthier, reducing your risk of heart disease and diabetes. Trying to bring your weight down to the normal range in the BMI is a terrific goal. But if you have a long way to go to get there, set some milestones for the road ahead. Reward yourself at each step, and don't get discouraged. Every little bit helps.

changeone.com Makes Losing Weight Even Easier

You've been reading about the *ChangeOne* program—now let us help you customize it to the way you live.

Increase your chances of weight-loss success with *ChangeOne* Online. Here are five great reasons to join today:

- ◼ You'll have access to hundreds of additional healthy, mouthwatering meals and recipes. We'll design you a meal plan with your weight-loss goals and preferences in mind.
- ◼ You'll get around-the-clock encouragement and advice from a caring community of other *ChangeOne* dieters to help you reach your weight-loss goals.
- ◼ You can use our calculators, weight tracker, food and activity journal and other interactive features to track your progress and get personalized feedback.
- ◼ You'll find the latest articles, news, and expert advice to keep you up to date on health, food, and fitness information.
- ◼ You'll receive weekly e-mail newsletters packed with delicious recipes, proven weight-loss tips, and lots more.

Sign up now: Go to changeone.com/newbook and get a *ChangeOne* program made for you.

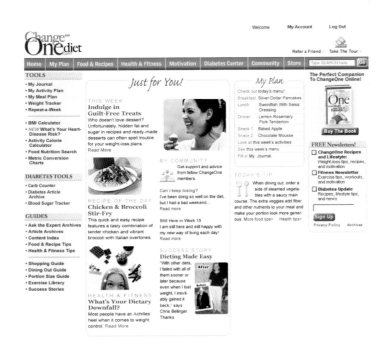

Recipe Index

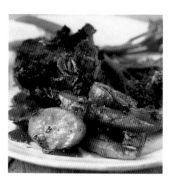
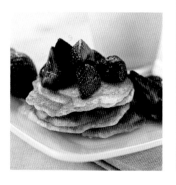

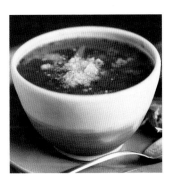

General Index